Benign Hematologic Disorders in Children

Editor

MICHAEL U. CALLAGHAN

PEDIATRIC CLINICS
OF NORTH AMERICA

www.pediatric.theclinics.com

Consulting Editor
BONITA F. STANTON

June 2018 • Volume 65 • Number 3

ELSEVIER

1600 John F. Kennedy Boulevard • Suite 1800 • Philadelphia, Pennsylvania, 19103-2899

http://www.theclinics.com

THE PEDIATRIC CLINICS OF NORTH AMERICA Volume 65, Number 3
June 2018 ISSN 0031-3955, ISBN-13: 978-0-323-58316-9

Editor: Kerry Holland
Developmental Editor: Casey Potter

The Pediatric Clinics of North America (ISSN 0031-3955) is published bimonthly by Elsevier Inc., 360 Park Avenue South, New York, NY 10010-1710. Months of issue are February, April, June, August, October, and December. Periodicals postage paid at New York, NY and additional mailing offices. Subscription prices are $216.00 per year (US individuals), $613.00 per year (US institutions), $292.00 per year (Canadian individuals), $816.00 per year (Canadian institutions), $338.00 per year (international individuals), $816.00 per year (international institutions), $100.00 per year (US students and residents), and $165.00 per year (international and Canadian residents and students). To receive students/resident rare, orders must be accompanied by name of affiliated institution, date of term, and the signature of program/residency coordinator on institution letterhead. Orders will be billed at individual rate until proof of status is received. Foreign air speed delivery is included in all *Clinics* subscription prices. All prices are subject to change without notice. **POSTMASTER:** Send address changes to *The Pediatric Clinics of North America*, Elsevier Health Sciences Division, Subscription Customer Service, 3251 Riverport Lane, Maryland Heights, MO 63043. **Customer Service: 1-800-654-2452 (US and Canada). From outside of the US and Canada: 1-314-447-8871. Fax: 1-314-447-8029. For print support, E-mail: JournalsCustomerService-usa@elsevier.com. For online support, E-mail: JournalsOnlineSupport-usa@elsevier.com.**

Reprints. For copies of 100 or more, of articles in this publication, please contact the Commercial Reprints Department, Elsevier Inc., 360 Park Avenue South, New York, NY 10010-1710. Tel.: 212-633-3874; Fax: 212-633-3820; E-mail: reprints@elsevier.com.

The Pediatric Clinics of North America is also published in Spanish by McGraw-Hill Inter-americana Editores S.A., Mexico City, Mexico; in Portuguese by Riechmann and Affonso Editores, Rua Comandante Coelho 1085, CEP 21250, Rio de Janeiro, Brazil; and in Greek by Althayia SA, Athens, Greece.

The Pediatric Clinics of North America is covered in *MEDLINE/PubMed (Index Medicus), Excerpta Medica, Current Contents, Current Contents/Clinical Medicine, Science Citation Index, ASCA, ISI/BIOMED,* and *BIOSIS.*

Printed in the United States of America.

Contributors

CONSULTING EDITOR

BONITA F. STANTON, MD
Founding Dean, Professor of Pediatrics, Hackensack Meridian School of Medicine at Seton Hall University, South Orange, New Jersey

EDITOR

MICHAEL U. CALLAGHAN, MD
Associate Professor of Pediatrics, Wayne State University, Children's Hospital of Michigan, Detroit, Michigan

AUTHORS

KHASHAYAR ARIANPOUR, BS
Department of Otolaryngology–Head and Neck Surgery, Wayne State University School of Medicine, Detroit, Michigan

STACY E. CROTEAU, MD, MMS
Director, Hemophilia/VWD Program, Boston Children's Hospital, Assistant Professor of Pediatrics, Harvard Medical School, Boston, Massachusetts

MICHAEL R. DeBAUN, MD, MPH
Department of Pediatrics, Division of Hematology/Oncology, Vanderbilt Center for Excellence in Sickle Cell Disease, Vanderbilt University Medical Center, Nashville, Tennessee

JORGE DI PAOLA, MD
Professor, Department of Pediatrics, Children's Hospital Colorado, Human Medical Genetics and Genomics, University of Colorado Denver, Aurora, Colorado

KATHRYN E. DICKERSON, MD
Assistant Instructor of Pediatrics, Division of Hematology/Oncology, University of Texas Southwestern, Dallas, Texas

BRADLEY P. DIXON, MD
Associate Professor, Department of Pediatrics, Renal Section, University of Colorado School of Medicine, Aurora, Colorado

BERTIL GLADER, MD, PhD
Department of Pediatrics (Hematology/Oncology), Stanford University School of Medicine, Lucile Packard Children's Hospital, Palo Alto, California

RACHAEL F. GRACE, MD, MMSc
Department of Pediatric Hematology/Oncology, Dana-Farber/Boston Children's Cancer and Blood Disorders Center, Harvard Medical School, Boston, Massachusetts

RALPH A. GRUPPO, MD
Professor of Clinical Pediatrics, Division of Hematology, Cancer and Blood Diseases Institute, Cincinnati Children's Hospital Medical Center, Cincinnati, Ohio

MATTHEW M. HEENEY, MD
Boston Children's Hospital, Harvard Medical School, Boston, Massachusetts

RAJESWARI JAYAVARADHAN, MS
Division of Experimental Hematology and Cancer Biology, Cancer and Blood Disease Institute (CBDI), Cincinnati Children's Hospital Medical Center (CCHMC), Pathobiology and Molecular Medicine Graduate Program, University of Cincinnati, Cincinnati, Ohio

SHAWN M. JOBE, MD, PhD
Director of Comprehensive Center for Bleeding Disorders, Blood Center of Wisconsin, Associate Investigator, Blood Research Institute, Associate Professor of Pediatrics and Cell Biology, Neurobiology, and Anatomy, Medical College of Wisconsin, Milwaukee, Wisconsin

PUNAM MALIK, MD
Professor of Pediatrics, Divisions of Experimental Hematology and Cancer Biology and Hematology, Cancer and Blood Disease Institute (CBDI), Cincinnati Children's Hospital Medical Center (CCHMC), Cincinnati, Ohio

EMILY RIEHM MEIER, MD, MSHS
Director, Sickle Cell Research, Indiana Hemophilia & Thrombosis Center, Indianapolis, Indiana; Adjunct Clinical Assistant Professor of Pediatrics and Human Development, Michigan State University College of Human Medicine, East Lansing, Michigan

NEETHU M. MENON, MD
Fellow, Pediatric Hematology Oncology, Division of Hematology/Oncology, University of Texas Southwestern, Dallas, Texas

SEAN MUTCHNICK, MD
Resident Physician, Department of Otolaryngology–Head and Neck Surgery, Wayne State University School of Medicine, Detroit, Michigan

CHRISTOPHER J. NG, MD
Assistant Professor, Department of Pediatrics, University of Colorado, Children's Hospital Colorado, Aurora, Colorado

JULIANA PEREZ BOTERO, MD
Associate Medical Director, BloodCenter of Wisconsin, Assistant Professor of Medicine, Medical College of Wisconsin, Milwaukee, Wisconsin

MADHVI RAJPURKAR, MD
Division of Pediatric Hematology Oncology, Carman and Ann Adams Department of Pediatrics, Wayne State University School of Medicine, Children's Hospital of Michigan, Detroit, Michigan

SARAH RAMIZ, MD
Division of Pediatric Hematology Oncology, Carman and Ann Adams Department of Pediatrics, Wayne State University School of Medicine, Children's Hospital of Michigan, Detroit, Michigan

SÜREYYA SAVAŞAN, MD
Professor of Pediatrics, Division of Hematology/Oncology, Pediatric Blood and Marrow Transplant Program, Children's Hospital of Michigan, Barbara Ann Karmanos Cancer Center, Wayne State University School of Medicine, Detroit, Michigan

RUCHIKA SHARMA, MD
Associate Medical Director, BloodCenter of Wisconsin, Assistant Professor of Pediatrics, Medical College of Wisconsin, Milwaukee, Wisconsin

PETER SVIDER, MD
Chief Resident, Department of Otolaryngology–Head and Neck Surgery, Wayne State University School of Medicine, Detroit, Michigan

SHAINA M. WILLEN, MD
Department of Pediatrics, Division of Hematology/Oncology, Vanderbilt Center for Excellence in Sickle Cell Disease, Vanderbilt University Medical Center, Nashville, Tennessee

AHMAR U. ZAIDI, MD
Department of Pediatrics, Division of Hematology/Oncology, Children's Hospital of Michigan, Wayne State University School of Medicine, Detroit, Michigan

AYESHA ZIA, MD
Assistant Professor of Pediatrics, Division of Hematology/Oncology, The University of Texas Southwestern, Dallas, Texas

RUCHIKA SHARMA, MD
Associate Medical Director, BloodCenter of Wisconsin, Assistant Professor of Pediatrics, Medical College of Wisconsin, Milwaukee, Wisconsin

PETER SVIDER, MD
Chief Resident, Department of Otolaryngology–Head and Neck Surgery, Wayne State University School of Medicine, Detroit, Michigan

SHANA M. WULTEN, MD
Department of Pediatrics, Division of Hematology/Oncology, Vanderbilt Center for excellence in Sickle Cell Disease, Vanderbilt University Medical Center, Nashville, Tennessee

AHMAR U. ZAIDI, MD
Department of Pediatrics, Division of Hematology/Oncology, Children's Hospital of Michigan, Wayne State University School of Medicine, Detroit, Michigan

AYESHA ZIA, MD
Assistant Professor of Pediatrics, Division of Hematology/Oncology, The University of Texas Southwestern, Dallas, Texas

Contents

> Rapid expansion of therapeutic options has increased the complexity of hemophilia care. Previously, on-demand therapy aimed to reduce morbidity and early mortality; however, now aggressive prophylaxis, particularly in children, encourages an active lifestyle. Accurate diagnosis, recognition of early threats to musculoskeletal health, and optimization of therapy are critical for both males and females affected by hemophilia. The diversity of emerging hemophilia therapies, from modified factor protein concentrates, to gene therapy, to nonfactor hemostatic strategies, provide an exciting opportunity to target unmet needs in the bleeding disorder community.

> Sickle cell disease (SCD) complications begin with the polymerization of sickle hemoglobin (HbS). Thus, SCD therapies are focused on preventing HbS production or reducing the circulating amount of HbS. Hydroxyurea treatment has become more widespread, whereas the number of evidence-based indications for erythrocyte transfusion is small. Hematopoietic stem cell transplant is a curative option for SCD, but less than 25% of patients have a suitable donor. This article focuses on supportive and preventive care improvements and the benefits of hydroxyurea. Indications for erythrocyte transfusion, hematopoietic stem cell transplant, and gene therapy trials are also summarized.

> We have entered an era of exploding interest in therapeutics for sickle cell disease. The expansion in our understanding of sickle cell disease pathophysiology has enhanced the range of potential therapeutic targets. From induction of fetal hemoglobin to antiadhesion molecules, we are potentially on the cusp of making life-altering modifications for individuals with sickle cell disease. This disease population cannot afford to let the current momentum wane. Studies exploring combinations of therapies affecting multiple steps in the pathophysiology and exploring novel and clinically relevant outcomes are incumbent.

Sickle cell disease is the most prevalent monogenic disorder worldwide, and curative therapies are limited to hematopoietic stem cell transplant to the few with matched donors. Gene therapy has curative potential, whereby autologous hematopoietic stem cells are genetically modified and transplanted, which would not be limited by matched donors, resulting in one-time, life-long correction devoid of immune side effects. Significant progress has been made to clinically translate gene therapy for sickle cell disease using lentivirus vectors carrying antisickling genes. This article focuses on the current state of the field, factors that determine clinical success, gene editing, and future prospects.

Although sickle cell disease and cystic fibrosis are two of the most common monogenic diseases presenting in childhood worldwide, cystic fibrosis and sickle cell disease enjoy vastly different funding and collaborative research efforts. Pulmonary complications in cystic fibrosis have well-established guidelines and multidisciplinary involvement focusing on comorbidities, routine monitoring, infectious complications, nutrition, and treatment recommendations. These guidelines can provide a framework on which to build knowledge of lung disease in sickle cell disease.

Pulmonary embolism (PE) in children is a rare condition with potential for high mortality. PE incidence is increasing owing to increased survival of children with predisposing conditions, increased use of central venous catheters, and improved awareness and recognition. Although pediatric PE is distinct from adult PE, management guidelines in children are extrapolated from the adult data. Treatment includes thrombolysis or thrombectomy, and pharmacologic anticoagulation. Ongoing clinical trials are evaluating the use of direct oral anticoagulants in children. Further research is required to develop pediatric-specific evidence-based guidelines for diagnosis and management of PE.

Atypical hemolytic uremic syndrome is a rare life-threatening disease of unregulated complement activation. When untreated, this condition has a generally poor prognosis; more than one-half of patients die or develop end-stage renal disease within 1 year. Atypical hemolytic uremic syndrome is characterized by thrombotic microangiopathy with evidence of hemolysis, thrombocytopenia, and renal impairment. This systemic disease affects the kidneys, brain, heart, lungs, gastrointestinal tract, pancreas, and skin. Acquired and genetic abnormalities of complement regulation may be identified in approximately 70% of patients. Plasma therapy is generally ineffective. Eculizumab blocks terminal complement activation, prevents complement-mediated organ damage, and is currently recommended as front-line therapy.

von Willebrand disease (VWD) is one of the most common inherited bleeding disorders. Since its first description in 1926, the diagnosis and management of VWD has significantly improved owing to increasing scientific knowledge of the genetics and biology of von Willebrand factor (VWF). This article reviews the molecular structure and function of VWF as well as the clinical symptoms, laboratory-based diagnostic workup, and classification schema for VWD. It highlights current treatment options and state-of-the art research in VWF and VWD.

Abnormal uterine bleeding is common in adolescents and is thought to affect 9% to 14% of women in their reproductive years. Certain unique aspects of underlying inherited or acquired blood disorders exacerbate the "expected" hormonal imbalance at this age, thereby increasing the morbidity of the underlying problem. A multifactorial etiology demands a collaborative approach between hematologists and gynecologists or adolescent medicine physicians to effectively manage abnormal uterine bleeding in young women with blood disorders.

Mucocutaneous bleeding symptoms and/or persistent thrombocytopenia occur in individuals with congenital disorders of platelet function and number. These disorders are often associated, apart from bleeding, with additional hematologic and clinical manifestations, including auditory, immunologic, and oncologic disease. Autosomal recessive, dominant, and X-linked inheritance patterns have been demonstrated. Precise delineation of the molecular cause of the platelet disorder can aid the pediatrician in the detection and prevention of specific disorder-associated manifestations and guide appropriate treatment and anticipatory care for the patient and family.

Mature red blood cells are anucleate, devoid of ribosomes and mitochondria, and reliant on both the glycolytic pathway for energy production and the hexose monophosphate shunt for cell protection from oxidative insults. Glucose-6-phosphate dehydrogenase deficiency is the most common red cell enzyme disorder worldwide. Clinical presentations include neonatal jaundice and episodic hemolysis in the setting of exposure to oxidative stress. Pyruvate kinase deficiency is the most common cause of congenital chronic nonspherocytic hemolytic anemia. Symptoms include neonatal jaundice, chronic hemolytic anemia, gallstones, and transfusion-related and transfusion-independent iron overload. Diagnosis is critical for appropriate supportive care, monitoring, and treatment.

Acquired aplastic anemia (aAA) characterized by peripheral pancytopenia and bone marrow aplasia is a rare and serious disorder. Differential diagnosis includes constitutional bone marrow failure syndromes and myelodysplastic disorders. Autoimmune reaction to altered hematopoietic stem cells highlights the underlying mechanism. Matched related donor allogeneic hematopoietic stem cell transplant is the ideal pediatric treatment; alternative approaches include immunosuppressive therapy and use of eltrombopag. Progression to clonal disorders can occur. Recently, alternative donor hematopoietic stem cell transplant outcomes have significantly improved. Despite advances, aAA continues to be a challenge for hematologists.

This article provides an organized foundation that facilitates the management of acute epistaxis and an understanding of features that merit further diagnostic workup. Prompt management, including measures such as holding pressure and using nasal packing, takes precedence over comprehensive diagnostic workup. Severe, recurrent, and posteriorly based bleeds should prompt consideration of alternate interventions and expert consultation.

PROGRAM OBJECTIVE
The goal of the *Pediatric Clinics of North America* is to keep practicing physicians and residents up to date with current clinical practice in pediatrics by providing timely articles reviewing the state-of-the-art in patient care.

TARGET AUDIENCE
All practicing pediatricians, physicians and healthcare professionals who provide patient care to pediatric patients.

LEARNING OBJECTIVES
Upon completion of this activity, participants will be able to:
1. Review treatment approaches in the management of epistaxis in Children
2. Discuss the evolving clinical management and treatment of Hemophilia
3. Recognize treatment options for sickle cell disease including novel drugs and generic therapies

ACCREDITATION
The Elsevier Office of Continuing Medical Education (EOCME) is accredited by the Accreditation Council for Continuing Medical Education (ACCME) to provide continuing medical education for physicians.

The EOCME designates this enduring material for a maximum of 15 *AMA PRA Category 1 Credit*(s)™. Physicians should claim only the credit commensurate with the extent of their participation in the activity.

All other healthcare professionals requesting continuing education credit for this enduring material will be issued a certificate of participation.

DISCLOSURE OF CONFLICTS OF INTEREST
The EOCME assesses conflict of interest with its instructors, faculty, planners, and other individuals who are in a position to control the content of CME activities. All relevant conflicts of interest that are identified are thoroughly vetted by EOCME for fair balance, scientific objectivity, and patient care recommendations. EOCME is committed to providing its learners with CME activities that promote improvements or quality in healthcare and not a specific proprietary business or a commercial interest.

The planning committee, staff, authors and editors listed below have identified no financial relationships or relationships to products or devices they or their spouse/life partner have with commercial interest related to the content of this CME activity:
Khashayar Arianpour, BS; Juliana Perez Botero, MD; Michael R. DeBaun, MD, MPH; Jorge Di Paola, MD; Kathryn E. Dickerson, MD; Ralph A. Gruppo, MD; Kerry Holland; Rajeswari Jayavaradhan, MS; Shawn M. Jobe, MD, PhD; Alison Kemp; Punam Malik, MD; Rajkumar Mayakrishnan; Neethu M. Menon, MD; Sean Mutchnick, MD; Sarah Ramiz, MD; Süreyya Savaşan, MD; Ruchika Sharma, MD; Bonita F. Stanton, MD; Peter Svider, MD; Shaina M. Willen, MD; Ahmar U. Zaidi, MD; Ayesha Zia, MD.

The planning committee, staff, authors and editors listed below have identified financial relationships or relationships to products or devices they or their spouse/life partner have with commercial interest related to the content of this CME activity:
Michael U. Callaghan, MD: participated in a speaker's burea for Novo Nordisk; owns stock in Alnylam Pharmaceuticals; has been a consultant/advisor for HEMA Biologics; has been a consultant/advisor and participated in speaker's bureau for Bayer AG, Genentech, Inc., and Shire. Dr. Callaghan has also been a consultant/advisor and received research support from Pfizer, Inc.
Stacy E. Croteau, MD, MMS: is a consultant/advisor for BioMarin Pharmaceutical, Bioverativ, Novo Nordisk, and CSL Behring. She has also received research support from Pfizer, Inc. and Spark Therapeutics. Dr. Croteau has been a consultant/advisor and received research support from Genentech, Inc. and Octapharma AG.
Bradley P. Dixon, MD: is a consultant/advisor for Achillion Pharmaceuticals, Inc and has received research support and has been a consultant/advisor for Alexion Pharmaceuticals, Inc.
Bertil Glader, MD, PhD: has received research support from Agios Pharmaceuticals.
Rachael F. Grace, MD, MMSc: has received research support and served as a consultant/advisor for Agios Pharmaceuticals.
Matthew M. Heeney, MD: has been a consultant/advisor for Novartis and receives/holds patents with UpToDate, Inc. He has been a consultant/advisor and received research support from AstraZeneneca, Pfizer, and Sancilio Pharmaceuticals Company, Inc.
Emily Riehm Meier, MD, MSHS: has received research support from Pfizer and has been a consultant/advisor for CVS Caremark

Christopher J. Ng, MD: has served as a consultant/advisor for CSL Behring and Shire.

Madhvi Rajpurkar, MD: has been a consultant/advisor for Shire, Novo Nordisk, HEMA Biologics, and Bayer Pharmaceuticals Healthcare LLC. Dr. Rajpurkar received research support from Bristol-Myers Squibb and has been a consultant/advisor and received research support from Pfizer.

UNAPPROVED/OFF-LABEL USE DISCLOSURE

The EOCME requires CME faculty to disclose to the participants:

1. When products or procedures being discussed are off-label, unlabelled, experimental, and/or investigational (not US Food and Drug Administration [FDA] approved); and

2. Any limitations on the information presented, such as data that are preliminary or that represent ongoing research, interim analyses, and/or unsupported opinions. Faculty may discuss information about pharmaceutical agents that is outside of FDA-approved labelling. This information is intended solely for CME and is not intended to promote off-label use of these medications. If you have any questions, contact the medical affairs department of the manufacturer for the most recent prescribing information.

TO ENROLL

To enroll in the *Pediatric Clinics of North America* Continuing Medical Education program, call customer service at 1-800-654-2452 or sign up online at http://www.theclinics.com/home/cme. The CME program is available to subscribers for an additional annual fee of USD 301.60.

METHOD OF PARTICIPATION

In order to claim credit, participants must complete the following:

1. Complete enrolment as indicated above.
2. Read the activity.
3. Complete the CME Test and Evaluation. Participants must achieve a score of 70% on the test. All CME Tests and Evaluations must be completed online.

CME INQUIRIES/SPECIAL NEEDS

For all CME inquiries or special needs, please contact elsevierCME@elsevier.com.

PEDIATRIC CLINICS OF NORTH AMERICA

ISSUE OF RELATED INTEREST

Clinics in Perinatology, September 2015 (Vol. 42, Issue 3)
Neonatal Hematology and Transfusion Medicine
Robert D. Christensen, Sandra E. Juul, and Antonio Del Vecchio, *Editors*

THE CLINICS ARE AVAILABLE ONLINE!
Access your subscription at:
www.theclinics.com

PEDIATRIC CLINICS OF
NORTH AMERICA

Foreword

Living up to Its Name: Advances in Benign Hematology

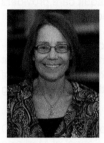

Bonita F. Stanton, MD
Consulting Editor

This issue of *Pediatric Clinics of North America* addresses a host of "benign" hematologic disorders. As part of the title to the *Pediatric Clinics of North America* issue, the term "benign" is used to specify those hematologic disorders that are not cancerous. The title does not imply that the disorders are without grave, even life-threatening, consequences. Nonetheless, Callaghan and his colleagues describe some of the many advances made in the twenty-first century that offer great hope that the adverse outcomes of these disorders are indeed becoming less common and less severe as our diagnostic and therapeutic opportunities increase both in the United States and globally.

Therapeutic options for hemophilia, affecting approximately 20,000 individuals in the United States and affecting all races, are increasing in important ways.[1] For example, new techniques have resulted in the prolongation of the replacement therapy of factors VIII and IX, thereby increasing the effectiveness and decreasing potential side effects of these therapies. Likewise, new approaches to producing replacement therapy are showing considerable promise in terms of duration of effect, means of administration, and alternatives in the face of antibodies.[2]

Sickle cell disease is the most common genetic blood disorder in the United States. In the United States, the incidence of the disease is approximately one per 500 African American births and one per 1000 to 1400 Hispanic American births. Estimates regarding sickle cell trait in the United States suggest that there are 73 cases per 1000 black newborns, 3 cases per 1000 white newborns, and 2.2 cases per 1000 Asian or Pacific Islander newborns. There are an estimated 7 cases per 1000 Hispanic newborns. An estimated 100,000 Americans are afflicted with sickle cell disease.[3,4] Despite its significant prevalence in the United States, approximately 74% of the world's annual 312,000 infants born with sickle cell disease reside in Sub-Saharan Africa,[5] underscoring the importance of a global perspective as we talk about new

Pediatr Clin N Am 65 (2018) xv–xvi
https://doi.org/10.1016/j.pcl.2018.03.002
0031-3955/18/© 2018 Published by Elsevier Inc.

treatment modalities available for this disease. Among the promising new modalities for treatment of sickle cell disease available over the last decade are new uses of hydroxyurea, drugs targeting mechanisms of the disorder (cell adhesion and inflammation), and genetic approaches. As well, the authors devote several articles to specific categories of advances and treatment advances for some of the greatest sources of morbidity and mortality among individuals with sickle cell disease.

As the most common inherited bleeding disorder (estimated at one in 1000 live births[6]), von Willebrand disease is of importance to pediatric and adult care providers across the globe. The authors describe several of the new diagnostic and treatment approaches that have become available over the past decade.

The remaining articles describe advances in clinical presentations of various diagnoses (epistaxis and uterine bleeding) and in clusters of abnormalities (platelet dysfunction, acquired aplastic anemia, and others) again underscoring the wealth of progress that has been made in recent years as well as advances that seem promising over the next decade.

Bonita F. Stanton, MD
School of Medicine
Seton Hall-Hackensack Meridian School of Medicine
Seton Hall University
400 South Orange Street
South Orange, NJ 07079, USA

E-mail address:
bonita.stanton@shu.edu

REFERENCES

1. Centers for Disease Control and Prevention. Hemophilia: homepage. Available at: https://www.cdc.gov/ncbddd/hemophilia/facts.html. Accessed March 24, 2015.
2. Ling G, Nathan AC, Tuddenham EGD. Recent advances in developing specific therapies for haemophilia. Br J Haematol, in press.
3. Centers for Disease Control and Prevention (CDC). Incidence of sickle cell trait–United States, 2010. MMWR Morb Mortal Wkly Rep 2014;63(49):1155–8.
4. Centers for Disease Control and Prevention. Sickle cell disease: homepage, data and statistics. Available at: https://www.cdc.gov/ncbddd/sicklecell/data.html. Accessed March 24, 2015.
5. Tewari S, Brousse V, Piel FB, et al. Environmental determinants of severity in sickle cell disease. Haematologica 2015;100:1108–16.
6. Sharma R, Flood VH. Advances in the diagnosis and treatment of Von Willebrand disease. Blood 2017;130:2386–91.

Preface

Benign Hematology

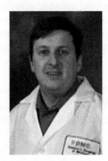

Michael U. Callaghan, MD
Editor

This April 2018 issue of *Pediatric Clinics of North America* focuses on the advancements in benign hematology. In 1590, in Holland, Hans and Zacharias Jannsen developed the compound microscope, and in the 1670s, Antonie van Leewenhoek examined blood using this device and observed red blood cells. For the next 200 years, the field progressed slowly until 1879, when, at the age of 25, Paul Ehrlich published his methods for staining blood cells and differential blood cell counting. This staining aided in Giulio Bizzozero's discovery of platelets in 1882. Since that time, disorders of the blood have been at the vanguard of clinical and basic science research. The easy access to samples and ability to monitor disease outcomes have attracted world class scientists to the study of diseases, such as hemophilia, von Willebrand disease, thrombotic disease, sickle cell anemia, red cell enzymopathies, and platelet disorders. The past few years have seen rapid advancement in the understanding of the genetics, pathophysiology, diagnosis, and treatment of hematologic disease. In this issue of *Pediatric Clinics of North America*, we review for the general pediatric practitioners some of these exciting advancements. Dr Croteau brings us up to speed on the rapidly advancing treatment of hemophilia and new treatment paradigms employing novel new agents and personalized pharmacokinetic-based regimen. The state-of-the-art in sickle cell disease is explored: Dr Meier updates us on the current standard of care; Drs Zaidi and Heeney summarize the protean pipeline approaches to sickle cell; Rajeswari Jayavaradhan and Dr Malik take us through the breakthroughs in gene therapy; and Drs Willen and DeBaun propose a better approach to pulmonary complications. Next, Drs Rajpurkar and Ramiz highlight the increasing prevalence of pulmonary embolism in pediatrics and lead us through our current therapies and knowledge gaps. The improving molecular understanding of and diagnostics and therapies for atypical hemolytic uremic syndrome are covered expertly by Drs Gruppo and Dixon, a hematologist and a nephrologist. The often related topics of heavy

Pediatr Clin N Am 65 (2018) xvii–xviii
https://doi.org/10.1016/j.pcl.2018.03.001
0031-3955/18/© 2018 Published by Elsevier Inc.

menstrual bleeding, von Willebrand disease, and platelet disorders are reviewed by Dr Zia, Drs Ng and DiPaola, and Drs Sharma, Botero, and Jobe, respectively. Each of these disorders has had major advancements in the past few years aided by genetic and clinical research. Drs Glader and Grace review the often overlooked enzyme disorders that are now the focus of active trials of new medication. In the penultimate article, Dr Savasan reviews the always challenging topic of acquired aplastic anemia, and this issue ends with a practical review for the practitioner of epistaxis, something frequently encountered in the pediatric clinic. While we were not able to cover all of the exciting breakthroughs in benign hematology, we hope this review helps practitioners at the front lines to identify and treat patients.

Michael U. Callaghan, MD
Wayne State University
Children's Hospital of Michigan
3901 Beaubien Street
Detroit, MI 48201, USA

E-mail address:
mcallagh@med.wayne.edu

Evolving Complexity in Hemophilia Management

Stacy E. Croteau, MD, MMS

KEYWORDS

- Bleeding • Hemarthrosis • Factor concentrate • Factor VIII • Factor IX • Inhibitors
- Gene therapy • Bispecific antibody

KEY POINTS

- The goals of hemophilia care, long-term outcomes, and expectations for burden of therapy are changing.
- Use of factor concentrates should be tailored to the needs of the individual patient. Musculoskeletal health, physical activity level, bleed frequency, and adherence must be considered.
- Nonfactor therapies are an exciting frontier in hemophilia, but attention to safe use in conjunction with factor replacement and bypassing therapies and interactions with standard coagulation assays must be incorporated into planning.
- Gene therapy for both factor VIII and factor IX deficiency is beginning to emerge as a potential cure or at least significant modulator of disease severity.

INTRODUCTION

Rapid expansion of therapeutic options has increased the complexity of hemophilia care. Previously, on-demand therapy aimed to reduce morbidity and early mortality; however, early initiation of prophylaxis decreases morbidity and encourages an active lifestyle. The integrated hemophilia care model available to patients in the United States and many developed countries globally is key to quality hemophilia management; ensuring accurate diagnosis, recognition of early threats to musculoskeletal health, and optimization of therapy for both males and females affected by hemophilia. The diversity of emerging hemophilia therapies, from modified factor proteins, to gene therapy, to nonfactor hemostatic strategies, provides an exciting opportunity to target unmet needs. Considerations for how these therap alter hemostasis, coagulation

Disclosure Statement: The author has received institutional grant/contracted research support from Pfizer, Baxalta, Octapharma, Dimension Therapeutics, Roche, Spark Therapeutics and Genentech, and has consulted or participated on a scientific advisory board of Aptevo, Bayer, BioMarin, Bioveritiv, CSL-Behring, Genentech, Novo Nordisk, and Octapharma.
Boston Children's Hospital, 300 Longwood Avenue, Boston, MA 02115, USA
E-mail address: stacy.croteau@childrens.harvard.edu

Pediatr Clin N Am 65 (2018) 407–425
https://doi.org/10.1016/j.pcl.2018.01.004
0031-3955/18/© 2018 Elsevier Inc. All rights reserved.

monitoring, patient safety, and long-term outcomes for all subpopulations, inhibitor patients, noninhibitor patients, previously untreated patients, and patients with mild hemophilia, are critical for hemophilia providers today.

FUNDAMENTALS OF HEMOPHILIA A AND B
Epidemiology

Hemophilia A (factor VIII [FVIII] deficiency) and hemophilia B (factor IX [FIX] deficiency) have an estimated US prevalence of 25,000 individuals and more than 400,000 individuals worldwide. The incidence of each is estimated at 1 in 5000 and 1 in 30,000 male births, respectively. No racial or ethnic predilection has been observed in disease incidence; however, polymorphisms of *F8* and *F9* have ethnic variation.[1,2] Characterization of clinically significant hemophilia in females has not yet been well-described. Increasingly, the burden of bleeding symptoms and the impact on musculoskeletal health in women are being recognized.[3,4] Efforts such as the Annual Global Survey and the World Bleeding Disorders Registry aim to improve data capture on the prevalence and clinical care of hemophilia and other rare bleeding disorders worldwide.[5–7]

Genetics

Both *F8* and *F9* are located on the distal end of the long arm of the X chromosome, at Xq28 and Xq27, respectively. Point mutations are the most common of the more than 4000 pathogenic variants identified.[8,9] Deletions, insertions, and rearrangements/inversions also occur, leading to reduced or absent functional clotting protein.[2,8] The most common *F8* pathogenic variant in severe FVIII deficiency is an intrachromosomal inversion resulting from homologous recombination in male germ cells (maternal grandfather), which separates exons 1 through 22 from 23 to 26 by inversion of intron 22.[10,11] In contrast, the most common pathogenic variant in severe FIX deficiency is single nucleotide substitution. De novo mutations arise in approximately one-third of patients with severe hemophilia.

Pathophysiology

The absence or reduction of functional FVIII or FIX results in impaired thrombin generation and less stable fibrin clots. FVIII, a glycoprotein cofactor, and activated FIX, a serine protease, amplify the rate of factor X activation, yielding about a 50,000-fold increase in thrombin generation. FVIII circulates as a trace plasma protein with its carrier protein, von Willebrand factor. The noncovalent interaction between FVIII and von Willebrand factor seems to play an important role in modulating the clearance of FVIII as well as its immunogenicity.[12] FVIII and FIX deficiency are generally considered to produce the same clinical phenotype, because of their shared role in the tenase complex. Some data suggest that those with FIX deficiency may experience less severe or less frequent bleed events; this supposition remains controversial.[13]

Clinical Features

The hallmark clinical feature of FVIII and FIX deficiency is hemarthrosis, with ankles, knees, and elbows being most frequently affected. Abnormal or excessive bleeding can occur in any organ or tissue, particularly after trauma. Musculoskeletal bleeding is characteristic in hemophilia, but mucosal bleeding, and epistaxis in particular, is common.

A male infant with FVIII or FIX deficiency may present with postcircumcision bleeding, soft tissue/muscular bleeding, cephalohematoma, or intracranial hemorrhage owing to minimal birth trauma or subsequent head injury.[14] Mild factor deficiency may not come to clinical attention until school age or adulthood, at the time of a trauma, dental procedure, or major surgery. Although patients with mild hemophilia are considered at low risk for chronic arthropathy, this may not be the case. A registry-based cohort study performed in Sweden noted a 16-fold increased incidence of arthropathy diagnosed in mild hemophilia patients born between 1984 and 2008 compared with the age-matched general population.[15]

Severity Classification

FVIII and FIX deficiency are divided into 3 severity levels which generally correlate with bleeding phenotype.[16]

- Severe: factor activity of less than 1 IU/dL.
- Moderate: factor activity of 1 to less than 5 IU/dL.
- Mild: factor activity of 5 to less than 50 IU/dL.

Both the 1-stage clotting assay (OSA) and chromogenic substrate assay (CSA) are commercially available for diagnostic evaluation and longitudinal assessment of patients with FVIII deficiency. OSA is presently more widely used in clinical coagulation laboratories. CSA for FIX is in development and available for research purposes. Although OSA and CSA typically produce concordant results, predictable discrepancies can arise. Debate over which assay is the most accurate for general clinical use continues; however, some clinical circumstances may warrant use of both assays (**Table 1**).[17,18]

- Mild hemophilia
- Specific *F8* genotypes
- High purity plasma-derived factor concentrate
- Modified FVIII concentrates (BDD, added moiety, etc)

Table 1
Discordant FVIII activity between OSA and CSA resulting from pathogenic variants in specific domains

Pathogenic Variant	CSA/OSA Ratio	Cause of Discrepancy
Missense pathogenic variants localized in the A1–A2–A3 domain interfaces	≤0.5	These pathogenic variants reduce stability of the FVIII heterodimer and FVIIIa heterotrimer
		• Because FVIIIa is produced all at once in OSA, the effect of this instability is minimized.
		• The incubation performed during the first step of the CSA favors a higher rate of A2 dissociation. This leads to a reduction in observed FVIII activity.
Pathogenic variants located close to or within thrombin cleavage, FIX- or vWF-binding sites	≥2.0	These pathogenic variants affect thrombin activation or FVIII binding to FIXa or VWF
		• The OSA is sensitive to alterations in thrombin binding or cleavage of FVIII.
		• The incubation phase of the CSA reduces the impact of the altered binding kinetics.

Abbreviations: CSA, chromogenic substrate assay; FVIII, factor VIII; OSA, 1-stage clotting assay; vWF, von Willebrand factor.
Adapted from Peyvandi F, Oldenburg J, Friedman KD. A critical appraisal of one-stage and chromogenic assays of factor VIII activity. J Thromb Haemost 2016;14:253; with permission.

FEMALES WITH HEMOPHILIA

The bleeding phenotype of carriers warrants consideration. Carriers are typically expected to have FVIII or FIX levels around 50 IU/dL, sufficient to confer a nonbleeding phenotype. Although many females are asymptomatic with normal factor levels, others have mild FVIII or FIX deficiency and clinically significant bleeding symptoms, such as heavy menstrual bleeding, postprocedure or postpartum bleeding requiring treatment.[4] Rarely, a female may have an unexpectedly low level in the moderate or severe deficiency range secondary to Turner syndrome, uniparental disomy, skewed lyonization, or compound heterozygous pathogenic variants.[2] Increasingly, bleeding symptoms in hemophilia carriers, joint health, and quality of life are being investigated. Retrospective evaluation of the hemophilia treatment center universal data collection dataset found that age and factor activity correlated with decrease in measured joint range of motion for hemophilia carriers compared with women who participated in the Normal Joint Study.[3] Although the clinical and functional significance is modest, these data highlight the importance of thoughtful investigation of the impact of mild factor deficiency and carrier status on long-term musculoskeletal and general health outcomes. Hemophilia carriers, even those with factor levels of 40% to 60%, seem to report more bleeding symptoms than controls.[3,19,20]

CONVENTIONAL HEMOPHILIA TREATMENT

The standard treatment for severe hemophilia patients is intravenous exogenous factor concentrate. Observational studies and randomized clinical trials have demonstrated the benefits of prophylaxis for both adults and children with severe hemophilia.[21–24] Despite this, data collected through the American Thrombosis and Hemostasis Network identified that only about 60% of US adult males and 70% to 80% school age children and adolescents with severe hemophilia use prophylaxis.[25]

The burden of frequent intravenous infusions, cost, and availability of factor concentrate contribute to less than ideal rates of continuous routine use of prophylaxis.[26] The dramatic decrease in total annual bleed events seen in the Joint Outcome Study (17.7 on-demand, 3.3 prophylaxis) required just over 3 times more factor concentrate. When Swedish physicians pioneered prophylaxis in the 1960s, the initial strategy of prophylaxis was to achieve trough factor levels of greater than 1 IU/dL. Empiric prophylaxis regimens emerged based on the mean adult half-life of FVIII and FIX concentrates and then modified as needed based on bleed events of the individual.[27]

A comparison of the intermediate dose prophylaxis used in the Netherlands (median, 2100 IU/kg per year) with the high-dose prophylaxis used in Sweden (median, 4000 IU/kg per year) revealed only a slight increase in the annual bleed rate. The median annual rate of joint bleeds on the intermediate regimen was 1.3 (interquartile range, 0.8–2.7) compared with 0 (interquartile range, 0.0–2.0) on the high-dose regimen. There was no detectable difference on reported social participation or quality of life. The annual cost of prophylaxis was 66% higher for the high-dose group, with an annual mean of $298,000 versus $180,000.[28] In areas with extreme limitation in hemophilia resources, even twice weekly low-dose prophylaxis seems to confer a clinical benefit compared with on-demand use.[29] The availability of factor concentrate to treat and prevent bleed events is essential for reducing hemophilia morbidity and mortality globally; however, the optimal prophylaxis regimen based on clinical need, desired joint outcomes, and pharmacoeconomics has not been well-defined.

PHARMACOKINETIC TAILORED PROPHYLAXIS

Traditional pharmacokinetic (PK) curves are labor intensive and impractical for routine clinical use. Classically, blood samples are collected at 11 time points over 48 to 72 hours for FVIII and 72 to 96 hours for FIX.[30] Morfini led early efforts in the 1970s to better characterize PK profiles of factor concentrates. Bjorkman and Collins[31] spear-headed the application of Bayesian analysis and population PK modeling, identifying strategies for use of a limited number of well-timed postinfusion blood samples to estimate a patient's PK profile and terminal half-life. This approach invigorated the concept of individualized PK in hemophilia, providing a practical clinical tool.[32]

Recently, licensed factor concentrates modified to extend the half-life of FVIII and FIX and others boasting a marginal increase in mean half-life compared with conventional factor concentrates have driven the interest of providers, payers, and patients in better understanding the usefulness of individual PK profile estimation. Increasingly, population PK models with the application of multiple factor concentrates are emerging.[33,34] The degree to which physician decision making and patient outcomes are positively impacted is under investigation.

EXTENDED HALF-LIFE FACTOR CONCENTRATES

Despite leveraging the same technologies of Fc fusion, pegylation, and albumin fusion, the effect on altering the circulating half-life of FVIII and FIX are remarkably different (**Table 2**). The dramatic half-life extension of FIX products provides the potential opportunity for reduced annual FIX product usage and infusions while maintaining trough levels of greater than 1 IU/dL. Albumin fusion and pegylated FIX concentrates may enable individuals to maintain a trough level of greater than 15 IU/dL with weekly infusions or less. With increasingly active hemophilia patients, the proportion of time per week spent within the mild deficiency range and not just the time greater than 1 IU/dL becomes an important consideration (**Fig. 1**).

Comparatively, FVIII extended half-life concentrates offer a modest improvement with half-life extensions 1.3 to 1.6 times an individual's baseline. For patients who have long half-lives at baseline, twice weekly infusions at typical prophylactic dosing may facilitate a less burdensome infusion schedule and reduced product use without loss of efficacy. For individuals with short half-lives and bleeding symptoms, despite adherence to an every other day regimen, the use of extended half-life concentrates may improve factor levels at the same infusion frequency.[35]

Alteration of FVIII or FIX with Fc fusion or pegylation can impact factor activity assessments by OSA and CSA (**Table 3**).[36] Knowledge of the activators and assays used by one's own coagulation laboratory is critical to correctly interpret activity levels.

Given the modest prolongation of FVIII half-life with current products, other technologies to extend the circulation time are under investigation. Attempts to use polysialic acid covalently bound to FVIII to significantly extend the half-life failed in phase I. Other approaches are focusing on the modification of the D'D3 domain from von Willebrand factor with albumin or through a combination of Fc fusion and XTEN technologies to reduce the clearance of FVIII.[37,38]

PREVIOUSLY UNTREATED OR MINIMALLY TREATED PATIENTS WITH SEVERE HEMOPHILIA

Currently, the most challenging complication of factor replacement is the development of neutralizing alloantibodies (inhibitors) to exogenous factor concentrate. Inhibitors occur in approximately 30% of patients with severe FVIII deficiency at a median of 12

Table 2
Recently licensed or anticipated factor concentrates for hemophilia A and B

Product *Trade Name*	Features	Cell Line	Mean Adult Half-Life ± SD (h), as Reported in US Package Insert
FVIII concentrates			
Novoeight *Turoctocog alfa*	B-domain truncated FVIII	CHO	10.8 ± 4.9
Afstyla *Ionoctocog alfa*	Single-chain, B-domain truncated FVIII FVIII activity by 1-stage clotting assay, multiply by conversion factor of 2	CHO	14.2 ± 3.7
Kovaltry Octocog alfa	Full-length FVIII, human chaperone protein heat shock protein 70 included to assist protein folding	BHK	14.3 ± 3.7
Adynovate *Rurioctocog alfa pegol*	Full-length FVIII, random pegylation with branched 20 kDa PEG, most covalently bind to the B-domain	CHO	14.7 ± 3.8
Nuwiq *Simoctocog alfa*	B-domain deleted FVIII	HEK-293	17.1 ± 11.2
Eloctate *Efmoroctocog alfa*	B-domain deleted FVIII, fusion with IgG1 Fc at carboxy-terminus	HEK-293	19.7 ± 2.3 (95% CI)
BAY 94-9027 *Damoctocog alfa pegol*	B-domain deleted FVIII, site-directed pegylation with 60 kDa PEG, linked to introduced cysteine residue	BHK	18.7 h (range: 12.1–30.0 h)*
Novoeight-GP *Turoctocog alfa pegol*	B-domain truncated FVIII, site-directed pegylation with 40 kDa PEG, conjugated to the 21 amino acid B-domain sequence	CHO	19 h (range: 11.6–27.3 h)*
FIX concentrates			
Ixinity *Trenonacog alfa*	rFIX, Thr-148 polymorphism	CHO	24.0 ± 6.0
Rixubis *Nonacog gamma*	rFIX	CHO	25.4 ± 6.9
Alprolix *Eftrenonacog alfa*	rFIX, fusion with IgG1 Fc at carboxy-terminus	HEK-293	86.5 ± 32.2
Idelvion *Albutrepenonacog alfa*	rFIX, fusion with recombinant human albumin at cleavable linker peptide	CHO	104.0 ± 18.7
Rebinyn *Nonacog beta pegol*	rFIX, site-directed pegylation with branched 40 kDa PEG at FIX activation peptide	CHO	111 (CV% 11.8)

Abbreviations: CI, confidence interval; CV%, coefficient of variance; FVIII, factor VIII; FIX, factor IX; IgG, immunoglobulin G; rFIX, recombinant factor IX.
* *Data from Refs.* [89,90]

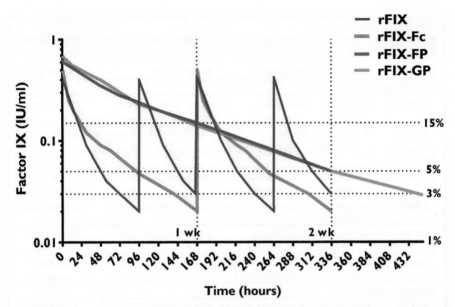

Fig. 1. Factor IX activity over time for conventional and extend the half-life factor IX concentrates following an infusion of 50 IU/kg, estimated from published pharmacokinetic profiles. rFIX, recombinant factor IX. (*Data from* Refs.[91–93])

exposure days compared with only 3% to 4% of patients with severe FIX deficiency.[39] Joint health, quality of life, and lifespan are markedly reduced for patients with persistent inhibitors compared with other hemophilia patients.[40,41] Elucidation of the pathophysiology of inhibitor development, risk assessment, opportunities to modify risk, and effective immune tolerance and bleed treatment strategies are areas of intense investigation.[42,43]

Inhibitor Risk and Opportunities for Risk Mitigation

Several risk factors for inhibitor development have been described (**Fig. 2**). The relative added risk or synergism among these factors are unknown. The Early Prophylaxis Immunologic Challenge (EPIC) study investigated early introduction (<1 year old) of low-dose (25 IU/kg/wk) prophylaxis and an effort to reduce immunologic danger signals to reduce inhibitor formation. Unfortunately, this study was stopped early for futility. This outcome may have reflected decision to incorporate all inhibitors, rather than focusing reduction of high-titer inhibitors.[44,45]

Publication of the Survey of Inhibitors in Plasma-Product Exposed Toddlers (SIPPET) trial sparked one of the most controversial considerations for inhibitor risk reduction. This global, randomized trial compared the rate of inhibitor development in previously untreated patients assigned to either a plasma-derived or recombinant concentrate available in their country. Although the incidence of inhibitors was 87% higher with recombinant concentrates (hazard ratio, 1.87; 95% confidence interval, 1.17–2.96), the 69% increase in high titer inhibitors was not statistically significant (hazard ratio, 1.69; 95% confidence interval, 0.96–2.98).[46] Some support initiating plasma-derived products in PUPs based on the potential for reduction in inhibitors; others counter that the generalizability of the data, owing to few regions contributing a disproportionate number of patients and concern with study and analysis methodology, do not support a practice change.[47–49]

Table 3
Summary of performance of different OSA activators and CSA for extended half-life factor concentrates

Activators	Ellagic Acid	Silica Based	Kaolin Based	Chromogenic
Fc fusion molecules				
rFVIII Fc	Acceptable recovery[a]	Acceptable recovery[a]	Acceptable recovery	Overestimates
rFIX Fc	Acceptable recovery	Slightly underestimates	Significantly underestimates	Not available
PEGylation				
BAY94-9027	Acceptable recovery	Significantly underestimates	Not available	Acceptable recovery
BAX855	Acceptable recovery	Acceptable recovery	Acceptable recovery	Overestimates
N8-GP	Acceptable recovery	Significantly underestimates[b]	Acceptable recovery	Acceptable recovery
N9-GP	Acceptable recovery	Significantly overestimates	Significantly underestimates	Acceptable recovery
Albumin fusion				
rFIX-FP	Not available	Acceptable recovery	Not available	Acceptable recovery

Abbreviations: CSA, chromogenic substrate assay; rFVIII, recombinant factor VIII; rFIX, recombinant factor IX; OSA, 1-stage clotting assay.
[a] Overestimates at medium and low concentrations.
[b] With most silica-based reagents.
Adapted from Pruthi RK. Laboratory monitoring of new hemostatic agents for hemophilia. Semin Hematol 2016;53(1):28–34.

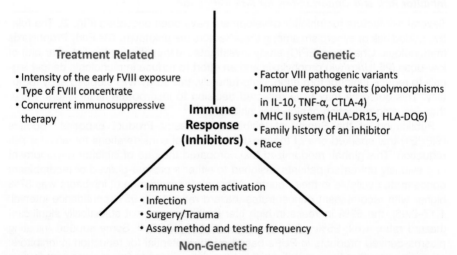

Treatment Related

• Intensity of the early FVIII exposure
• Type of FVIII concentrate
• Concurrent immunosuppressive therapy

Immune Response (Inhibitors)

Genetic

• Factor VIII pathogenic variants
• Immune response traits (polymorphisms in IL-10, TNF-α, CTLA-4)
• MHC II system (HLA-DR15, HLA-DQ6)
• Family history of an inhibitor
• Race

• Immune system activation
• Infection
• Surgery/Trauma
• Assay method and testing frequency

Non-Genetic

Fig. 2. Risk factors for inhibitor development. CTLA-4, cytotoxic T-lymphocyte antigen 4; FVIII, factor VIII; IL-10, interleukin 10; MHC, major histocompatibility complex; TNF-α, tumor necrosis factor-α.

Immune Tolerance Induction

All current hemophilia inhibitor guidelines agree that eradication of high-titer (>5 BU) FVIII inhibitors should be attempted using immune tolerance induction (ITI).[39,50–52] The nuances of ITI for FIX inhibitors are more complex. Although ITI successfully eliminates 70% to 80% of FVIII inhibitors, the impact on FIX inhibitors is much less. Dosing and infusion frequency for ITI are not standardized. The International ITI study randomized favorable risk high-titer inhibitor patients to either a low-dose (50 IU/kg per dose 3 times a week) or a high-dose (200 IU/kg/d) ITI regimen. Although the overall success of ITI did not differ between the groups, the time to tolerance milestones, namely, the time to negative titer and time to normal recovery, were delayed in the low-dose group. Correspondingly, this group had a higher bleed rate resulting in early termination of the study.[53]

Bleed Treatment and Prophylaxis in the Setting of High-Titer Inhibitors

High-titer inhibitors neutralize the hemostatic effect of exogenous factor, necessitating use of activated prothrombin complex concentrates or activated recombinant factor VII.[54] In some settings, concomitant use of FVIII may be beneficial owing to variable inhibitor kinetics.[55] Challenges with the use of bypassing agents include reduced efficacy compared with simple factor replacement, need for either frequent infusion (up to every 2 hours for activated recombinant factor VII) or large infusion volume (20–50 mL for activated prothrombin complex concentrate), and no validated assay to quantify the hemostatic effect. The prophylactic use of bypassing agents in children and adults not undergoing ITI has been demonstrated to have a clinical benefit.[56,57]

Modifications intended extend the half-life of activated recombinant factor VII are under investigation.[58] A recombinant porcine FVIII concentrate has been licensed for acquired hemophilia A in adults and has undergone limited investigation in congenital FVIII deficiency with inhibitors.[59–61]

EMERGING THERAPIES

Frequent infusion requirement, inhibitor risk, need for IV infusion, and difficult access to factor concentrates in some regions has heightened the interest in alternate hemophilia therapies.[62] For several decades, these monogenic X-linked disorders have aspired for a gene therapy cure. Despite slow early progress, recent success has spurred a surge in interest and resources invested in hemophilia gene therapy.[63–66] Emerging nonfactor replacement strategies may provide novel therapeutic options for patients with FVIII and FIX deficiency and potentially those with other rare bleeding disorders. Because these nonfactor small molecules and biologics are not substrates for FVIII or FIX neutralizing alloantibodies, these investigational therapies are particularly exciting for patients with inhibitors.

GENE THERAPY AND GENE EDITING

Nathwani and colleagues[67,68] published the first sustained success and subsequently data from several other groups have emerged (**Table 4**).[69,70] Attention to vector selection and design, codon optimized transgenes, promoter selection, and target cell (myocyte, hepatocyte, hematopoietic stem cell) have all proven to be critical elements to success.

Although gene therapy has been generally well tolerated, several challenges to successful AAV-mediated gene therapy remain:

Table 4
Gene therapy/gene editing trials for FVIII and FIX deficiency

Product (Sponsor)	Vector	Promotor Transgene	ClinicalTrials.gov Identifier	Released Trial Results to Date
Factor VIII				Dose Level, Participants Enrolled, Outcome
BMN 270 (BioMarin Pharmaceutical)	AAV5	B-domain deleted FVIII	NCT02576795 (phase I/II, not recruiting)	6×10^{12} vg/kg, n = 1, FVIII activity <1% at 20 wk 2×10^{13} vg/kg, n = 1, FVIII activity 2% at 16 wk 4×10^{13} vg/kg, n = 6, FVIII activity 7%–45% at 20 wk 6×10^{13} vg/kg, n = 7, FVIII activity 19%–164% with minimum of 52 wk of follow-up, prophylactic corticosteroids initiated
SPK-8011 (Spark Therapeutics)	AAV-Spark 200	HLP-FVIII-V3	NCT03003533 (phase I/II, recruiting)	5×10^{11} vg/kg, n = 2, FVIII activity 6%–37% with minimum 30 wk follow-up 1×10^{12} vg/kg, n = 2, 7%–24% with minimum of 14 wk follow-up
GO-8 (University College, Lyndon)	scAAV2/8	B-domain deleted FVIII	NCT03001830 (phase I, recruiting)	No results posted to date
SB-525 (Sangamo Therapeutics)	AAV2/6	B-domain deleted FVIII	NCT03061201 (phase I/II, recruiting)	No results posted to date
SHP654 (Shire)	AAV8	B-domain deleted FVIII, CpG depleted, codon optimized	Announced	Not yet recruiting
DTX-201 (REGENXBIO)	AAVRh10	B-domain deleted FVIII	Announced	Not yet recruiting

Factor IX				
SPK-9001 (Spark Therapeutics)	AAV-Spark 100	FIXR338L	NCT02484092 (phase I/II, recruiting)	5×10^{11} vg/kg/n = 10/FIX activity 14%–81% with minimum 52 wk of follow-up
scAAV2/8-LP1-hFIXco (St. Jude Children's Research Hospital)	scAAV2/8	LP1-hFIXco	NCT00979238	Ten patients dosed in 3 dosing cohorts, mean steady state FIX activity 2.9%–7.2% with follow-up of $\geq$16 mo
AskBio009 (Baxalta/Shire)	scAAV8	TTR-FIXR338L	NCT01687608 (phase I/II, not recruiting)	2×10^{11} vg/kg/n = 2/sustained FIX activity achieved <3%; 1×10^{12} vg/kg/n = 4/1 patient with FIX activity 25% at 2 y; 3×10^{12} vg/kg/n = 2/sustained FIX activity achieved <3%
DTX101 (Dimension Therapeutics)	AAVrh10	hFIX	NCT02618915 (phase I, not recruiting)	1.6×10^{12} gc/kg/n = 3/3%–4% with minimum 24 wk of follow-up; 5×10^{12} gc/kg/n = 3/5–8% with minimum 7 wk of follow-up
AMT-060 (UniQure Biopharma)	AAV5	LP1-hFIXco	NCT02396342 (phase I/2, not recruiting) Announced clinical program proceeding with AMT-061.	5×10^{12} gc/kg/n = 5/FIX = 36.5% with minimum 52 wk of follow-up; 2×10^{13} gc/kg/n = 5/FIX = 3.1%–12.7% with minimum 26 wk follow-up
SB-FIX (Sangamo Therapeutics)	AAV2/6	ZNF mediated gene editing (ZFN1, ZFN2, and FIX cDNA donor)	NCT02695160 (phase I, recruiting)	No results posted to date

Abbreviations: FVIII, factor VIII; FIX, factor IX.

- Presence of preexisting antibodies to AAV reduce patient eligibility;
- Achieving consistent factor levels within target range (ideally normal range);
- Understanding immune response that results in loss of transgene expression, typically with asymptomatic alanine aminotransferase elevation; and
- Long-term longitudinal data on persistence of gene expression and safety.

The leading wave of gene therapy programs are anchored in liver-directed AAV vector technology; however, cell-based approaches are entering early phase trials.[71–73] Interest in gene editing technology to correct or place functional gene copy in a safe harbor are also emerging.[74–76]

EMICIZUMAB (HemLibra, ACE910)

A recombinant, humanized bispecific monoclonal antibody, emicizumab (ACE910, Roche, Switzerland), substitutes for the cofactor function of activated FVIII, binding FIXa and factor X on a phospholipid membrane.[77] The lack of structural homology between emicizumab and FVIII prevents emicizumab from being neutralized by FVIII inhibitors or from being acted on by physiologic regulatory proteins. Investigation of the safety and efficacy of emicizumab, administered as a weekly subcutaneous injection, has been pursued in FVIII deficiency both with and without inhibitors.[78,79] Initial results from a phase III study targeting patients with inhibitors requiring bypassing agents use demonstrated a 79% bleed reduction for patients on emicizumab compared with pre-study on bypassing agent prophylaxis. For those using on-demand bypassing agents before study enrollment, the annualized bleeding rate decreased by 87% in aggregate.[80] These data led to approval of emicizumab by the US Food and Drug Administration in late 2017.

Safety Considerations

Overall, emicizumab has been well-tolerated with mild injection site reactions being the most common adverse event reported.[80] There have not yet been neutralizing antidrug antibodies reported. Four serious adverse events of thrombosis and thrombotic microangiopathy occurred in the setting of emicizumab and multiple doses of activated prothrombin complex concentrate to treat bleeding. One patient with evidence of resolving thrombotic microangiopathy died in the context of persistent gastrointestinal bleeding and a refusal of blood transfusion. Safety and efficacy studies in patients with noninhibitor FVIII deficiency are under way.

Laboratory Monitoring Considerations

The binding characteristics of even small (nontherapeutic) amounts of emicizumab in plasma normalize the activated partial thromboplastin time (aPTT), rendering the activated partial thromboplastin time and assays based on this assay, including the 1-stage FVIII assay and modified Nijmegen-Bethesda assay, inaccurate. Additionally, because emicizumab is a humanized antibody, it does not assay appropriately with chromogenic assay kits that use bovine reagents. How the plasma concentration of emicizumab and a human chromogenic FVIII activity assessment correlate with in vivo hemostasis has not yet been described.

REDUCTION OF ANTICOAGULANT PROTEINS

Inspired by the observation that severe hemophilia patients with coinheritance of heterozygous thrombophilia pathogenic variants such as factor V Leiden seem to have a less severe bleeding phenotype, the idea of "rebalancing" the procoagulation and anticoagulation protein levels was pursued as an approach to hemophilia therapy (**Fig. 3**).[81,82] Small molecules and biologics to reduce proteins responsible for inhibiting the coagulation cascade such as antithrombin (AT), tissue factor pathway inhibitor (TFPI), and activated protein C are all in development.[83–85]

Fitusiran

Fitusiran decreases hepatocyte production of AT by interfering with AT messenger RNA production encoded by SERPINC1.[85] A phase I trial investigating weekly and monthly subcutaneous injection schedules demonstrated a dose-dependent AT reduction of up to 88%.[86] As expected, the decrease in AT resulted in an increase in thrombin generation. Participants in the monthly dose cohort had an 85% reduction in their annualized bleed rate compared with before the study using on-demand factor replacement. Initially, no significant adverse events had been observed, but recently a fatal cerebral venous sinus thrombosis was reported in a subject in the phase II open-label extension study.

Tissue Factor Pathway Inhibitor Inhibition

TFPI, a Kunitz-type serine protease inhibitor, plays a key role in modulating activation of tissue factor-factor VIIa and prothrombinase. Blocking the function of TFPI serves to amplify procoagulation signaling and the thrombin burst. Both aptamers and monoclonal antibodies have been developed to interfere with TFPI function. Unfortunately, in humans the anti-TFPI aptamer resulted in increased bleeding owing to an unexpected increase in full-length TFPI plasma levels. Development was discontinued.[87]

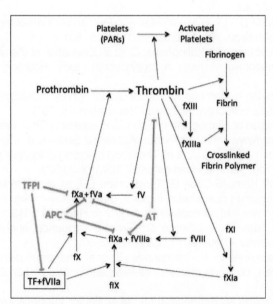

Fig. 3. Schematic of coagulation highlighting major endogenous anticoagulant proteins targeted for investigation as hemophilia therapy (*red*). The aim of each of these therapies is to boost thrombin generation and improve fibrin formation. APC, activated protein C; AT, antithrombin; f, factor; TF, tissue factor; TFPI, tissue factor pathway inhibitor. (*From* Polderdijk SGI, Baglin TP, Huntington JA. Targeting activated protein C to treat hemophilia. Curr Opin Hematol 2017;24(5):447; with permission.)

Several TFPI monoclonal antibodies are presently in early phase development. Safety, pharmacokinetic, and pharmacodynamic data were recently released on concizumab, a humanized high-affinity monoclonal antibody directed against the Kunitz-type protease inhibitor 2 domain.[88] The double-blinded multiple-dose escalation trial in 24 patients reported no serious adverse events or antidrug antibodies. The phase I trial for BAY 1093884 and a phase II trial for PF-06741086 are recruiting (NCT02571569 and NCT02974855, respectively).

SUMMARY

Assurance of access to safe factor concentrates and the institution of prophylaxis as standard of care dramatically ameliorated the disease burden of hemophilia in many parts of the world. Expansion of the availability of basic diagnostics and treatment to resource-limited settings (representing nearly 75% of the global hemophilia population) is essential. The next frontier of hemophilia therapies aim to further reduce the burden of treatment by supporting effective hemostasis with less frequent infusions, easier administration, or perhaps the elimination of any need for prophylactic treatment altogether. The integration of these novel therapies into routine hemophilia care will require thoughtful conversations among providers, patients, payers, and manufacturers to ensure therapeutic goals are safely met.

REFERENCES

1. Mannucci PM, Tuddenham EG. The hemophilias–from royal genes to gene therapy. N Engl J Med 2001;344(23):1773–9.
2. Bowen DJ. Haemophilia A and haemophilia B: molecular insights. Mol Pathol 2002;55(2):127–44.
3. Sidonio RF, Mili FD, Li T, et al. Females with FVIII and FIX deficiency have reduced joint range of motion. Am J Hematol 2014;89(8):831–6.
4. James PD, Mahlangu J, Bidlingmaier C, et al. Evaluation of the utility of the ISTH-BAT in haemophilia carriers: a multinational study. Haemophilia 2016;22(6): 912–8.
5. World Federation of Hemophilia Annual Global Survey. Available at: https://www.wfh.org/en/data-collection. Accessed September 15, 2017.
6. World Federation of Hemophilia (WFH) World Bleeding Disorders Registry. Available at: https://www.wfh.org/en/wbdr. Accessed September 15, 2017.
7. Pierce GF, Iorio A, O'Hara J, et al. The world bleeding disorders registry: the pilot study. Res Pract Thromb Haemost 2017;1(Suppl. 1):803.
8. Rallapalli PM, Kemball-Cook G, Tuddenham EG, et al. An interactive mutation database for human coagulation factor IX provides novel insights into the phenotypes and genetics of hemophilia B. J Thromb Haemost 2013;11(7):1329–40.
9. Peyvandi F, Kunicki T, Lillicrap D. Genetic sequence analysis of inherited bleeding diseases. Blood 2013;122(20):3423–31.
10. Lakich D, Kazazian HH Jr, Antonarakis SE, et al. Inversions disrupting the factor VIII gene are a common cause of severe haemophilia A. Nat Genet 1993;5(3): 236–41.
11. Rossiter JP, Young M, Kimberland ML, et al. Factor VIII gene inversions causing severe hemophilia A originate almost exclusively in male germ cells. Hum Mol Genet 1994;3(7):1035–9.
12. Pipe SW, Montgomery RR, Pratt KP, et al. Life in the shadow of a dominant partner: the FVIII-VWF association and its clinical implications for hemophilia A. Blood 2016;128(16):2007–16.

13. Escobar M, Sallah S. Hemophilia A and hemophilia B: focus on arthropathy and variables affecting bleeding severity and prophylaxis. J Thromb Haemost 2013; 11(8):1449–53.
14. Kulkarni R, Presley RJ, Lusher JM, et al. Complications of haemophilia in babies (first two years of life): a report from the centers for disease control and prevention universal data collection system. Haemophilia 2017;23(2):207–14.
15. Osooli M, Lovdahl S, Steen Carlsson K, et al. Comparative burden of arthropathy in mild haemophilia: a register-based study in Sweden. Haemophilia 2017;23(2): e79–86.
16. Den Uijl IE, Mauser Bunschoten EP, Roosendaal G, et al. Clinical severity of haemophilia A: does the classification of the 1950s still stand? Haemophilia 2011; 17(6):849–53.
17. Peyvandi F, Oldenburg J, Friedman KD. A critical appraisal of one-stage and chromogenic assays of factor VIII activity. J Thromb Haemost 2016;14(2):248–61.
18. Pavlova A, Delev D, Pezeshkpoor B, et al. Haemophilia A mutations in patients with non-severe phenotype associated with a discrepancy between one-stage and chromogenic factor VIII activity assays. Thromb Haemost 2014;111(5): 851–61.
19. Di Michele DM, Gibb C, Lefkowitz JM, et al. Severe and moderate haemophilia A and B in US females. Haemophilia 2014;20(2):e136–43.
20. Plug I, Mauser-Bunschoten EP, Brocker-Vriends AH, et al. Bleeding in carriers of hemophilia. Blood 2006;108(1):52–6.
21. Aledort LM, Haschmeyer RH, Pettersson H. A longitudinal study of orthopaedic outcomes for severe factor-VIII-deficient haemophiliacs. The orthopaedic outcome study group. J Intern Med 1994;236(4):391–9.
22. Tagliaferri A, Feola G, Molinari AC, et al. Benefits of prophylaxis versus on-demand treatment in adolescents and adults with severe haemophilia A: the POTTER study. Thromb Haemost 2015;114(1):35–45.
23. Manco-Johnson MJ, Abshire TC, Shapiro AD, et al. Prophylaxis versus episodic treatment to prevent joint disease in boys with severe hemophilia. N Engl J Med 2007;357(6):535–44.
24. Manco-Johnson MJ, Kempton CL, Reding MT, et al. Randomized, controlled, parallel-group trial of routine prophylaxis vs. on-demand treatment with sucrose-formulated recombinant factor VIII in adults with severe hemophilia A (SPINART). J Thromb Haemost 2013;11(6):1119–27.
25. American Thrombosis and Hemostatic Network (ATHN) Research Report Brief 12.31. 2016. Available at: https://athn.org/content/resource-center/. Accessed September 15, 2017.
26. Valentino LA. Considerations in individualizing prophylaxis in patients with haemophilia A. Haemophilia 2014;20(5):607–15.
27. Coppola A, Di Capua M, Di Minno MN, et al. Treatment of hemophilia: a review of current advances and ongoing issues. J Blood Med 2010;1:183–95.
28. Fischer K, Steen Carlsson K, Petrini P, et al. Intermediate-dose versus high-dose prophylaxis for severe hemophilia: comparing outcome and costs since the 1970s. Blood 2013;122(7):1129–36.
29. Verma SP, Dutta TK, Mahadevan S, et al. A randomized study of very low-dose factor VIII prophylaxis in severe haemophilia - a success story from a resource limited country. Haemophilia 2016;22(3):342–8.
30. Morfini M. Pharmacokinetic studies: international guidelines for the conduct and interpretation of such studies. Haemophilia 2006;12:6–11.

31. Bjorkman S, Collins P, Project on Factor VI I I/Factor IX Pharmacokinetics of the Factor VIII/Factor IX Scientific and Standardization Committee of The ISTH. Measurement of factor VIII pharmacokinetics in routine clinical practice. J Thromb Haemost 2013;11(1):180–2.

32. Collins PW, Fischer K, Morfini M, et al, International Prophylaxis Study Group Pharmacokinetics Expert Working Group. Implications of coagulation factor VIII and IX pharmacokinetics in the prophylactic treatment of haemophilia. Haemophilia 2011;17(1):2–10.

33. Hazendonk HC, van Moort I, Fijnvandraat K, et al. The "OPTI-CLOT" trial. A randomised controlled trial on periOperative PharmacokineTIc-guided dosing of CLOTting factor concentrate in haemophilia A. Thromb Haemost 2015;114(3): 639–44.

34. Iorio A, Keepanasseril A, Foster G, et al. Development of a web-accessible population pharmacokinetic service-hemophilia (WAPPS-Hemo): study protocol. JMIR Res Protoc 2016;5(4):e239.

35. Croteau SE, Neufeld EJ. Transition considerations for extended half-life factor products. Haemophilia 2015;21(3):285–8.

36. Pruthi RK. Laboratory monitoring of new hemostatic agents for hemophilia. Semin Hematol 2016;53(1):28–34.

37. Pestel S, Raquet E, Mischnik M, et al. Half-life extension of FVIII by coadministration of a recombinant D'D3 albumin fusion protein. Res Pract Thromb Haemost 2017;1(Suppl. 1):143.

38. Aleman M, Kistanova E, Seth-Chhabra E, et al. Recombinant FVIIIFc-VWF-XTEN promotes normal fibrin formation, structure and stability. Res Pract Thromb Haemost 2017;1(Suppl. 1):374.

39. DiMichele DM, Hoots WK, Pipe SW, et al. International workshop on immune tolerance induction: consensus recommendations. Haemophilia 2007;13(Suppl 1): 1–22.

40. Brown TM, Lee WC, Joshi AV, et al. Health-related quality of life and productivity impact in haemophilia patients with inhibitors. Haemophilia 2009;15(4):911–7.

41. Walsh CE, Soucie JM, Miller CH, United States Hemophilia Treatment Center Network. Impact of inhibitors on hemophilia A mortality in the United States. Am J Hematol 2015;90(5):400–5.

42. Astermark J. Why do inhibitors develop? Principles of and factors influencing the risk for inhibitor development in haemophilia. Haemophilia 2006;12(Suppl 3): 52–60.

43. Astermark J. FVIII inhibitors: pathogenesis and avoidance. Blood 2015;125(13): 2045–51.

44. Kurnik K, Bidlingmaier C, Engl W, et al. New early prophylaxis regimen that avoids immunological danger signals can reduce FVIII inhibitor development. Haemophilia 2010;16(2):256–62.

45. Auerswald G, Kurnik K, Aledort LM, et al. The EPIC study: a lesson to learn. Haemophilia 2015;21(5):622–8.

46. Peyvandi F, Mannucci PM, Garagiola I, et al. A randomized trial of factor VIII and neutralizing antibodies in hemophilia A. N Engl J Med 2016;374(21):2054–64.

47. van den Berg HM, Pipe S, Ljung R. Plasma products do not solve the inhibitor problem. Haemophilia 2017;23(3):346–7.

48. Iorio A. Research and policy implications of a recently published controlled study in previously untreated haemophilia patients at high risk of inhibitor development. Haemophilia 2017;23(3):350–2.

49. Peyvandi F, Mannucci PM, Palla R, et al. SIPPET: methodology, analysis and generalizability. Haemophilia 2017;23(3):353–61.

50. Collins PW, Chalmers E, Hart DP, et al. Diagnosis and treatment of factor VIII and IX inhibitors in congenital haemophilia: (4th edition). UK Haemophilia Centre Doctors Organization. Br J Haematol 2013;160(2):153–70.

51. Astermark J, Morado M, Rocino A, et al. Current European practice in immune tolerance induction therapy in patients with haemophilia and inhibitors. Haemophilia 2006;12(4):363–71.

52. Valentino LA, Kempton CL, Kruse-Jarres R, et al. US guidelines for immune tolerance induction in patients with haemophilia a and inhibitors. Haemophilia 2015; 21(5):559–67.

53. Hay CR, DiMichele DM, International Immune Tolerance Study. The principal results of the International Immune Tolerance Study: a randomized dose comparison. Blood 2012;119(6):1335–44.

54. Astermark J, Donfield SM, DiMichele DM, et al. A randomized comparison of bypassing agents in hemophilia complicated by an inhibitor: the FEIBA NovoSeven Comparative (FENOC) Study. Blood 2007;109(2):546–51.

55. Doshi BS, Gangadharan B, Doering CB, et al. Potentiation of thrombin generation in hemophilia A plasma by coagulation factor VIII and characterization of antibody-specific inhibition. PLoS One 2012;7(10):e48172.

56. Leissinger C, Gringeri A, Antmen B, et al. Anti-inhibitor coagulant complex prophylaxis in hemophilia with inhibitors. N Engl J Med 2011;365(18):1684–92.

57. Konkle BA, Ebbesen LS, Erhardtsen E, et al. Randomized, prospective clinical trial of recombinant factor VIIa for secondary prophylaxis in hemophilia patients with inhibitors. J Thromb Haemost 2007;5(9):1904–13.

58. Young G, Quon DV, Escobar MA, et al. CP-5-001: A phase 1/2a, open-label, multicenter, dose escalation study to assess the safety, pharmacokinetics and pharmacodynamics profile of a long-acting recombinant factor VIIa (MOD-5014) in adult men with hemophilia A or B. Res Pract Thromb Haemost 2017; 1(Suppl. 1):391.

59. Kempton CL, Abshire TC, Deveras RA, et al. Pharmacokinetics and safety of OBI-1, a recombinant B domain-deleted porcine factor VIII, in subjects with haemophilia A. Haemophilia 2012;18(5):798–804.

60. Kruse-Jarres R, St-Louis J, Greist A, et al. Efficacy and safety of OBI-1, an anti-haemophilic factor VIII (recombinant), porcine sequence, in subjects with acquired haemophilia A. Haemophilia 2015;21(2):162–70.

61. Croteau SE, Abajas YL, Wolberg AS, et al. Recombinant porcine factor VIII for high-risk surgery in paediatric congenital haemophilia A with high-titre inhibitor. Haemophilia 2017;23(2):e93–8.

62. Hartmann J, Croteau SE. 2017 Clinical trials update: Innovations in hemophilia therapy. Am J Hematol 2016;91(12):1252–60.

63. Buchlis G, Podsakoff GM, Radu A, et al. Factor IX expression in skeletal muscle of a severe hemophilia B patient 10 years after AAV-mediated gene transfer. Blood 2012;119(13):3038–41.

64. High KA, Anguela XM. Adeno-associated viral vectors for the treatment of hemophilia. Hum Mol Genet 2016;25(R1):R36–41.

65. Manno CS, Chew AJ, Hutchison S, et al. AAV-mediated factor IX gene transfer to skeletal muscle in patients with severe hemophilia B. Blood 2003;101(8): 2963–72.

66. Manno CS, Pierce GF, Arruda VR, et al. Successful transduction of liver in hemophilia by AAV-factor IX and limitations imposed by the host immune response. Nat Med 2006;12(3):342–7.

67. Nathwani AC, Tuddenham EG, Rangarajan S, et al. Adenovirus-associated virus vector-mediated gene transfer in hemophilia B. N Engl J Med 2011;365(25): 2357–65.

68. Nathwani AC, Reiss UM, Tuddenham EG, et al. Long-term safety and efficacy of factor IX gene therapy in hemophilia B. N Engl J Med 2014;371(21):1994–2004.

69. George LA, Sullivan SK, Giermasz A, et al. Hemophilia B gene therapy with a high-specific-activity factor IX variant. N Engl J Med 2017;377(23):2215–27.

70. Rangarajan S, Walsh L, Lester W, et al. AAV5-factor VIII gene transfer in severe hemophilia A. N Engl J Med 2017;377(26):2519–30.

71. Chen Y, Schroeder JA, Kuether EL, et al. Platelet gene therapy by lentiviral gene delivery to hematopoietic stem cells restores hemostasis and induces humoral immune tolerance in FIX(null) mice. Mol Ther 2014;22(1):169–77.

72. Kuether EL, Schroeder JA, Fahs SA, et al. Lentivirus-mediated platelet gene therapy of murine hemophilia A with pre-existing anti-factor VIII immunity. J Thromb Haemost 2012;10(8):1570–80.

73. Shi Q, Wilcox DA, Fahs SA, et al. Factor VIII ectopically targeted to platelets is therapeutic in hemophilia A with high-titer inhibitory antibodies. J Clin Invest 2006;116(7):1974–82.

74. Anguela XM, Sharma R, Doyon Y, et al. Robust ZFN-mediated genome editing in adult hemophilic mice. Blood 2013;122(19):3283–7.

75. Park CY, Kim DH, Son JS, et al. Functional correction of large factor VIII gene chromosomal inversions in hemophilia A patient-derived iPSCs using CRISPR-Cas9. Cell Stem Cell 2015;17(2):213–20.

76. Sharma R, Anguela XM, Doyon Y, et al. In vivo genome editing of the albumin locus as a platform for protein replacement therapy. Blood 2015;126(15):1777–84.

77. Kitazawa T, Igawa T, Sampei Z, et al. A bispecific antibody to factors IXa and X restores factor VIII hemostatic activity in a hemophilia A model. Nat Med 2012; 18(10):1570–4.

78. Shima M, Hanabusa H, Taki M, et al. Factor VIII-mimetic function of humanized bispecific antibody in hemophilia A. N Engl J Med 2016;374(21):2044–53.

79. Uchida N, Sambe T, Yoneyama K, et al. A first-in-human phase 1 study of ACE910, a novel factor VIII-mimetic bispecific antibody, in healthy subjects. Blood 2016;127(13):1633–41.

80. Oldenburg J, Mahlangu JN, Kim B, et al. Emicizumab prophylaxis in hemophilia A with inhibitors. N Engl J Med 2017;377(9):809–18.

81. Franchini M, Lippi G. Factor V Leiden and hemophilia. Thromb Res 2010;125(2): 119–23.

82. Shetty S, Vora S, Kulkarni B, et al. Contribution of natural anticoagulant and fibrinolytic factors in modulating the clinical severity of haemophilia patients. Br J Haematol 2007;138(4):541–4.

83. Polderdijk SG, Adams TE, Ivanciu L, et al. Design and characterization of an APC-specific serpin for the treatment of hemophilia. Blood 2017;129(1):105–13.

84. Maroney SA, Mast AE. New insights into the biology of tissue factor pathway inhibitor. J Thromb Haemost 2015;13(Suppl 1):S200–7.

85. Sehgal A, Barros S, Ivanciu L, et al. An RNAi therapeutic targeting antithrombin to rebalance the coagulation system and promote hemostasis in hemophilia. Nat Med 2015;21(5):492–7.

86. Pasi KJ, Rangarajan S, Georgiev P, et al. Targeting of antithrombin in hemophilia A or B with RNAi therapy. N Engl J Med 2017;377(9):819–28.
87. Dockal M, Pachlinger R, Hartmann R, et al. Biological explanation of clinically observed elevation of TFPI plasma levels after treatment with TFPI-antagonistic aptamer BAX 499. Blood 2012;120(21):1104.
88. Eichler H, Angchaisuksiri P, Kavakli KK, et al. Evaluation of safety and establishment of a PK/PD relationship of concizumab in hemophilia A patients. Res Pract Thromb Haemost 2017;1(Suppl. 2):1.
89. Coyle TE, Reding ME, Lin JC, et al. Phase I study of BAY 94-9027, a PEGylated B-domain-deleted recombinant factor VIII with an extended half-life, in subjects with hemophilia A. J Thromb Haemost 2014;12(4):488–96.
90. Tiede A, Brand B, Fischer R, et al. Enhancing the pharmacokinetic properties of recombinant factor VIII: first-in-human trial of glycoPEGylated recombinant factor VIII in patients with hemophilia A. J Thromb Haemost 2013;11(4):670–8.
91. Powell JS, Pasi KJ, Ragni MV, et al. Phase 3 study of recombinant factor IX Fc fusion protein in hemophilia B. N Engl J Med 2013;369:2313–23.
92. Negrier C, Knobe K, Tiede A, et al. Enhanced pharmacokinetic properties of a glycoPEGylated recombinant factor IX: a first human dose trial in patients with hemophilia B. Blood 2011;118(10):2695–701.
93. Santagostino E, Martinowitz U, Lissitchkov T, et al. Long-acting recombinant coagulation factor IX albumin fusion protein (rIX-FP) in hemophilia B: results of a phase 3 trial. Blood 2016;127(14):1761–9.

Treatment Options for Sickle Cell Disease

Emily Riehm Meier, MD, MSHS

KEYWORDS

- Sickle cell disease • Hydroxyurea • Transfusion
- Hematopoietic stem cell transplant • Fetal hemoglobin

KEY POINTS

- Hydroxyurea is well tolerated and effective in reducing the number of sickle cell–related complications in all ages of people with HbSS and HbSβ⁰thalassemia.
- Erythrocyte transfusions have a limited number of indications in treating people with sickle cell disease.
- The overall survival for matched sibling donor hematopoietic stem cell transplantation exceeds 90%, but less than 20% of people with sickle cell disease have a matched sibling donor available.

INTRODUCTION

Since the description of the first case of sickle cell disease (SCD) in 1910 by James Herrick and Ernest Irons, much has been learned about the disorder and improvements in care have increased survival in childhood.[1] Despite these advances, the average life expectancy for individuals with SCD has not changed in the past 30 years and remains half that of the average American.[2,3]

SCD is used to describe individuals who have hemoglobin S (HbS) as the predominant form of hemoglobin. HbS is caused by a single point mutation in the beta globin gene substituting a hydrophobic valine amino acid for glutamic acid at position 6 of the beta chain, making HbS molecules much more likely to polymerize in states of dehydration or acidosis. HbS polymerization causes the characteristic sickle shape change and downstream effects of sickling that include anemia, vaso-occlusion, cell adhesion, and vasoconstriction (**Fig. 1**). Inability of rigid, sickled cells to pass through the microvasculature leads to hypoxia of the tissues and painful vaso-occlusive episodes (VOE). Intrasplenic sickling leads to eventual splenic autoinfarction, which is responsible for an increased risk of infection with encapsulated organisms in individuals with SCD. Sickled erythrocytes and reticulocytes have adhesion proteins on

Disclosure Statement: Research funding from Pfizer (ASPIRE IIR #WI222809); Consultancy – CVS Caremark.

Sickle Cell Research, Indiana Hemophilia and Thrombosis Center, 8326 Naab Road, Indianapolis, IN 46260, USA

E-mail address: emeier@ihtc.org

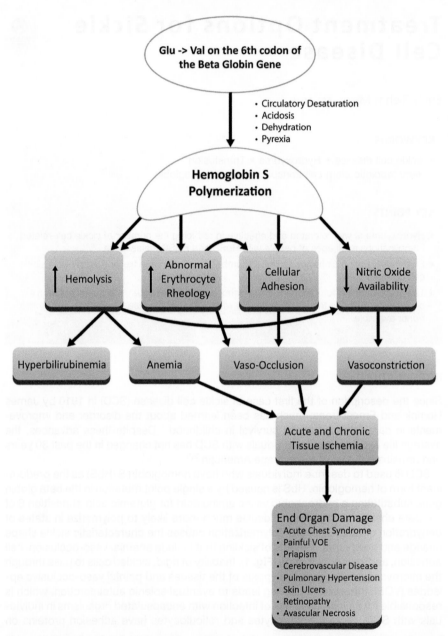

Fig. 1. Sickle cell pathophysiology. The pathophysiology of sickle cell disease is complex and stems from the polymerization of HbS that occurs during periods of hypoxemia, dehydration, acidosis, and pyrexia. Polymers of sickle hemoglobin cause the characteristic shape change of the erythrocyte and lead to hemolysis, abnormal rheology, cellular adhesion, and decreased nitric oxide availability. These changes result in anemia, vaso-occlusion, and vasoconstriction that are the cause of SCD-associated end organ damage. VOE, vaso-occlusive episode. (*From* Meier ER, Rampersad A. Pediatric sickle cell disease: past successes and future challenges. Pediatr Res 2017;81(1-2):249–58; with permission.)

their surface that damage vascular endothelium, leading to vasculopathy and vaso-spasm.[4,5] Endogenous nitric oxide, produced in the endothelium from arginine maintains patent vessel walls. In individuals with SCD, nitric oxide is consumed by plasma-free hemoglobin and degraded by arginase, which is released from hemolyzed sickle erythrocytes.[6] More recently, altered interactions between the vascular endothelium, neutrophils, platelet, and sickled erythrocytes have been identified as direct promoters of sickle vaso-occlusion and inducers of a chronic inflammatory state in people with SCD.[7] Recently an association between menses and sickle cell pain has also been noted (See Shaina M. Willen and Michael DeBaun's article, "The Epidemiology and Management of Lung Diseases in Sickle Cell Disease: Lessons Learned from Acute and Chronic Lung Disease in Cystic Fibrosis," in this issue).

Because HbS polymerization is the initiating factor of the cascade of pathophysiologic causes of the clinical complications that individuals with SCD experience, reducing HbS concentration is the mainstay of therapy for the disease. Thus, hydroxyurea (HU) and transfusions and the recently Food and Drug Administration (FDA)-approved L-glutamine are the focus of this article. Supportive care initiatives that have led to improved survival for children with SCD in developed countries are also discussed. Finally, recent breakthroughs in curative therapies for SCD, hematopoietic stem cell transplant (HSCT) and gene therapy, are highlighted. Pipeline therapies are reviewed elsewhere in this issue (See Ahmar U. Zaidi and Matthew M. Heeney's article, "A Scientific Renaissance: Novel Drugs in Sickle Cell Disease," in this issue.)

SUPPORTIVE CARE THERAPIES
Infection Prophylaxis and Fever Management

Before universal newborn screening, penicillin prophylaxis, and vaccination against encapsulated organisms, infection was a common cause of death in children with SCD. The randomized, placebo-controlled trial of prophylactic penicillin (PROPS) revealed that twice daily administration of prophylactic penicillin in children with SCD less than 5 years of age drastically reduced the rate of invasive pneumococcal disease.[8] The risk of invasive pneumococcal disease in children with SCD has decreased 70% to 90% since the addition of the protein-conjugated pneumococcal vaccine series (Prevnar) in early infancy.[9] The PROPS study included children with HbSS and HbSβ[0]thalassemia, the two sickle genotypes with the highest risk of pneumococcal infection because of splenic autoinfarction. Children with HbSC and HbSβ[+]thalassemia have less splenic dysfunction and, therefore, a decreased risk of invasive pneumococcal disease, leading the National Heart, Lung, and Blood Institute (NHLBI) Evidence Based Disease Management Guidelines Committee to state that practitioners should "consider withholding penicillin from children with HbSC and HbSβ[+]thalassemia unless they have had a splenectomy."[10]

All people with SCD, regardless of genotype, should be considered functionally asplenic because of the autoinfarction of the spleen that occurs at a young age from recurrent intravascular sickling. Education of families and patients about the importance of emergency evaluation for fevers greater than or equal to 101°F[10] and the appropriate management with blood culture and timely administration of an antibiotic (eg, ceftriaxone) effective against *Streptococcus pneumoniae*, *Haemophilus influenza*, and other encapsulated, rapidly multiplying organisms has further decreased the morbidity and mortality from infection.[11,12]

Folate Supplementation

The sickled erythrocyte has an average life span of 12 to 16 days, one-tenth that of a healthy erythrocyte containing normal adult hemoglobin (HbA), which results in an increased erythropoietic drive in affected individuals.[13,14] The increased erythrocyte production could place individuals with SCD at risk of folate deficiency. However, no differences in hematologic indices or clinical complications were found during the only placebo-controlled study of folic acid supplementation, although those study participants who received folic acid had higher serum folate levels than control subjects.[15] This study was completed before the FDA mandated the fortification of grains with folic acid to decrease the number of infants born with neural tube defects.[16] A recent comparison of children with HbSS or HbSβ⁰thalassemia, most of whom were being treated with HU, found no differences between erythrocyte folate levels and hematologic indices in those receiving folate supplementation versus those who were not.[16] The authors concluded that folic acid supplementation is not necessary in children with SCD, and folic acid is only mentioned in the 2014 National Institutes of Health Evidence Based Management Guidelines for SCD in reference to preventing neural tube defects.[10]

DISEASE-MODIFYING THERAPIES
Hydroxyurea

Fetal hemoglobin (HbF) contains two α chains and two γ globin chains. In healthy infants, HbF production is silenced postnatally and HbA becomes the predominant hemoglobin.[17] In infants with SCD, however, HbF is replaced by HbS during the postnatal hemoglobin switch. Individuals with SCD whose erythrocytes still contain a high concentration of HbF have a milder clinical SCD course than those who have low intraerythrocytic HbF concentrations. HU, a once daily oral medication that is rapidly absorbed, alters the kinetics of erythropoiesis by inhibiting ribonucleotide reductase, which prevents cells from leaving the G1/S phase of the cell cycle.[18,19] Thus, HU increases HbF levels, thereby decreasing HbS concentration within the erythrocyte and preventing HbS polymerization, thus decreasing erythrocyte sickling and subsequent hemolysis.[20] Additional mechanisms of HU action include reduction of the neutrophil and platelet count, which ameliorates the abnormal cell adhesion-inflammation pathways, and correction of the nitric oxide deficiency state brought about by SCD-associated hemolysis.[21–23]

The Multi-Center Study of Hydroxyurea (MSH) was a randomized, double-blind, placebo-controlled trial to determine if daily HU could decrease the frequency of painful VOEs in adults with SCD. To be eligible for the study, adults had to have had three or more VOEs in the year preceding study enrollment. The trial was stopped early by the data safety and monitoring board because interim data analysis revealed that HU treatment resulted in a 44% reduction of VOE.[24] Additional clinical benefits of HU in this study were fewer episodes of acute chest syndrome (ACS) and fewer unscheduled erythrocyte transfusions; laboratory benefits included higher hemoglobin and HbF levels, and lower reticulocyte, neutrophil, and platelet counts.[24] Because of the remarkable results from the MSH study, the FDA approved HU in 1998 for use in adults with symptomatic SCD. Individuals enrolled in MSH were offered open-label HU and participation in a long-term follow-up study. Those who continued to take HU had improved survival compared with those individuals who did not take HU, which was confirmed in a longitudinal observational study in Greece.[25,26]

HU was approved as a treatment for children ages 2 years and older in December 2017. Prior to receiving FDA approval, however, the number of children with SCD being treated with HU is steadily increasing after studies similar to the MSH were published. The BABY HUG study (multicenter randomized, placebo-controlled trial of HU in young children with HbSS or HbSβ⁰thalassemia) enrolled children between 9 and 18 months of age.[27] Unlike the MSH, infants enrolled in the BABY HUG study were not required to have had SCD-associated symptoms like VOE. Similar to all other studies of HU treatment in adults, adolescents, and children with SCD, rates of VOE, ACS, and unscheduled erythrocyte transfusions decreased in those BABY HUG participants who received HU.[28–30] Importantly, the growth, development, or risk of genotoxicity did not differ between the placebo and HU groups in the BABY-HUG study.[28,31,32] Based on these results, the 2014 NHLBI Evidence Based Management Guidelines for SCD recommend that all infants 9 months of age and older with HbSS or HbSβ⁰thalassemia be offered HU as treatment, regardless of the frequency or severity of disease complications.[10]

Two recent studies have compared the efficacy of the standard therapy (chronic erythrocyte transfusions and chelation) for primary or secondary stroke prevention to HU and phlebotomy (alternate therapy). The study of secondary stroke prevention, Stroke With Transfusion Changing to Hydroxyurea (SWiTCH), was stopped early by the study's data safety and monitoring board when a scheduled interim analysis revealed statistical futility for reaching the composite primary end point of both recurrent stroke rate and improved transfusional hematochromatosis. The study design allowed for an increased rate of stroke in the alternate treatment group, provided that iron burden was improved because transfusional hematochromatosis can cause significant organ damage. The stroke rate in the alternative arm was higher (n = 7; 10%) than the standard treatment arm (n = 0; 0%) as expected, but phlebotomy was inferior to chelation at improving iron overload, so the composite end point was not reached. Because of the inferior results on SWiTCH's HU/phlebotomy arm, chronic transfusion plus chelation remains the mainstay of secondary stroke prevention in children with SCA.[33]

HU and phlebotomy was recently found to be an acceptable alternative to standard treatment (transfusion/chelation therapy) for primary stroke prevention in children with abnormal transcranial Doppler ultrasound (TCD) flow velocities without evidence of severe vasculopathy on brain MRI/MRA.[34] Before the recently published Abnormal TCD with Transfusions Changing to HU (TWiTCH) trial, small cohort studies indicated that HU may reduce TCD velocities from abnormal or conditional to normal.[35,36] TCD is a noninvasive screening tool to identify children with HbSS or HbSβ⁰thalassemia who may be at increased risk for stroke. TCD measures the flow velocity through the cerebral arterial circulation, particularly the internal carotid and middle cerebral arteries. Increased flow velocity correlates with the presence of a narrowed vessel or segment; velocities of greater than or equal to 200 cm/s are strongly associated with increased risk of stroke.[37] The Stroke Prevention Trial in Sickle Cell Anemia (STOP) trial decreased the stroke rate from 10% to less than 1% when children with two consecutive abnormal TCD studies (usually performed 2–4 weeks apart) started prophylactic chronic monthly blood transfusions to reduce HbS concentration to 30% or less.[38] Before the publication of the TWiTCH study results in 2016, transfusions and chelation therapy were continued indefinitely because the Optimizing Primary Stroke Prevention in Sickle Cell Anemia (STOP 2) trial showed that discontinuation of transfusions caused reversion to abnormal TCD values and, in some cases, overt stroke.[39]

The TWiTCH trial randomized children with abnormal TCDs who had received at least 1 year of chronic transfusion therapy and who did not have severe cerebral vasculopathy[34] to either continue transfusion therapy and iron chelation with deferasirox or change to HU and phlebotomy. In the alternate HU plus phlebotomy study arm, transfusions were weaned over 4 to 9 months as HU doses were escalated to maximum tolerated dose (MTD), based on absolute neutrophil count. Phlebotomy commenced once transfusions had stopped, and patients were monitored by TCD every 3 months to ensure that TCD velocities did not revert to abnormal. The first scheduled interim analysis showed noninferiority of the alternative therapy arm. After 50% of participants had exited the study, repeat analyses supported these findings and the study was terminated by the NHLBI.[40] These findings support HU and phlebotomy as an acceptable substitute for standard treatment in children with abnormal TCD but without severe vasculopathy who have received at least 1 year of chronic transfusion therapy.

Initiating hydroxyurea

HU elevates HbF production that increases erythrocyte life span, decreases the rate of hemolysis, and by default, decreases reticulocyte count and is generally well tolerated with few irreversible side effects. Because of the direct effect of HU on the bone marrow, myelosuppression is the most common side effect and can affect all three cell lines. Thus, close laboratory monitoring, especially after treatment initiation and during dose escalation, is paramount (**Table 1**). Baseline evaluation before HU initiation should include a detailed history and physical examination, laboratory evaluations including complete blood count (CBC), HbF quantitation, liver and renal function testing, and urine pregnancy test if indicated. Although HU has not been shown to be a carcinogen, animal studies have demonstrated it to be a mutagen and teratogen.[41] No birth defects have been reported in children born to women being

Table 1 HU dosing strategy			
Weeks After HU Initiated	HU Dose (mg/kg/d)[a]	Weeks Until Next CBC/Reticulocyte count[b]	Dose Adjustment
0	20	2	None
2	20	2	None
4	20	4	None
8	20	2	Increase by 5 mg/kg/d
10	25	2	None
12	25	4	None
16	25	2	Increase by 5 mg/kg/d
18	30	2	None
20	30	4	None
24	30	2	Increase by 5 mg/kg/d
26	35	2	None
28	35	4	None
32	35	8	None
40	35	8–12	None
48–52	35	8–12	None[c]

[a] 20 mg/kg/d is the usual starting dose for children and infants; 15 mg/kg/d is the usual starting dose for adults. Patients with concomitant chronic renal disease should have their starting dose decreased to 5 to 10 mg/kg/d.

[b] Liver and kidney function tests and a hemoglobin electrophoresis should be obtained every 3 to 6 mo.

[c] Once MTD is reached, dose should be adjusted for weight gain.

treated with HU during pregnancy or fathered by men taking HU.[26,42] Randomized controlled trials on the reproductive effects of HU are lacking, so individuals of child-bearing potential should be counseled at each clinic visit to use effective contraception while taking HU. HU should be discontinued 3 to 6 months before conception is attempted and mothers should continue to hold HU therapy while breastfeeding. Other side effects of HU include skin changes (hyperpigmentation, darkening of the nailbeds, hair thinning), nausea, headache, and small increases in creatinine because HU is cleared by the kidneys.[43] No evidence exists that HU increases leukemia risk in individuals treated with HU.[44] A discussion of the risks and benefits of HU treatment should be had with the patient and their family members, and questions and concerns should be addressed before initiating treatment.

Hydroxyurea dose escalation

In children 9 months of age and greater, HU should be started at 20 mg/kg in a single daily dose rounded to the nearest 10 mg. Because clinical response to HU is dose dependent and attaining MTD is beneficial for individuals with SCD,[45] HU dose should be escalated every 8 weeks in the absence of dose-limiting cytopenias (see **Table 1**; **Table 2**) until MTD is achieved. MTD is defined as 35 mg/kg/d or the dose beyond which two episodes of drug toxicity have occurred.[46] CBC and reticulocyte count should be checked every 4 weeks while in dose escalation and 2 weeks after every dose change. If neutropenia or thrombocytopenia occur, hold HU and repeat CBC with differential in 2 weeks. If toxicity is associated with illness and subsequently resolves, HU should be restarted at previous dose and dose escalation may continue. If there is no associated illness, restart HU at 5 mg/kg/d lower than the dose associated with cytopenias. Once MTD has been achieved, laboratory monitoring should include CBC with differential and reticulocyte count every 2 to 3 months. Complete metabolic panel (electrolytes, renal and liver function tests) should be obtained every 3-6 months. Pregnancy testing should be obtained routinely in sexually active adolescents and adults as clinically indicated. Increases in hemoglobin, mean corpuscular volume and HbF levels and decreased white blood cell, absolute neutrophil, platelet, and reticulocyte counts indicate an appropriate laboratory response to HU. Patients and their families should be advised that clinical benefit may not be evident for at least 1 month and possibly not for 3 to 6 months after HU initiation because it can take that long for HbF levels to increase to a high enough level to prevent HbS polymerization and subsequent hemolysis. Therefore, a 6-month trial of HU at the MTD is recommended before considering discontinuation of HU. Although poor adherence is the most common cause of treatment failure, a proportion of patients are biologically resistant to HU.[47] They should also be reminded that HU has to be taken on a daily basis and that its beneficial effects are lost if it is discontinued.

During monitoring visits, providers should elicit symptoms of toxicity and reiterate adherence, advising patients not to take extra doses if a dose is missed and to continue to take HU when sick or hospitalized unless instructed by a physician.

Table 2
HU dose-limiting toxicities

Laboratory Value	Toxicity Definition
Absolute neutrophil count	<1.5 K/µL
Hemoglobin	20% decrease or <4.5 g/dL
Platelet count	<80 K/µL
Absolute reticulocyte count	<80 K/µL unless hemoglobin ≥9.0 g/dL

Contraceptive counseling before HU initiation and at follow-up visits should also be provided to patients of both genders.

Hydroxyurea is underused

Despite its proven benefits in preventing SCD-related complications, only 30% of eligible patients are receiving HU.[48] This low utilization rate is caused by provider and patient factors. Many providers are unaware of HU as a treatment option for SCD or, if aware of HU, are not convinced of its therapeutic benefit.[49] Some providers are concerned about the side effects of HU or being able to obtain laboratory results at recommended intervals to monitor for myelosuppression.[49,50] When providers offer HU as a therapeutic option, more than 20% of families decline, citing concern about side effects or unwillingness to adhere to laboratory screening schedule.[51]

HU use has been extended to patients who have hemoglobinopathies other than HbSS or HbSβ⁰thalassemia, such as HbSC or HbSβ⁺ thalassemia with frequent VOE or recurrent ACS. However, their responses to HU are extremely variable and there is also considerable variation in the dose of drug that individual patients are able to tolerate; some experience myelotoxicity at only 7.5 mg/kg/d and others are able to take up to 30 mg/kg/d.[52]

Transfusion Therapy

Blood transfusions are used for management of acute conditions and prevention of complications associated with SCD.[53] The main goal in transfusing individuals with SCD is to reduce the concentration of circulating HbS. Therefore, only sickle-negative erythrocytes should be transfused.[53] The method of transfusion depends on the underlying goal of therapy. Indications for episodic erythrocyte transfusion

Table 3
Indications for erythrocyte transfusions in individuals with SCD

Indication	Preferred Transfusion Method
Need to increase oxygen-carrying capacity	
Acute, symptomatic anemia	Simple
Aplastic crisis	Simple
Before surgery requiring general anesthesia	Simple
Need to improve microvascular perfusion	
Acute or impending cerebrovascular event	Exchange transfusion
Symptomatic acute chest syndrome + hemoglobin more than 1 g/dL lower than baseline	Simple
Symptomatic severe acute chest syndrome (O_2 sat <90% with supplemental oxygen)	Exchange
Acute splenic sequestration + severe anemia	Simple
Hepatic sequestration	Exchange or simple
Intrahepatic cholestasis	Exchange or simple
Multisystem organ failure	Exchange or simple
Transfusion is not indicated	
Uncomplicated VOE	
Priapism	
Asymptomatic anemia	
Acute kidney injury	

from the 2014 NHLBI Evidence Based Management Guidelines are found in **Table 3**.[10] Chronic erythrocyte transfusion therapy is only indicated for children who have had an overt stroke or abnormal TCD in these guidelines.

- *Simple transfusion* involves transfusing erythrocytes without removing any of the patient's own blood. The amount of blood to be transfused should be calculated based on the child's body weight, current hemoglobin level, and indication for transfusion. Simple transfusion usually consists of giving 10 to 15 mL/kg of packed red blood cells (pRBCs) over 3 to 4 hours. Children who are not receiving chronic, monthly erythrocyte transfusions likely have high HbS percentages, so the goal post-transfusion hemoglobin should not exceed 10 g/dL because of the risk of hyperviscosity. Sickled erythrocytes are rigid and inherently increase blood viscosity; thus, raising the hematocrit to more than 30% without first reducing HbS concentration places patients at risk of hyperviscosity-related complications, such as hypertension and cerebral hemorrhage.[54]
- *Partial manual exchange transfusion* usually involves pretransfusion phlebotomy of 5 to 10 mL/kg of whole blood (depending on the hematocrit at the start of the procedure and patient's hemodynamic stability) followed by transfusion of 10 to 15 mL/kg pRBCs.
- *Automated red cell exchange transfusion* uses continuous flow instrumentation to efficiently and effectively replace the patient's whole blood with donor pRBCs. The goal fraction of cells remaining is 25% to 30%, roughly equivalent to a HbS level of 30% and is accomplished by exchanging equal volumes of 50 to 80 mL/kg of donor pRBCs for the patient's whole blood. This method rapidly and substantially reduces the concentration of HbS without increasing the overall hematocrit or blood viscosity, and is the preferred method of transfusion for children who present with an acute stroke.[55] Automated red cell exchange reduces transfusional hematochromatosis in children who need chronic transfusion therapy compared with partial manual exchange and simple transfusion.[56] Limitations of automated red cell exchange include the need for adequate venous access for the procedure, and many individuals who require chronic erythrocytapheresis have indwelling venous catheters.

Risks of transfusion therapy

- *Alloimmunization*: Between 20% and 40% of individuals with SCD who receive erythrocyte transfusion develop alloantibodies with standard ABO and Rh matched erythrocytes.[57] Limited phenotyping for C, E, and Kell reduces alloimmunization rates to less than 15% and should be performed for all patients with SCD.[10] Extended antigenically matched erythrocytes should be provided for patients with known alloantibodies to less frequently occurring antigens (eg, Duffy or Kidd).[58,59]
- *Transfusional Hematochromatosis* is generally defined as serum ferritin levels greater than or equal to 1000 ng/mL on two measurements separated by at least 1 month. Iron overload typically occurs within 2 years of initiating chronic transfusion therapy or after 10 to 20 pRBC transfusions (~120 mL/kg of pRBC).[53] Chronically transfused patients are at risk for iron overload because of the low rate of iron excretion in humans (1–2 mg/d) compared with the amount of iron in each milliliter of pRBCs (0.75 mg of iron in each milliliter of transfused blood).[53] Because untreated iron overload can result in cardiac, hepatic, and endocrine abnormalities, chronically transfused patients should be monitored with serum

ferritin levels monthly. Liver iron content is measured with specialized MRI techniques that are preferred over the more invasive liver biopsy.[60] Cardiac iron burden can also be measured with MRI, although patients with SCD have a lower prevalence of cardiac iron overload than patients with transfusion-dependent thalassemia. Thyroid and pituitary function laboratory values should be obtained annually. Chelation therapy with deferasirox is indicated when two consecutive ferritin levels exceed 1000 ng/mL. Two preparations of derferasirox are available, Exjade (recommended dosage 20–40 mg/kg/d) or Jadenu (recommended dosage 14–28 mg/kg/d). These oral iron chelators are preferable to desferal, which requires daily subcutaneous administration, although adherence to chelation continues to be an issue.[61]

L-Glutamine

In July 2017, L-glutamine became the first new oral medication approved by the FDA to treat people with SCD in almost 20 years. Although the exact mechanism of action for L-glutamine has not been fully elucidated, glutamine is an amino acid that is a known precursor for nicotinamide adenine dinucleotide (NAD+) synthesis.[62] Sickled erythrocytes are more susceptible to oxidative damage, which may lead to ongoing hemolysis and VOE. Increased levels of NAD+ help to prevent oxidative damage, thereby decreasing hemolysis and vaso-occlusion. Early studies demonstrated a severalfold increase in the uptake of L-glutamine by sickle erythrocytes compared with healthy control erythrocytes; the L-glutamine was primarily used to produce NAD+.[62] Because of the shortened erythrocyte lifespan, children with SCD have higher protein turnover than healthy children and were found to have glutamine levels 47% lower than healthy children.[63,64]

Seventy people with SCD, 5 years of age and older, were enrolled in a phase 2 study of pharmaceutical grade L-glutamine.[65] Hospitalizations were significantly decreased compared with the placebo group, and the number of VOEs was lower in those receiving L-glutamine, although the difference between groups was not statistically significant. The number of VOEs in the phase 3 double-blind, placebo-controlled trial of L-glutamine was reduced by 25% in the L-glutamine group compared with placebo (average of three VOEs in the L-glutamine arm vs mean of four VOEs in the placebo group). Nearly three-quarters of the people enrolled in the phase 3 study were being treated with HU.[66] L-Glutamine powder is available in 5-g packets and should be mixed in 8 ounces of cold or room temperature liquid (water, milk, or apple juice are listed as examples in the package insert) or 4 to 6 ounces of pudding or applesauce and ingested immediately. Dosing is based on weight: people less than 30 kg should take 5 g twice daily, those between 30 and 65 kg should take 10 g twice daily, and those greater than 65 kg should take 15 g twice daily. Gastrointestinal side effects (constipation, abdominal pain, nausea) had the greatest frequency in the phase 3 trial.[66]

CURATIVE TREATMENT OPTIONS
Hematopoietic Stem Cell Transplantation

The only currently available cure for SCD is HSCT. Matched sibling donor (MSD) transplants in patients with SCD have the highest overall survival (OS) rates (93%–97%), disease-free survival (DFS) rates (82%–100%), and lowest rates of graft rejection (8%–18%) and graft-versus-host disease (GVHD) (6%–35%).[67,68] Unfortunately, less than 20% of people with SCD have an MSD, so just over 1000 transplants for SCD have been documented in the literature.[68,69] Most of the MSD HSCT that have been performed to date used myeloablative condition regimens that are associated with end-organ toxicities, including gonadal toxicities that frequently result in sterility, a concern for patients and families.[70,71] Because of these concerns, most HSCT trials for SCD now use reduced intensity conditioning regimens that have recently been shown to have similar rates of OS (93%), event free survival (EFS) (90.7%), and GVHD (23% acute GVHD, 13% chronic GVHD).[72] An analysis of all MSD HSCT performed for SCD in the United States and Europe revealed that conditioning regimen had no effect on OS or EFS.[68] However, increasing age was associated with worsened OS and EFS; people 16 years of age and older had an OS of 81% and EFS of 85% compared with an OS of 95% and EFS of 93% for children younger than 16 ($P<.001$ for OS and EFS).[68] A continuous relationship between death and age was observed with every year of increasing age, increasing the risk of graft failure or death by 10%.[68] Similarly, rates of GVHD were significantly lower in children less than 16 years of age compared with older adolescents and adults.

Given the paucity of available MSD for patients with SCD, studies evaluating alternative donor HSCT using stem cells from matched unrelated donors (MUD) or haploidentical donors are ongoing and have shown mixed results. Haploidentical HSCT have low rates of GVHD, but high rates (40%–50%) of graft rejection.[73] Comparatively, MUD HSCT have low rates of rejection, but higher rates of GHVD.[74] Results from the first unrelated donor-reduced intensity HSCT for children with SCD (the SCURT trial, NCT00745420) were published in 2016. The umbilical cord arm of the study was closed several years earlier because of high rates of graft rejection, which met the predetermined stopping rule.[74] Two-year OS and EFS rates were lower than MSD (79% and 69%, respectively). Almost 40% of SCURT trial participants developed chronic GVHD, the leading cause of mortality in the study.[75] Similar to MSD HSCT, increasing age was associated to decreased survival; all but one death in the SCURT trial occurred in a person 16 years or older. Thus, alternative donor HSCT using stem cells from MUD or haploidentical donors should only be performed in the context of a research study, and studies are ongoing to determine the conditioning regimens and GVHD prophylaxis strategies that provide the best OS and EFS without increasing late effects.

Eligibility for ongoing HSCT trials to patients who do not meet the severity criteria listed in **Box 1** is a source of ongoing discussion among hematologists, HSCT physicians, and medical ethicists, given what is known about the early mortality in adults with SCD and reduced quality of life.[3,76,77] One of the most fascinating and frustrating

---

Box 1
Indications for MSD hematopoietic stem cell transplant

Overstroke

Abnormal TCD

Frequent VOE (at least 3/y for the preceding 2 years) despite HU

Recurrent ACS despite supportive care/disease-modifying therapy with HU

More than three combined ACS + VOE annually for the past 3 years

Pulmonary hypertension

Recurrent priapism

Sickle nephropathy

Adapted from King A, Shenoy S. Evidence-based focused review of the status of hematopoietic stem cell transplantation as treatment of sickle cell disease and thalassemia. Blood 2014;123(20):3090. Reproduced with permission of American Society of Hematology; permission conveyed through Copyright Clearance Center, Inc.

aspects of SCD care is how people with the same single amino acid substitution can have different clinical complications of differing severity that occur at different times in their lives. The search for a predictor of SCD severity has been ongoing for more than 30 years, and the only currently available validated predictor of a severe SCD outcome is TCD, which only identifies children at highest risk for stroke; predictors for recurrent VOE or ACS are not currently available. HbF levels and alpha globin gene number have frequently been studied as possible early predictors of severe SCD, but results of these studies have varied depending on outcome variables and study sample sizes.[78] Absolute reticulocyte count greater than 200 K/μL between the ages of 2 and 6 months is associated with triple the risk of hospitalization before age 3 years and higher rates of stroke and death in a historical SCD newborn cohort. Absolute reticulocyte count was the only predictor studied before infants developed SCD-related symptomatology, allowing it to function as a true predictor of SCD severity.[78]

Risk stratification would be beneficial as patients and families weigh the risks and benefits of HSCT compared with disease-modifying therapy with HU. In addition to the risks of GVHD and graft rejection mentioned previously, the rates of intra-HSCT complications are higher for people with SCD than other nonmalignant conditions, particularly intracranial hemorrhage. Aggressive supportive care with pRBC and platelet transfusions is necessary and transfusion thresholds are higher.[79] Additionally, avoidance of hypertension and hypomagnesemia protects HSCT recipients from neurologic sequelae in the immediate post-HSCT period.[80] Referral to HSCT centers with experience in performing HSCT for people with SCD is imperative to minimize risks to patients.

Gene Therapy

Because the monogenetic defect that causes SCD has been well characterized since its discovery, SCD is an excellent candidate for gene-modifying or replacement therapies. Gene therapy is also an attractive curative option because less than 20% of people with SCD have an MSD for HSCT. Gene therapy strategies for SCD include replacement of the abnormal beta globin gene, augmenting HbF production by manipulation of the gamma globin gene, or reactivating silenced gamma globin genes.[81–83] For gene therapy to be effective in curing SCD, gene transfer to the hematopoietic stem cell population must be efficient and provide long-term gene expression. The first report of gene therapy used to treat an adolescent with SCD was published in early 2017.[84] There are several open gene therapy trials for adults with SCD in the United States (NCT02186418, NCT02247843, NCT02151526, and NCT02140554). Two comprehensive reviews on gene therapy in SCD provide more in-depth information.[82,83]

SUMMARY

The clinical complications of SCD result from a cascade of events that starts with the polymerization of HbS. Thus, the goal of disease-modifying therapies is to decrease HbS concentration, either by increasing HbF levels (HU) or increasing HbA levels (transfusion). Curative options, such as HSCT and gene therapy, strive to eliminate the production of HbS. Supportive therapies, such as antibiotic prophylaxis, have increased survival of children by preventing death from overwhelming infection, but have not increased overall life expectancy for people living with SCD. With the increasingly widespread use of disease-modifying and curative therapies, it is hoped that life expectancy will increase and approach that of the average American in the near future.

REFERENCES

1. Herrick JB. Peculiar elongated and sickle-shaped red blood corpuscles in a case of severe anemia. JAMA 2014;312(10):1063.
2. Platt OS, Brambilla DJ, Rosse WF, et al. Mortality in sickle cell disease. Life expectancy and risk factors for early death. N Engl J Med 1994;330(23):1639–44.
3. Lanzkron S, Carroll CP, Haywood C Jr. Mortality rates and age at death from sickle cell disease: U.S., 1979-2005. Public Health Rep 2013;128(2):110–6.
4. Zennadi R, Whalen EJ, Soderblom EJ, et al. Erythrocyte plasma membrane-bound ERK1/2 activation promotes ICAM-4-mediated sickle red cell adhesion to endothelium. Blood 2012;119(5):1217–27.
5. Vilas-Boas W, Figueiredo CV, Pitanga TN, et al. Endothelial nitric oxide synthase (-786T>C) and Endothelin-1 (5665G>T) gene polymorphisms as vascular dysfunction risk factors in sickle cell anemia. Gene Regul Syst Bio 2016;10:67–72.
6. Bakshi N, Morris CR. The role of the arginine metabolome in pain: implications for sickle cell disease. J Pain Res 2016;9:167–75.
7. Zhang D, Xu C, Manwani D, et al. Neutrophils, platelets, and inflammatory pathways at the nexus of sickle cell disease pathophysiology. Blood 2016;127(7): 801–9.
8. Gaston MH, Verter JI, Woods G, et al. Prophylaxis with oral penicillin in children with sickle cell anemia. A randomized trial. N Engl J Med 1986;314(25):1593–9.
9. Adamkiewicz TV, Silk BJ, Howgate J, et al. Effectiveness of the 7-valent pneumococcal conjugate vaccine in children with sickle cell disease in the first decade of life. Pediatrics 2008;121(3):562–9.
10. National Heart Lung and Blood Institute (NHLBI). Evidence-based management of sickle cell disease: expert panel report, 2014. 2014. Available at: http://www.nhlbi.nih.gov/health-pro/guidelines/sickle-cell-disease-guidelines. Accessed September 14, 2017.
11. Baskin MN, Goh XL, Heeney MM, et al. Bacteremia risk and outpatient management of febrile patients with sickle cell disease. Pediatrics 2013;131(6):1035–41.
12. Rubin LG, Schaffner W. Clinical practice. Care of the asplenic patient. N Engl J Med 2014;371(4):349–56.
13. Franco RS. The measurement and importance of red cell survival. Am J Hematol 2009;84(2):109–14.
14. Franco RS, Yasin Z, Palascak MB, et al. The effect of fetal hemoglobin on the survival characteristics of sickle cells. Blood 2006;108(3):1073–6.
15. Dixit R, Nettem S, Madan SS, et al. Folate supplementation in people with sickle cell disease. Cochrane Database Syst Rev 2016;(2):CD011130.
16. Nguyen GT, Lewis A, Goldener C, et al. Discontinuation of folic acid supplementation in young patients with sickle cell anemia. J Pediatr Hematol Oncol 2017; 39(6):470–2.
17. Oneal PA, Gantt NM, Schwartz JD, et al. Fetal hemoglobin silencing in humans. Blood 2006;108(6):2081–6.
18. Yarbro JW. Mechanism of action of hydroxyurea. Semin Oncol 1992;19(3 Suppl 9):1–10.
19. From the Centers for Disease Control and Prevention. Mortality among children with sickle cell disease identified by newborn screening during 1990-1994: California, Illinois, and New York. JAMA 1998;279(14):1059–60.
20. Noguchi CT, Rodgers GP, Serjeant G, et al. Levels of fetal hemoglobin necessary for treatment of sickle cell disease. N Engl J Med 1988;318(2):96–9.

21. Saleh AW, Hillen HF, Duits AJ. Levels of endothelial, neutrophil and platelet-specific factors in sickle cell anemia patients during hydroxyurea therapy. Acta Haematol 1999;102(1):31–7.

22. Nahavandi M, Wyche MQ, Perlin E, et al. Nitric oxide metabolites in sickle cell anemia patients after oral administration of hydroxyurea; hemoglobinopathy. Hematology 2000;5(4):335–9.

23. Charache S. Mechanism of action of hydroxyurea in the management of sickle cell anemia in adults. Semin Hematol 1997;34(3 Suppl 3):15–21.

24. Charache S, Terrin ML, Moore RD, et al. Effect of hydroxyurea on the frequency of painful crises in sickle cell anemia. Investigators of the multicenter study of hydroxyurea in sickle cell anemia. N Engl J Med 1995;332(20):1317–22.

25. Steinberg MH, Barton F, Castro O, et al. Effect of hydroxyurea on mortality and morbidity in adult sickle cell anemia: risks and benefits up to 9 years of treatment. JAMA 2003;289(13):1645–51.

26. Voskaridou E, Christoulas D, Bilalis A, et al. The effect of prolonged administration of hydroxyurea on morbidity and mortality in adult patients with sickle cell syndromes: results of a 17-year, single-center trial (LaSHS). Blood 2010;115(12):2354–63.

27. Wynn L, Miller S, Faughnan L, et al. Recruitment of infants with sickle cell anemia to a phase III trial: data from the BABY HUG study. Contemp Clin Trials 2010; 31(6):558–63.

28. Wang WC, Ware RE, Miller ST, et al. Hydroxycarbamide in very young children with sickle-cell anaemia: a multicentre, randomised, controlled trial (BABY HUG). Lancet 2011;377(9778):1663–72.

29. Nottage KA, Hankins JS, Smeltzer M, et al. Hydroxyurea use and hospitalization trends in a comprehensive pediatric sickle cell program. PLoS One 2013;8(8): e72077.

30. Thornburg CD, Files BA, Luo Z, et al. Impact of hydroxyurea on clinical events in the BABY HUG trial. Blood 2012;120(22):4304–10 [quiz: 4448].

31. Rana S, Houston PE, Wang WC, et al. Hydroxyurea and growth in young children with sickle cell disease. Pediatrics 2014;134(3):465–72.

32. McGann PT, Flanagan JM, Howard TA, et al. Genotoxicity associated with hydroxyurea exposure in infants with sickle cell anemia: results from the BABY-HUG Phase III Clinical Trial. Pediatr Blood Cancer 2012;59(2):254–7.

33. Ware RE, Helms RW. Stroke with transfusions changing to hydroxyurea (SWiTCH). Blood 2012;119(17):3925–32.

34. Helton KJ, Adams RJ, Kesler KL, et al. Magnetic resonance imaging/angiography and transcranial Doppler velocities in sickle cell anemia: results from the SWiTCH trial. Blood 2014;124(6):891–8.

35. Kratovil T, Bulas D, Driscoll MC, et al. Hydroxyurea therapy lowers TCD velocities in children with sickle cell disease. Pediatr Blood Cancer 2006;47(7):894–900.

36. Zimmerman SA, Schultz WH, Burgett S, et al. Hydroxyurea therapy lowers transcranial Doppler flow velocities in children with sickle cell anemia. Blood 2007; 110(3):1043–7.

37. Adams R, McKie V, Nichols F, et al. The use of transcranial ultrasonography to predict stroke in sickle cell disease. N Engl J Med 1992;326(9):605–10.

38. Adams RJ, McKie VC, Hsu L, et al. Prevention of a first stroke by transfusions in children with sickle cell anemia and abnormal results on transcranial Doppler ultrasonography. N Engl J Med 1998;339(1):5–11.

39. Adams RJ, Brambilla D. Discontinuing prophylactic transfusions used to prevent stroke in sickle cell disease. N Engl J Med 2005;353(26):2769–78.

40. Ware RE, Davis BR, Schultz WH, et al. Hydroxycarbamide versus chronic trans-
    fusion for maintenance of transcranial doppler flow velocities in children with
    sickle cell anaemia-TCD with transfusions changing to hydroxyurea (TWiTCH):
    a multicentre, open-label, phase 3, non-inferiority trial. Lancet (London, England)
    2016;387(10019):661–70.
41. Santos JL, Bosquesi PL, Almeida AE, et al. Mutagenic and genotoxic effect of hy-
    droxyurea. Int J Biomed Sci 2011;7(4):263–7.
42. Ballas SK, McCarthy WF, Guo N, et al. Exposure to hydroxyurea and pregnancy
    outcomes in patients with sickle cell anemia. J Natl Med Assoc 2009;101(10):
    1046–51.
43. McGann PT, Ware RE. Hydroxyurea therapy for sickle cell anemia. Expert Opin
    Drug Saf 2015;14(11):1749–58.
44. Castro O, Nouraie M, Oneal P. Hydroxycarbamide treatment in sickle cell dis-
    ease: estimates of possible leukaemia risk and of hospitalization survival benefit.
    Br J Haematol 2014;167(5):687–91.
45. Zimmerman SA, Schultz WH, Davis JS, et al. Sustained long-term hematologic ef-
    ficacy of hydroxyurea at maximum tolerated dose in children with sickle cell dis-
    ease. Blood 2004;103(6):2039–45.
46. Ware RE. How I use hydroxyurea to treat young patients with sickle cell anemia.
    Blood 2010;115(26):5300–11.
47. Halsey C, Roberts IA. The role of hydroxyurea in sickle cell disease. Br J Haema-
    tol 2003;120(2):177–86.
48. Lanzkron S, Haywood C Jr, Segal JB, et al. Hospitalization rates and costs of care
    of patients with sickle-cell anemia in the state of Maryland in the era of hydroxy-
    urea. Am J Hematol 2006;81(12):927–32.
49. Lanzkron S, Haywood C Jr, Hassell KL, et al. Provider barriers to hydroxyurea use
    in adults with sickle cell disease: a survey of the sickle cell disease adult provider
    network. J Natl Med Assoc 2008;100(8):968–73.
50. Brandow AM, Jirovec DL, Panepinto JA. Hydroxyurea in children with sickle cell
    disease: practice patterns and barriers to utilization. Am J Hematol 2010;85(8):
    611–3.
51. Brandow AM, Panepinto JA. Hydroxyurea use in sickle cell disease: the battle
    with low prescription rates, poor patient compliance and fears of toxicities. Expert
    Rev Hematol 2010;3(3):255–60.
52. Luchtman-Jones L, Pressel S, Hilliard L, et al. Effects of hydroxyurea treatment for
    patients with hemoglobin SC disease. Am J Hematol 2016;91(2):238–42.
53. Chou ST, Fasano RM. Management of patients with sickle cell disease using
    transfusion therapy: guidelines and complications. Hematol Oncol Clin North
    Am 2016;30(3):591–608.
54. Johnson CS. Arterial blood pressure and hyperviscosity in sickle cell disease.
    Hematol Oncol Clin North Am 2005;19(5):827–37, vi.
55. Hulbert ML, Scothorn DJ, Panepinto JA, et al. Exchange blood transfusion
    compared with simple transfusion for first overt stroke is associated with a lower
    risk of subsequent stroke: a retrospective cohort study of 137 children with sickle
    cell anemia. J Pediatr 2006;149(5):710–2.
56. Fasano RM, Leong T, Kaushal M, et al. Effectiveness of red blood cell exchange,
    partial manual exchange, and simple transfusion concurrently with iron chelation
    therapy in reducing iron overload in chronically transfused sickle cell anemia pa-
    tients. Transfusion 2016;56(7):1707–15.
57. Hendrickson JE, Tormey CA. Red blood cell antibodies in hematology/oncology
    patients: interpretation of immunohematologic tests and clinical significance of

detected antibodies. Hematology/oncology Clin North America 2016;30(3): 635–51.

58. Sins JW, Biemond BJ, van den Bersselaar SM, et al. Early occurrence of red blood cell alloimmunization in patients with sickle cell disease. Am J Hematol 2016;91(8):763–9.

59. Wang CJ, Kavanagh PL, Little AA, et al. Quality-of-care indicators for children with sickle cell disease. Pediatrics 2011;128(3):484–93.

60. Quinn CT, St Pierre TG. MRI measurements of iron load in transfusion-dependent patients: implementation, challenges, and pitfalls. Pediatr Blood Cancer 2016; 63(5):773–80.

61. Coates TD, Wood JC. How we manage iron overload in sickle cell patients. Br J Haematol 2017;177(5):703–16.

62. Niihara Y, Zerez CR, Akiyama DS, et al. Oral L-glutamine therapy for sickle cell anemia: I. Subjective clinical improvement and favorable change in red cell NAD redox potential. Am J Hematol 1998;58(2):117–21.

63. Salman EK, Haymond MW, Bayne E, et al. Protein and energy metabolism in pre-pubertal children with sickle cell anemia. Pediatr Res 1996;40(1):34–40.

64. Hibbert JM, Creary MS, Gee BE, et al. Erythropoiesis and myocardial energy re-quirements contribute to the hypermetabolism of childhood sickle cell anemia. J Pediatr Gastroenterol Nutr 2006;43(5):680–7.

65. Niihara Y, Macan H, Eckman JR, et al. L-glutamine therapy reduces hospitaliza-tion for sickle cell anemia and sickleB0-thalassemia patients at six months: a phase II randomized trial. Clin Pharmacol Biopharm 2014;3(1):1–5.

66. Administration FD. Endari package insert. 2017. Available at: https://www. accessdata.fda.gov/scripts/cder/daf/index.cfm?event=overview.process&Appl No=208587. Accessed September 14, 2017.

67. King A, Shenoy S. Evidence-based focused review of the status of hematopoietic stem cell transplantation as treatment of sickle cell disease and thalassemia. Blood 2014;123(20):3089–94 [quiz: 3210].

68. Gluckman E, Cappelli B, Bernaudin F, et al. Sickle cell disease: an international survey of results of HLA-identical sibling hematopoietic stem cell transplantation. Blood 2017;129(11):1548–56.

69. Justus D, Perez-Albuerne E, Dioguardi J, et al. Allogeneic donor availability for hematopoietic stem cell transplantation in children with sickle cell disease. Pe-diatr Blood Cancer 2015;62(7):1285–7.

70. Walters MC, Hardy K, Edwards S, et al. Pulmonary, gonadal, and central nervous system status after bone marrow transplantation for sickle cell disease. Biol Blood Marrow Transplant 2010;16(2):263–72.

71. Meier ER, Dioguardi JV, Kamani N. Current attitudes of parents and patients to-ward hematopoietic stem cell transplantation for sickle cell anemia. Pediatr Blood Cancer 2015;62(7):1277–84.

72. King AA, Kamani N, Bunin N, et al. Successful matched sibling donor marrow transplantation following reduced intensity conditioning in children with hemoglo-binopathies. Am J Hematol 2015;90(12):1093–8.

73. Bolanos-Meade J, Fuchs EJ, Luznik L, et al. HLA-haploidentical bone marrow transplantation with posttransplant cyclophosphamide expands the donor pool for patients with sickle cell disease. Blood 2012;120(22):4285–91.

74. Kamani NR, Walters MC, Carter S, et al. Unrelated donor cord blood transplanta-tion for children with severe sickle cell disease: results of one cohort from the phase II study from the Blood and Marrow Transplant Clinical Trials Network (BMT CTN). Biol Blood Marrow Transplant 2012;18(8):1265–72.

75. Shenoy S, Eapen M, Panepinto JA, et al. A trial of unrelated donor marrow transplantation for children with severe sickle cell disease. Blood 2016;128(21): 2561–7.
76. Nickel RS, Hendrickson JE, Haight AE. The ethics of a proposed study of hematopoietic stem cell transplant for children with "less severe" sickle cell disease. Blood 2014;124(6):861–6.
77. Panepinto JA. Health-related quality of life in patients with hemoglobinopathies. Hematology Am Soc Hematol Educ Program 2012;2012:284–9.
78. Meier ER, Fasano RM, Levett PR. A systematic review of the literature for severity predictors in children with sickle cell anemia. Blood Cells Mol Dis 2017;65:86–94.
79. Arnold SD, Bhatia M, Horan J, et al. Haematopoietic stem cell transplantation for sickle cell disease: current practice and new approaches. Br J Haematol 2016; 174(4):515–25.
80. Bernaudin F, Socie G, Kuentz M, et al. Long-term results of related myeloablative stem-cell transplantation to cure sickle cell disease. Blood 2007;110(7):2749–56.
81. Negre O, Eggimann AV, Beuzard Y, et al. Gene therapy of the beta-hemoglobinopathies by lentiviral transfer of the beta(A(T87Q))-Globin Gene. Hum Gene Ther 2016;27(2):148–65.
82. Hoban MD, Orkin SH, Bauer DE. Genetic treatment of a molecular disorder: gene therapy approaches to sickle cell disease. Blood 2016;127(7):839–48.
83. Orkin SH. Recent advances in globin research using genome-wide association studies and gene editing. Ann N Y Acad Sci 2016;1368(1):5–10.
84. Ribeil JA, Hacein-Bey-Abina S, Payen E, et al. Gene therapy in a patient with sickle cell disease. N Engl J Med 2017;376(9):848–55.

A Scientific Renaissance
Novel Drugs in Sickle Cell Disease

Ahmar U. Zaidi, MD[a],*, Matthew M. Heeney, MD[b]

KEYWORDS

- Sickle cell disease • Therapeutic targets • Pathophysiology
- Induction of fetal hemoglobin • Antiadhesion molecules

KEY POINTS

- We have entered an era of exploding interest in therapeutics for sickle cell disease.
- The expansion in our understanding of sickle cell disease pathophysiology has enhanced the range of potential therapeutic targets.
- From induction of fetal hemoglobin to antiadhesion molecules, we are potentially on the cusp of making life-altering modifications for individuals with sickle cell disease.
- This disease population cannot afford to let the current momentum wane.
- Studies exploring combinations of therapies affecting multiple steps in the pathophysiology and exploring novel and clinically relevant outcomes are incumbent.

INTRODUCTION

It has been 2 decades since hydroxyurea was approved by the US Food and Drug Administration (FDA) for the treatment of sickle cell disease (SCD) in adults, and until recently it remained the only approved medication for this disease. Up until the last 5 years, there has been minimal progress in drug development to improve the survival and quality of life of children with SCD (**Fig. 1**).

The eruption of recent activity in drug development for this population can be linked to changes in legislation promoting pharmaceutical research in orphan diseases and children, and the evolution of our understanding of the pathophysiology of SCD. Over the past few decades, investigators have identified novel pathways in the complex pathophysiology of this disease.[1] Although the polymerization of deoxygenated hemoglobin S (HbS) remains the initiating event in the pathophysiology of SCD, our understanding of how cellular adhesion (leukocytes, platelets, and endothelial cells), oxidative damage, vascular reactivity, nitric oxide (NO), inflammation, and the coagulation system contribute to vasoocclusion and the broader phenotype of the disease

[a] Children's Hospital of Michigan, Wayne State University School of Medicine, Department of Pediatrics, Division of Hematology/Oncology, 3901 Beaubien, Detroit, MI 48201, USA; [b] Boston Children's Hospital, Harvard Medical School, 300 Longwood Avenue, Boston, MA 02115, USA
* Corresponding author.
E-mail address: ahmar@wayne.edu

Pediatr Clin N Am 65 (2018) 445–464
https://doi.org/10.1016/j.pcl.2018.01.006
0031-3955/18/© 2018 Elsevier Inc. All rights reserved.

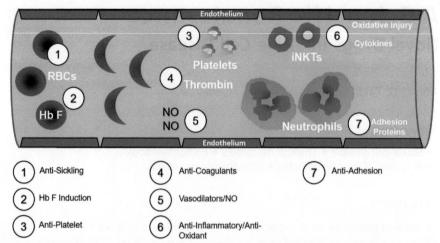

Fig. 1. Various targets of new drugs in sickle cell disease. iNKTs, invariant natural killer T cells; NO, nitric oxide; RBCs, red blood cells.

have provided novel targets whose exploration is providing hope for more disease modifying treatments. The investigation and recent FDA approval of L-glutamine, only the second drug labeled for SCD, was the result of thinking beyond hemoglobin and red blood cells.

Although significant strides are being made in drug development, the conduct of clinical trials in SCD remains challenging with respect to choice of meaningful clinical endpoints and rate of enrollment that may require more centers and costs. Many recent trials have developed novel endpoints, and have included enrollment in regions of the world with a high disease burden. In this review, we aim to discuss the current state of drug development in SCD. Owing to the expansive nature of current research in SCD, we highlight some drugs within the text of the article, but have included tables with a complete list of compounds under investigation.

THERAPEUTIC STRATEGIES FOR SICKLE CELL DISEASE
Agents That Induce Fetal Hemoglobin or Modulate Hemoglobin

The polymerization of deoxygenated HbS can be interfered with through a variety of mechanisms. Recognition that naturally occurring high levels of fetal hemoglobin (HbF) improve mortality in SCD,[2] increasing the proportion of HbF is a clear therapeutic opportunity to improve SCD phenotypes. Deoxygenation of HbS reveals the substituted hydrophobic valine residue that participates in HbS polymerization. Therefore, efforts to increase HbS oxygen affinity or interfere with polymerization directly have also drawn interest. Finally, epigenetic mechanisms such as histone deacetylation and DNA methylation do play an important role in the silencing of the gamma globin genes, and provide yet another pathway being targeted by investigators. There are several drugs that are being actively studied for their ability to increase the proportion of HbF or modulate hemoglobin to prevent sickling (**Table 1**).

Hemoglobin-Modifying Agents

GBT440
Global Blood Therapeutics is developing a novel oral small molecule hemoglobin modifier for SCD that binds to alpha globin and increases hemoglobin oxygen affinity.

Table 1
Hemoglobin F induction and anti-sickling agents

Drug Name	ClinicalTrials.gov Identifier	Target/Mechanism	Route	Category	Phase	Sponsor
Hemoglobin-modifying agents						
GBT440	NCT02850406	Increases Hb affinity for oxygen	PO	Anti-sickling	Phase II/III	Global Blood Therapeutics
SCD-101	NCT02380079	Hemoglobin modifier	PO	Anti-sickling	Phase I	Ivenux, LLC
4,4'-Di(1,2,3-triazolyl) disulfide (TD-3)	—	Increases Hb affinity for oxygen	—	Anti-sickling	Preclinical	Massachusetts General Hospital
VZHE-039	—	Allosteric effector of hemoglobin	—	Anti-sickling	Preclinical	Virginia Commonwealth University
HbF inducers						
HQK-1001 (sodium dimethylbutyrate)	NCT00842088	Promoter-targeted fetal globin gene-inducing agent	PO	HbF induction	Completed phase II	HemaQuest Pharmaceuticals Inc
Pomalidomide	NCT01522547	Increased HbF by transcriptional mechanism	PO	HbF induction	Completed phase I	Celgene Corporation
Metformin	NCT02981329	Increased HbF	PO	HbF Induction	Early phase I	Baylor College of Medicine
INCB059872	NCT03132324	LSD-1 inhibitor	PO	HbF Induction	Phase I	Incyte Corporation
Decitabine and tetrahydrouridine	NCT01685515	DNMT1	PO	HbF Induction	Phase I	Cleveland Clinic
Panobinostat (LBH589)	NCT01245179	HDAC inhibitor	PO	HbF induction	Phase I	Novartis Pharmaceuticals

(continued on next page)

Table 1
(continued)

Drug Name	ClinicalTrials.gov Identifier	Target/Mechanism	Route	Category	Phase	Sponsor
ACY-957	—	HDAC inhibition	—	HbF induction	Preclinical	Acetylon Pharmaceuticals
RN-1	—	LSD-1 inhibitor	—	HbF induction	Preclinical	NIH
Dimethyl fumarate	—	Gamma-globin induction	—	HbF induction	Preclinical	Biogen
gg1-VP64	—	Zinc-finger gamma-globin activator	—	HbF induction	Preclinical	Georgia Regents University
Other anti-sickling mechanism						
Memantine hydrochloride	NCT03247218	NMDA receptor blocker → decrease intracellular calcium	PO	Anti-sickling	Phase II	HaEmek Medical Center, Israel
Warmed saline	NCT02316366	Temperature regulation	IV	Anti-sickling	—	Nationwide Children's Hospital

Abbreviations: DNMT1, DNA methyltransferase; Hb, hemoglobin; HbF, fetal hemoglobin; HDAC, histone deacetylase; IV, intravenous; LSD-1, lysine-specific demethylase 1; NMDA, N-methyl-D-aspartate; PO, by mouth.

Adult patients are being enrolled in the Phase II HOPE (Hemoglobin Oxygen Affinity Modulation to Inhibit HbS PolymErization) Study, and children are being enrolled in phase II studies.[3] Preliminary phase I/II studies did not only show that the drug is well-tolerated, but have shown rapid reduction in markers of hemolysis and improved oxygen delivery.[4]

5-Hydroxymethyl-2-furfural

This botanically derived aromatic aldehyde is one of several similar compounds that act allosterically with HbS to increase oxygen affinity and reduce polymer formation.[5] 5-Hydroxymethyl-2-furfural (SCD-101) stabilizes the R-state hemoglobin by interaction of its aldehyde moiety with the N-terminal of hemoglobin. This drug is currently undergoing dose-escalation and efficacy studies in a phase I trial.

4,4'-Di(1,2,3-triazolyl)disulfide

A preclinical compound from the investigators at Massachusetts General Hospital has displayed some encouraging data. By targeting the thiol group of Hb β-Cys93, TD-3 increases hemoglobin's affinity for oxygen by destabilizing the T-state and stabilizing the R-state. Furthermore, it seems that this site may be involved in polymer formation and its alteration could diminish sickling. The compound was well-tolerated in murine models and was able to increase the affinity of oxygen to hemoglobin.[6,7]

VZHE-039

This novel allosteric effector of hemoglobin is a substituted benzaldehyde with potent in vitro antipolymerization activity. Studies are preclinical and further studies to investigate the solubility, bioavailability, kinetics, and biological activity of this agent are ongoing.[8]

Fetal Hemoglobin Inducers

Sodium dimethylbutyrate

Short chain fatty acids have been investigated in beta globin disorders for their ability to induce HbF by an unclear mechanism. HemaQuest Pharmaceutical's compound Sodium dimethylbutyrate (HQK-1001), an oral butyrate derivative had a proposed mechanism of increased HbF production by promoter targeting.[9] A phase II trial studied the compound in 76 subjects over 48 weeks. Unfortunately, the study was prematurely closed owing to an interim analysis showing no significant increase in HbF and more pain in the study arm.[10]

Pomalidomide

This derivative of thalidomide upregulates HbF production by a transcriptional mechanism that is not completely understood. Pomalidomide is being studied for maximum tolerated dose, safety and ability to induce HbF. Results of the phase I trial show that the drug is well-tolerated and increases HbF, F-cells, and total Hb. A phase II study is planned.[11–13]

Metformin

Investigators at the Baylor College of Medicine showed that knockdown of FOXO3 resulted in reduced gamma globin expression, suggesting that it was a regulator of gamma globin. Metformin is known to increase FOXO3 expression and the investigators showed a dose-dependent increased gamma globin levels in primary erythroid cells with metformin. Coculture with hydroxyurea revealed additive effects on gamma globin expression in the same system. A phase I study of metformin is actively enrolling.[14]

Decitabine and tetrahydrouridine

DNA methyltransferase is a key element in the modulation of chromatin responsible for suppression of gamma globin production; this makes it an attractive target in SCD. The hypomethylating agent, decitabine, has the ability to deplete DNA methyltransferase; however, when used alone, it is rapidly metabolized by cytidine deaminase. The cytidine deaminase inhibitor, tetrahydrouridine, has been added to decitabine by investigators in an attempt to prolong its effect. A phase I results of this combination showed clinically relevant HbF elevation and an acceptable safety profile.[15]

Panobinostat and vorinostat

Histone deacetylase inhibitors function by expanding the acetylation of lysine residues in histones, which results in a decreased association of basic core histone proteins with DNA. The net effect is the amplified availability of certain genes, including gamma globin, to be more accessible for transcription.[16] Therefore, the histone deacetylase inhibitors are a promising class of agents for investigation in SCD. Vorinostat was investigated in a small phase I/II trial and found to be tolerated well with modest HbF induction, but with concerns about underdosing.[17] Preliminary data from patients with hematologic malignancies receiving panobinostat have shown augmentation of HbF levels.[18] Novartis Pharmaceuticals is conducting phase I trials of pabinostat in SCD.

ACY-957

ACY-957 is a selective chemical inhibitor of histone deacetylase 1 and 2 that is capable of inducing HbF. Preclinical studies reveal that erythroid progenitors treated with ACY-957 develop changes in gene expression of GATA2 by histone acetylation-induced activation.[19,20]

Lysine specific demethylase-1 inhibitors

Lysine specific demethylase-1 is an enzyme that reduces gamma globin expression by removal of monomethyl and dimethyl residues from lysine 4 residues of histone H3. There has been some excitement around this pathway, and there are 2 drugs under investigation currently: INCB059872 (phase I) and RN-1 (preclinical). Murine studies show a promising effect on sickle cell pathology and HbF induction.[21]

Dimethyl fumarate

Dimethyl fumarate is a small molecule agonist of nuclear factor (erythroid derived-2)-like 2 (Nrf2). Nrf2 is a basic leucine zipper protein that has been shown to increase HbF levels as well as generate antioxidant and inflammatory-protective compounds. Murine models exposed to dimethyl fumarate showed a 3- to 4-fold increase in F cells.[22] Additional murine and nonhuman primate models showed similar results.[23]

gg1-VP64

gg1-VP64 is an artificial zinc-finger transcription factor that was designed to interact with proximal gamma globin promoters. Induction of up to 20% HbF in erythroblasts was demonstrated in the preclinical setting using an in vitro culture model of human erythropoiesis.[24,25]

Other Anti-Sickling Mechanisms

Memantine hydrochloride

N-Methyl-D-aspartate receptors are highly upregulated on SCD erythrocytes. Induction of HbS polymerization in vitro by placing cells in a low oxygen setting revealed that calcium uptake, cellular dehydration, and polymerization could all be drastically reduced by inhibiting N-methyl-D-aspartate receptors. Inhibition of this receptor has been explored in both Israel and Germany.[26]

Agents That Interfere with Coagulation

It is established that, even during steady state, patients with SCD show evidence of platelet activation, an activated coagulation cascade with thrombin generation, and activated fibrinolytic system that result in an overall prothrombotic phenotype.[27–29] These disturbances in these coagulation pathways likely contribute to the pathophysiology of SCD and, therefore, have been an attractive target to investigators hoping to improve the phenotype of SCD. Furthermore, the pathogenesis of sickle vasoocclusion includes the activation of endothelial cells and their interaction with various plasma proteins and intercellular adhesion molecules, including selectins, many of which contain heparin-binding sites.[30] In this section, we review agents in production that affect various points along these pathways (**Table 2**).

Coagulation cascade disrupters

Rivaroxaban and apixaban Sparkenbaugh and colleagues[31] examined the contribution of factor Xa to the inflammatory process in murine models of SCD. Serine proteases in the coagulation cascade are capable of generating a multiple cellular effects. Notably, activation via protease activated receptors contributes to the inflammation of many vascular disorders.[32] Thus, the disrupting the activation of factor Xa could limit the activation of protease activated receptors and downstream inflammation. The novel direct factor Xa inhibitor rivaroxaban is undergoing phase II investigation to examine its effects on vascular cell adhesion molecule-1 and interleukin-6 levels in adult SCD patients. Another direct factor Xa inhibitor, apixaban, is currently in phase III investigation to evaluate the effect on mean daily pain score in outpatients with SCD. Results from the trials are not yet published.

N-Acetylcysteine N-Acetylcysteine is an antioxidant drug with an established safety profile that has been studied over the past 2 decades in SCD. Its contribution to the disruption of the pathophysiology of SCD is thought to relate to its diminution of oxidative damage. A recent phase III study investigated oral N-acetylcysteine in SCD, and established that there was no significant improvement in SCD-related pain in the treatment arm.[33] However, after adjustment for a high rate of nonadherence, there was a trend toward reduction of pain. Another group is investigating the effect intravenous N-acetylcysteine in a phase II trial to reduce the von Willebrand factor–associated contribution to hemolysis during acute vasoocclusive pain; results from the first 2 patients were presented at the 2017 American Society of Hematology Annual meeting and showed safety and tolerability.[34]

Heparins

Low-molecular-weight heparin and unfractionated heparin Low-molecular-weight heparin and unfractionated heparin exert their anticoagulant effect by potentiating antithrombin's inactivation of factors IIa and Xa. Microfluidics studies have established that sickle erythrocyte adhesion to endothelial cells via very late antigen 4 and vascular cell adhesion molecule-1, is interrupted by low-molecular-weight heparin.[35] Furthermore, low-molecular-weight heparin is also suggested to exert antiinflammatory effects by suppression of tumor necrosis factor, and this effect may be further beneficial to the pathogenesis of SCD and pain.[36] Investigators at the University of Pittsburgh are involved in a phase II study of unfractionated heparin based on initial findings by Matsui and colleagues,[37] which described inhibition of sickle cell and P-selectin adhesion in a clinically attainable concentration. The low-molecular-weight heparins tinzaparin and dalteparin have been evaluated for the treatment of acute vasoocclusive pain with some possible benefit.[38] Tinzaparin being currently

Table 2
Coagulation-interrupting agents

Drug Name	ClinicalTrials.gov Identifier	Target/Mechanism	Route	Category	Phase	Sponsor
Coagulation cascade disrupters						
Apixaban	NCT02179177	Direct factor Xa inhibitor	PO	Anticoagulants	Phase III	Bristol-Myers Squibb
Rivaroxaban	NCT02072668	Direct factor Xa inhibitor	PO	Anticoagulants	Phase II	University of North Carolina, Chapel Hill
N-acetylcysteine	NCT01800526	NAC decreases VWF	IV	Anticoagulants	Phase II	Bloodworks (Puget Sound Blood Center)
Heparins						
Unfractionated heparin	NCT02098993	Inactivation of factors Xa and IIa	IV	Anticoagulants	Phase II	University of Pittsburgh
Low-molecular-weight heparin	NCT02580773	Inactivation of factor Xa	SQ	Anticoagulants	Phase III	Assistance Publique - Hôpitaux de Paris
Sevuparin	NCT02515838	Chemically modified heparin with low anticoagulant activity	IV	Anticoagulants	Phase II	Modus Therapeutics AB
Antiplatelet agents						
Ticagrelor	NCT02482298	P2Y(12) antagonist with antiplatelet activity	PO	Antiplatelet	Completed phase II	AstraZeneca

Abbreviations: IV, intravenous; NAC, *N*-acetylcysteine; PO, by mouth; SQ, subcutaneously; VWF, von Willebrand factor.

being studied by French investigators in a phase III trial for the sickle cell complication of acute chest syndrome.

Sevuparin Sevuparin is a negatively charged polysaccharide derived from heparin, but with the antithrombin-binding pentasaccharide sequence deleted. Therefore, the drug has low anticoagulant activity but maintains the antiadhesive properties of heparins through blockade of intercellular adhesion molecules and plasma factors involved in vasoocclusive crisis in vitro and animal models of SCD.[39] Sevuparin is now undergoing an international phase II trial.

Antiplatelet agents

The platelets of SCD patients are activated during steady state and are further activated during vasoocclusion. Clinical trials of antiplatelet medications had been small and inconclusive,[40] until a large pediatric trial of prasugrel an irreversible platelet ADP $P2Y_{12}$ receptor antagonist to inhibit ADP-mediated platelet activation revealed no significant reduction in vasoocclusive pain episodes.[41]

Ticagrelor Ticagrelor is also a ADP $P2Y_{12}$ receptor antagonist; however, it differs from parasugrel in that it does not require metabolic activation, is reversible, and has the additional potential benefit of increasing local adenosine with vasodilatory and antiinflammatory effects.[1,41] Ticagrelor recently completed phase II trial and results are pending.

Agents That Cause Vasodilation

Chronic hemolytic anemias can result in elevated plasma hemoglobin that depletes NO, an endothelial-derived effector of vasodilation, and beneficial pleiotropic effects on the adhesion of circulating blood cells key to the pathophysiology of SCD. NO production is also compromised by oxidative damage from ischemia-reperfusion injury and by the consumption of the NO synthase (NOS) substrate arginine through the release of the intraerythrocyte enzyme arginase.[42] NO activates smooth muscle soluble guanylyl cyclase that results in increased intracellular cyclic guanosine monophosphate, smooth muscle relaxation, vasodilation, and increased local blood flow. Without NO vasodilation and blood flow is reduced. Phosphodiesterase-9 inhibitors produce their effect by facilitating increased cellular cyclic guanosine monophosphate levels by inhibiting its degradation. In this section, we review Phosphodiesterase-9 inhibitors as well as other products being investigated that directly alter the vasodilation in SCD (**Table 3**).

Phosphodiesterase-9 inhibitors

PF-04447943 PF-04447943 is an oral agent that selectively inhibits phosphodiesterase-9 and is in phase I trial. Murine studies were presented at the American Society of Hematology Meeting in 2016 and showed a reduction in leukocyte–platelet aggregates and soluble E-selectin with chronic treatment.[43]

IMR-687 IMR-687 is in phase I investigations and murine studies have shown augmented HbF levels, reduction of sickling, leukocytosis, and microvascular stasis.[44]

Soluble guanylate cyclase stimulators

IW-1701 This orally available soluble guanylate cyclase stimulator binds to sGC and enhances NO signaling. A phase Ib dose study was conducted, and showed tolerability in healthy subjects. Pharmacodynamic results showed acceptable levels of plasma cyclic guanosine monophosphate levels.[45] The phase II study, "A Study of the Effect of IW-1701, a Stimulator of Soluble Guanylate Cyclase (sGC), on Patients with Sickle Cell Disease (SCD) (STRONG-SCD)" is planned for the end of the year.

Table 3
Vasodilating agents

Drug Name	ClinicalTrials.gov Identifier	Target/Mechanism	Route	Category	Phase	Sponsor
PDE9is						
IMR-687	NCT02998450	PDE9i	PO	Vasodilator	Phase I	Imara Inc
PF-04447943	NCT02114203	PDE9i	PO	Vasodilator	Phase I	Pfizer
Stimulators of soluble guanylate cyclase						
Riociguat	NCT02633397	Soluble guanylate cyclase stimulator	PO	Vasodilator	Phase II	University of Pittsburgh
IW-1701	NCT03285178	Soluble guanylate cyclase stimulator	PO	Vasodilator	Phase II	Ironwood Pharmaceuticals, Inc
Additional enhancers of the NO pathway						
Magnesium sulfate	NCT01197417	Inhibition of calcium in the vascular smooth-muscle/endothelial dependent release of NO	IV	Vasodilator	Completed phase III	Medical College of Wisconsin
6R-BH4 (sapropterin dihydrochloride)	NCT00445978	6R-isomer of tetrahydrobiopterin/NO pathway	PO	Vasodilator	Completed phase II	BioMarin Pharmaceutical
Inhaled NO	NCT01089439	Local NO donor	Inhaled	Vasodilator	Completed phase II	Assistance Publique - Hôpitaux de Paris
Arginine	NCT02536170	L-Arg – (NOS) → citrulline + NO	IV	Vasodilator	Phase II	Emory University
Topical sodium nitrite	NCT02863068	Sodium nitrite → local donor of NO	Topical	Vasodilator	Phase II	Montefiore Medical Center
Nitrous oxide 50%	NCT01891812	Local NO donor	Inhaled	Vasodilator	Phase II	Columbia University
L-citrulline (PO)	NCT02659644	L-Arg – (NOS) → citrulline + NO	PO	Vasodilator	Phase I	University of Mississippi Medical Center
L-citrulline (IV)	NCT02697240	L-Arg – (NOS) → citrulline + NO	IV	Vasodilator	Phase I	University of Mississippi Medical Center

Abbreviations: IV, intravenous; NO, nitric oxide; NOS, nitric oxide synthase; PDE9i, phosphodiesterase-9 inhibitor; PO, by mouth.

Additional enhancers of the nitric oxide pathway

6R-BH4 (sapropterin dihydrochloride) 6R-BH4, also known as BH4 or tetrahydrobiopterin, is a cofactor for the production of NO by NOSs. Deficiency of this cofactor can result in loss of normal NO production by the vascular endothelium. BioMarin Pharmaceutical completed phase II investigation, and results are yet to be published.

Inhaled nitric oxide In 2011, Gladwin and colleagues[46] published the results of a phase II, randomized, double-blind, placebo-controlled, multicenter study of NO inhalation for up to 72 hours in 50 participants with SCD presenting with a vasoocclusive crisis. They showed no significant difference in either arm. A recently completed phase II trial in Paris investigating the use of inhaled NO in acute chest syndrome has yet to publish results.

Arginine and L-citrulline The potential value of arginine and L-citrulline stem from their roles in the NO synthesis pathway. Arginine is converted into citrulline and NO via NOS enzymes. The effectiveness of arginine in vasoocclusive pain was studied in a single-center, prospective, randomized, double-blind, placebo-controlled phase II trial and was completed in 2013.[47] The trial demonstrated a significant reduction in opioid use. Supplementation with citrulline is hypothesized to be a more effective way of accumulating plasma and tissue arginine.[48] Citrulline, as opposed to arginine, is not subject to degradation by arginase in the gastrointestinal system and, once absorbed, is converted to arginine. L-Citrulline, both oral and intravenous, is being studied in phase I by investigators at the University of Mississippi Medical Center. Supplementation with NOS substrates remains a fascinating stratagem with as-yet unpublished results.

Agents That Reduce Inflammation

The role of inflammation in the pathophysiology of SCD has increased exponentially in the past decade with a variety of cells and molecules being implicated in these pathways.[1] The activation of endothelial cells by free heme can initiate a waterfall of proinflammatory cytokines. Sickle erythrocytes and platelets can activate endothelial cells in a similar fashion.[1] This proinflammatory state has direct contribution to the SCD phenotype and, as such, has been an exciting area for study for investigators. We review some of the compounds under investigation to modify the inflammatory consequences of SCD (**Table 4**).

Nonspecific antiinflammatory agents

L-Glutamine With the ability to augment the redox potential in the human body by generation of glutathione, L-glutamine showed a decrease in pain episodes in a phase III investigation by Emmaus Medical, Inc. Although phase III trial results have not been published yet, L-glutamine was recently approved by the FDA for treatment of SCD.

Simvastatin and atorvastatin The statin family of drugs have many pleiotropic effects that could be beneficial in SCD. In particular, statins have antiinflammatory effects and enhance NO production.[49] A pilot study in 2011 evaluating markers of vascular dysfunction in SCD showed that simvastatin increased NO levels, and decreased C-reactive protein and interleukin-6 in a dose-dependent manner. A phase II study of simvastatin was recently completed, with unpublished results as of yet.[50] Atorvastatin is currently undergoing phase II investigation.

Inhaled budesonide/mometasone These agonists of glucocorticoid receptors are commonly used in asthma and were recently trialed in a phase I investigation for budesonide and phase II for mometasone, with as-yet unpublished results.

Table 4
Anti-inflammatory agents

Drug Name	ClinicalTrials.gov Identifier	Target/Mechanism	Route	Category	Phase	Sponsor
Nonspecific antiinflammatory agents						
L-Glutamine	NCT01179217	Increase NAD redox potential	PO	Antiinflammatory	Completed phase III	Emmaus Medical, Inc
Simvastatin	NCT00508027, NCT01702246	Increase endothelial NO and decrease inflammation	PO	Antiinflammatory	Completed phase II	Children's Hospital & Research Center Oakland
Atorvastatin	NCT01732718	Improve endothelial dysfunction	PO	Antiinflammatory	Phase II	University of North Carolina, Chapel Hill
Inhaled mometasone	NCT02061202	Inhaled corticosteroid	Inhaled	Antiinflammatory	Phase II	Icahn School of Medicine at Mount Sinai
Vitamin D	NCT01443728	Vitamin D_3	PO	Antiinflammatory	Phase II	Columbia University
Budesonide	NCT02187445	Inhaled corticosteroid	Inhaled	Antiinflammatory	Completed phase I	Vanderbilt University
Omega-3 fatty acid supplementation						
SC411	NCT02973360	DHA/EPA	PO	Antiinflammatory	Phase II, phase III	Sancilio and Company, Inc
SCD-Omegatex (DHA/EPA)	NCT02947100	DHA/EPA	PO	Antiinflammatory	Phase II	National Institute of General Medical Sciences (NIGMS), Thomas Jefferson University, Solutex GC, S.L.

Immune pathway targeting agents						
ACZ885 (canakinumab)	NCT02961218	Monoclonal antibody to IL-1 beta	SQ	Antiinflammatory	Phase II	Novartis Pharmaceuticals
Regadenoson	NCT01788631	iNKT cell reduction	IV	Antiinflammatory	Phase II	Dana Farber Cancer Institute
NKTT120	NCT01783691	Monoclonal antibody directed to invariant TCR of iNKT	IV	Antiinflammatory	Completed phase I	NKT Therapeutics
TAK242	—	TLR4 inhibitor	—	Antiinflammatory	Preclinical	University of Minnesota
Keap1ASO	—	ASO against Keap1	—	Antiinflammatory	Preclinical	Ionis Pharmaceuticals
Leukotriene Down-Regulator						
Zileuton	NCT01136941	Inhibitor of 5-lipoxygenase	PO	Antiinflammatory	Completed phase I	Children's Hospital Medical Center, Cincinnati

Abbreviations: ASO, antisense oligonucleotide; DHA, docosahexaenoic acid; EPA, eicosapentaenoic acid; IL, interleukin; iNKT, invariant natural killer T cells; IV, intravenous; NAD, Nicotinamide adenine dinucleotide; NO, nitric oxide; PO, by mouth; SQ, subcutaneous; TCR, T-cell receptor; TLR4, Toll-like receptor 4.

Omega-3 fatty acid supplementation

SCD-Omegatex/SC411 (eicosapentaenoic and docosahexaenoic acids) In murine models, omega-3 fatty acid supplementation showed reduced systemic inflammatory biomarkers.[51] Small studies of fish oil supplementation containing omega-3 fatty acids (eicosapentaenoic acid/docosahexaenoic acid) reducing pain episodes in SCD. Most recently, Daak and colleagues[52] confirmed the previous studies in a phase III trial in Sudan. SCD-Omegatex is in phase I/II trials. Sancilio & Co. recently completed phase II trial of SC411, a docosahexaenoic acid–enriched omega-3 formulated to increase bioavailability and reduce food-effect and results are pending. A phase III trial of SC411 is planned.

Immune pathway targeting agents

NKTT120/regadenoson Invariant natural killer T cells (iNKTs) are rapidly activated and generate a large immune response, and are thought to be an important part of the pathophysiology of SCD.[53,54] NKTT120 is a humanized monoclonal antibody that targets iNKTs. A phase I study was completed recently showing that, in high doses, iNKTs were not detectable in peripheral blood for 2 to 5 months without serious adverse events.[54] A trial to determine an effect on vasoocclusive pain is being planned. Another compound targeting iNKTs is regadenoson, an adenosine A_{2A} receptor agonist.[55,56] A phase II trial of a low-dose infusion of regadenoson did not reduce iNKT activation or show clinical efficacy.[57]

TAK242 Mast cell activation contributes to inflammation and pain, and these cells often show increased Toll-like receptor 4 on their surface.[58] A therapeutic approach targeting TAK242 has been developed and tested in murine models with promising results; TAK242 resulted in decreased acute pain induced by hypoxia/reoxygenation.[59]

Keap1-ASO Nuclear factor erythroid 2-related factor 2 (Nrf2) regulates the expression of genes that protect cells from oxidative stress. The switch to activate this protection is maintained by a protein known as the Kelch-like ECH-associated protein1 or Keap1. As oxidative damage is sensed by the cells, Keap1 is inactivated and the transcription of proteins that enhance the antioxidant potential of the cell is augmented.[60] The production and testing of an antisense oligonucleotide against Keap1, which would inactivate it, showed decreased organ damage in murine models.[61]

Leukotriene downregulator

Zileuton (N-(1-benzo[b]thien-2-ylethyl)-N-hydroxyurea) The inhibition of 5-lipoxygenase is the mechanism of this drug, which is currently approved for use in asthma. This drug works by dampening the inflammatory response, which has the potential to benefit a variety of outcomes in SCD. 5-Lipoxygenase is paramount in the production of leukotrienes, which are potent inducers of cytokines.[62] Furthermore, zileuton, a hydroxyurea-containing molecule, has also been shown to induce the production of HbF.[63] Phase I studies showed safety and tolerability for high doses of this compound.[64]

Agents That Reduce Adhesion

Interactions between blood cells and the endothelium have been well-characterized in SCD during steady state and vasoocclusion, and are characterized by a myriad of cellular and endothelial proteins.[65,66] There are distinct families of proteins with clear functions and sites of action that, when dysregulated, may cause pathologic sequelae. Of particular interest have been the family of adhesion proteins known as selectins,

Table 5
Anti-adhesion agents

Drug Name	ClinicalTrials.gov Identifier	Target/Mechanism	Route	Category	Phase	Sponsor
Poloxamer 188 (MST - 188)	NCT01737814	Purified surfactant	IV	Antiadhesion	Completed phase III	Mast Therapeutics
Rivipansel (GMI-1070)	NCT02433158	Pan-selectin inhibitor (E > P)	IV	Antiadhesion	Phase III	Pfizer
Crizanlizumab	NCT01895361	Monoclonal antibody to P-selectin	IV	Antiadhesion	Completed phase II	Novartis
Propranolol	NCT01077921	Nonselective beta-blocker	PO	Antiadhesion	Completed phase II	Duke University Medical Center
Intravenous Gammaglobulin (Gamunex)	NCT01757418	Inhibition of neutrophil adhesion	IV	Antiadhesion	Phase II	Albert Einstein College of Medicine, Inc
Montelukast	NCT01960413	Leukotriene receptor antagonist	PO	Antiadhesion	Phase II	Vanderbilt University Medical Center
PSI697	—	P-selectin inhibitor	—	Antiadhesion	Preclinical	Pfizer

Abbreviations: IV, intravenous; PO, by mouth.

specifically P- and E-selectin.[67–69] In this section, we briefly discuss some encouraging agents targeting intercellular adhesion (**Table 5**).

GMI-1070/Rivipansel

GMI-1070 is a small molecule pan-selectin inhibitor that was specifically designed to mimic the carbohydrate structures of selectin antagonists and inhibit the disease-related contribution of selectins. Inhibition of selectin-mediated endothelial and leukocyte adhesions with GMI-1070 infusion reduced vasoocclusive pain intensity and increased survival in preclinical studies in murine models. A phase II trial in acute SCD related vasoocclusive pain produced a "clinically meaningful" reduction in time to vasoocclusive pain resolution and a statistically significant reduction in intravenous opioid usage.[70] A large phase III trial for the treatment of acute vasoocclusive pain is currently under way.

SelG1/SEG101/crizanlizumab

Crizanlizumab is a humanized monoclonal antibody that specifically inhibits adhesion of P-selectin to P-selectin glycoprotein ligand-1. In a phase II trial of repeated dosing over 1 year to prevent vasoocclusive pain, crizanlizumab significantly reduced the rate of vasoocclusive pain and increased the time to first and second pain events with few adverse events.[71] The plan for phase III or other trials is pending.

Propranolol

Propranolol is a nonspecific beta-blocker in SCD that decreased sickle erythrocyte adhesiveness in a murine model of SCD when the mice were treated with propranolol before epinephrine exposure. These investigators from Duke University Medical Center also presented a phase I dose escalation study of propranolol in SCD patients and revealed a dose-dependent decrease in human sickle erythrocyte adhesion to endothelium in vitro with no adverse events.[72] Phase II studies were completed recently by the same investigators, but results do not seem to have been published.

PSI697

This is a small molecule antagonist of P-selectin that inhibits the binding of P-selectin to P-selectin glycoprotein ligand-1. In a murine model of SCD, animals treated with PSI-697 showed a 55% decrease in adherent neutrophils and a 78% decrease in the number of neutrophil-platelet aggregates compared with controls.[73] These preclinical data suggest that further investigation is warranted.

Intravenous gamma globulin

Although there is much focus on the selectins, activated macrophage-1 antigen on neutrophils is an attractive target for sickle cell therapies. Murine model studies showed a tremendous improvement in erythrocyte–white blood cell adhesiveness, along with improved microcirculatory blood flow.[74] Phase I studies showed similar results with an excellent safety profile, and phase II studies are ongoing.[75]

SUMMARY

We have entered an era of exploding interest in therapeutics for SCD. The expansion in our understanding of SCD pathophysiology has enhanced the range of potential therapeutic targets. From induction of HbF to antiadhesion molecules, we are potentially on the cusp of making life-altering modifications for individuals with SCD. This disease population cannot afford to let the current momentum wane. Studies exploring combinations of therapies affecting multiple steps in the pathophysiology and exploring novel and clinically relevant outcomes are incumbent.

REFERENCES

1. Zhang D, Xu C, Manwani D, et al. Neutrophils, platelets, and inflammatory pathways at the nexus of sickle cell disease pathophysiology. Blood 2016;127(7):801–9.
2. Platt OS, Thorington BD, Brambilla DJ, et al. Pain in sickle cell disease. Rates and risk factors. N Engl J Med 1991;325:11–6.
3. Lehrer-Graiwer J, Howard J, Hemmaway CJ, et al. GBT440, a potent anti-sickling hemoglobin modifier reduces hemolysis, improves anemia and nearly eliminates sickle cells in peripheral blood of patients with sickle cell disease. Blood 2015;126.
4. Lehrer-Graiwer J, Howard J, Hemmaway CJ, et al. Long-term dosing in sickle cell disease subjects with GBT440, a novel HbS polymerization inhibitor. Blood 2016;128.
5. Xu GG, Pagare PP, Ghatge MS, et al. Design, synthesis, and biological evaluation of ester and ether derivatives of antisickling agent 5-HMF for the treatment of sickle cell disease. Mol Pharm 2017;14(10):3499–511.
6. Nakagawa A, Lui FE, Wassaf D, et al. Identification of a small molecule that increases hemoglobin oxygen affinity and reduces SS erythrocyte sickling. ACS Chem Biol 2014;9:2318–25.
7. Nakagawa A, Michele F, Liu C, et al. Development of a triazolyldisulfide compound that increases the affinity of hemoglobin for oxygen and reduces hypoxic sickling of sickle cells. Blood 2016;128.
8. Safo MK, Xu G, Ghatge M, et al. Vzhe-039, a novel structurally-enhanced allosteric hemoglobin effector inhibits sickling of SS erythrocytes in vitro, and exhibits improved pharmacologic properties In Vivo. Blood 2016;128.
9. Kutlar A, Ataga K, Reid M, et al. A phase 1/2 trial of HQK-1001, an oral fetal globin inducer, in sickle cell disease. Am J Hematol 2012;87:1017–21.
10. Reid ME, El Beshlawy A, Inati A, et al. A double-blind, placebo-controlled phase II study of the efficacy and safety of 2,2-dimethylbutyrate (HQK-1001), an oral fetal globin inducer, in sickle cell disease. Am J Hematol 2014;89:709–13.
11. Moutouh-De Parseval LA, Verhelle D, Glezer E, et al. Pomalidomide and lenalidomide regulate erythropoiesis and fetal hemoglobin production in human CD34 + cells. J Clin Invest 2008;118(1):248–58.
12. Meiler SE, Wade M, Kutlar F, et al. Pomalidomide augments fetal hemoglobin production without the myelosuppressive effects of hydroxyurea in transgenic sickle cell mice. Blood 2011;118:1109–12.
13. Kutlar A, Swerdlow PS, Meiler SE, et al. Pomalidomide in sickle cell disease: phase I study of a novel anti-switching agent. Blood 2013;122.
14. Zhang Y, Weiss M, Sumazin P, et al. Metformin induces FOXO3-dependent fetal hemoglobin production in primary erythroid cells. Blood 2016;128.
15. Molokie R, Lavelle D, Gowhari M, et al. Oral tetrahydrouridine and decitabine for non-cytotoxic epigenetic gene regulation in sickle cell disease: a randomized phase 1 study. PLoS Med 2017;14:e1002382.
16. Esrick EB, McConkey M, Lin K, et al. Inactivation of HDAC1 or HDAC2 induces gamma globin expression without altering cell cycle or proliferation. Am J Hematol 2015;90:624–8.
17. Okam MM, Esrick EB, Mandell E, et al. Phase 1/2 trial of vorinostat in patients with sickle cell disease who have not benefitted from hydroxyurea. Blood 2015;125:3668–9.
18. Kutlar A, Patel N, Ustun C, et al. LBH589 (panobinostat): a potential novel anti-switching therapy. Blood 2015;114.

19. Shearstone JR, Chonkar A, Bhol K, et al. The histone deacetylase 1 and 2 (HDAC1/2) Inhibitor ACY-957 Increases Epsilon (HbE) and Gamma (HbG) Globin mRNA in the peripheral blood of non-anemic rats and monkeys. Blood 2015;126.

20. Shearstone JR, Golonzhka O, Chonkar A, et al. Chemical inhibition of histone deacetylases 1 and 2 induces fetal hemoglobin through activation of GATA2. PLoS One 2016;11:e0153767.

21. Cui S, Sangerman J, Nouraie SM, et al. Activity of RN-1, an LSD-1 inhibitor, on fetal globin expression in sickle mice and sickle erythroid progenitors. Blood 2015;126.

22. Krishnamoorthy S, Gupta D, Sturtevant S, et al. Dimethyl fumarate induces fetal hemoglobin in sickle cell disease. Blood 2015;126.

23. Krishnamoorthy S, Pace B, Gupta D, et al. Dimethyl fumarate increases fetal hemoglobin, provides heme detoxification, and corrects anemia in sickle cell disease. JCI Insight 2017;2(20) [pii:96409].

24. Costa FC, Fedosyuk H, Neades R, et al. Induction of fetal hemoglobin in vivo mediated by a synthetic gamma-globin zinc finger activator. Anemia 2012; 2012:507894.

25. Wilber A, Tschulena U, Hargrove PW, et al. A zinc-finger transcriptional activator designed to interact with the gamma-globin gene promoters enhances fetal hemoglobin production in primary human adult erythroblasts. Blood 2010; 115(15):3033–41.

26. Hänggi P, Makhro A, Gassmann M, et al. Red blood cells of sickle cell disease patients exhibit abnormally high abundance of N-methyl D-aspartate receptors mediating excessive calcium uptake. Br J Haematol 2014;167:252–64.

27. Francis RB. Platelets, coagulation, and fibrinolysis in sickle cell disease: their possible role in vascular occlusion. Blood Coagul Fibrinolysis 1991;2:341–53.

28. Noubouossie D, Key NS, Ataga KI. Coagulation abnormalities of sickle cell disease: relationship with clinical outcomes and the effect of disease modifying therapies. Blood Rev 2016;30:245–56.

29. Ataga KI, Brittain JE, Desai P, et al. Association of coagulation activation with clinical complications in sickle cell disease. PLoS One 2012;7:e29786.

30. Telen MJ, Batchvarova M, Shan S, et al. Sevuparin binds to multiple adhesive ligands and reduces sickle red blood cell-induced vaso-occlusion. Br J Haematol 2016;175:935–48.

31. Sparkenbaugh EM, Chantrathammachart P, Mickelson J, et al. Differential contribution of FXa and thrombin to vascular inflammation in a mouse model of sickle cell disease. Blood 2014;123(11):1747–56.

32. Rothmeier AS, Ruf W. Protease-activated receptor 2 signaling in inflammation. Semin Immunopathol 2012;34:133–49.

33. Sins JWR, Fijnvandraat K, Rijneveld AW, et al. Effect of N-acetylcysteine on pain in daily life in patients with sickle cell disease: a randomised clinical trial. Br J Haematol 2017. https://doi.org/10.1111/bjh.14809.

34. Ozpolat H, Chen J, Fu X, et al. Effects of N-acetylcysteine infusion in patients with sickle cell disease during vaso-occlusive crises. Presented at the American Society of Hematology 59th Annual Meeting and exposition. Atlanta (GA), 2017.

35. Lancelot M, White J, Sarnaik S, et al. Low molecular weight heparin inhibits sickle erythrocyte adhesion to VCAM-1 through VLA-4 blockade in a standardized microfluidic flow adhesion assay. Br J Haematol 2017;178:479–81.

36. Carr JA, Cho J-S. Low molecular weight heparin suppresses tumor necrosis factor expression from deep vein thrombosis. Ann Vasc Surg 2007;21:50–5.

37. Matsui NM, Varki A, Embury SH. Heparin inhibits the flow adhesion of sickle red blood cells to P-selectin. Blood 2002;100:3790–6.

38. van Zuuren EJ, Fedorowicz Z. Low-molecular-weight heparins for managing vaso-occlusive crises in people with sickle cell disease. In: van Zuuren EJ, editor. Cochrane database of systematic reviews. Chichester (UK): John Wiley & Sons, Ltd; 2015. https://doi.org/10.1002/14651858.CD010155.pub3.

39. Lindgren M, White J, Liu K, et al. Sevuparin blocks sickle blood cell adhesion and sickle-leukocyte rolling on immobilized l-selectin in a dose dependent manner. Blood 2016;128.

40. Charneski L, Congdon HB. Effects of antiplatelet and anticoagulant medications on the vasoocclusive and thrombotic complications of sickle cell disease: a review of the literature. Am J Health Syst Pharm 2010;67:895–900.

41. Heeney MM, Hoppe CC, Abboud MR, et al. A multinational trial of prasugrel for sickle cell vaso-occlusive events. N Engl J Med 2016;374:625–35.

42. Morris CR. Vascular risk assessment in patients with sickle cell disease. Haematologica 2011;96:1–5.

43. Jasuja R, Parks E, Murphy JE, et al. Chronic administration of the PDE9 inhibitor PF-04447943 reduces leukocyte-platelet aggregates and markers of endothelial activation in a mouse model of sickle cell disease. Blood 2016; 128.

44. McArthur JG, Maciel T, Chen C, et al. A novel, highly potent and selective PDE9 inhibitor for the treatment of sickle cell disease. Blood 2016;128.

45. Mittleman R, Wilson P, Sykes K, et al. 3533 multiple-ascending-dose study of the soluble guanylate cyclase stimulator, IW-1701, in healthy subjects. Presented at the American Society of Hematology 59th Annual Meeting and Exposition. Atlanta (GA), 2017.

46. Gladwin MT, Kato GJ, Weiner D, et al. Nitric oxide for inhalation in the acute treatment of sickle cell pain crisis: a randomized controlled trial. JAMA 2011;305: 893–902.

47. Morris CR, Kuypers FA, Lavrisha L, et al. A randomized, placebo-controlled trial of arginine therapy for the treatment of children with sickle cell disease hospitalized with vaso-occlusive pain episodes. Haematologica 2013;98:1375–82.

48. Mccarty MF. Potential utility of full-spectrum antioxidant therapy, citrulline, and dietary nitrate in the management of sickle cell disease. Med Hypotheses 2010;74: 1055–8.

49. Ataga KI. Novel therapies in sickle cell disease. Hematol Am Soc Hematol Educ Program 2009;2009:54–61.

50. Hoppe C, Jacob E, Styles L, et al. Simvastatin reduces vaso-occlusive pain in sickle cell anaemia: a pilot efficacy trial. Br J Haematol 2017;177(4):620–9.

51. Kalish BT, Matte A, Andolfo I, et al. Dietary ω-3 fatty acids protect against vasculopathy in a transgenic mouse model of sickle cell disease. Haematologica 2015; 100:870–80.

52. Daak A, Ghebremeskel K, Hassan Z, et al. Effect of omega-3 (n 2 3) fatty acid supplementation in patients with sickle cell anemia: randomized, double-blind, placebo-controlled. Am J Clin Nutr 2013;3:37–44.

53. Field JJ. Can selectin and iNKT cell therapies meet the needs of people with sickle cell disease? Hematology 2015;2015:426–32.

54. Field JJ, Majerus E, Ataga KI, et al. NNKTT120, an anti-iNKT cell monoclonal antibody, produces rapid and sustained iNKT cell depletion in adults with sickle cell disease. PLoS One 2017;12:e0171067.

55. Field JJ, Lin G, Okam MM, et al. Sickle cell vaso-occlusion causes activation of iNKT cells that is decreased by the adenosine A2A receptor agonist regadenoson. Blood 2013;121:3329–34.

56. Nathan DG, Field J, Lin G, et al. Sickle cell disease (SCD), iNKT cells, and regadenoson infusion. Trans Am Clin Climatol Assoc 2012;123:312–7 [discussion: 317–8].

57. Field JJ, Majerus E, Gordeuk VR, et al. Randomized phase 2 trial of regadenoson for treatment of acute vaso-occlusive crises in sickle cell disease. Blood Adv 2017;1:1645–9.

58. Vincent L, Vang D, Nguyen J, et al. Mast cell activation contributes to sickle cell pathobiology and pain in mice. Blood 2013;122:1853–62.

59. Lei J, Wang Y, Paul J, et al. Pharmacological inhibition of TLR4 reduces mast cell activation, neuroinflammation and hyperalgesia in sickle mice. Blood 2015;126.

60. Keleku-Lukwete N, Suzuki M, Otsuki A, et al. Keap1-Nrf2 system: potential role in prevention of sickle cell disease organs damages and inflammation. Blood 2015;126.

61. Nettleton M, Almeida LE, Kamimura S, et al. Antisense oligonucleotide against Kelch-Like ECH-associated protein1 ameliorates liver injury in sickle cell mice. Blood 2016;128.

62. Kuvibidila S, Warrier RP, Haynes J, et al. Hydroxyurea and zileuton differentially modulate cell proliferation and interleukin-2 secretion by murine spleen cells: possible implication on the immune function and risk of pain crisis in patients with sickle cell disease. Ochsner J 2015;15(3):241–7.

63. Haynes J, Surendra Baliga B, Obiako B, et al. Zileuton induces hemoglobin F synthesis in erythroid progenitors: role of the L-arginine–nitric oxide signaling pathway. Blood 2004;103(10):3945–50.

64. Quarmyne M-O, Rayes O, Gonsalves C, et al. A phase I trial of zileuton in sickle cell disease. Blood 2013;122.

65. Shiu Y-T, Udden MM, Mcintire LV. Perfusion with sickle erythrocytes up-regulates ICAM-1 and VCAM-1 gene expression in cultured human endothelial cells. Blood 2000;95(10):3232–41.

66. Zennadi R, Chien A, Xu K, et al. Sickle red cells induce adhesion of lymphocytes and monocytes to endothelium. Blood 2008;112(8):3474–83.

67. Embury SH, Matsui NM, Ramanujam S, et al. The contribution of endothelial cell P-selectin to the microvascular flow of mouse sickle erythrocytes in vivo. Blood 2004;104:3378–85.

68. Matsui NM, Borsig L, Rosen SD, et al. P-selectin mediates the adhesion of sickle erythrocytes to the endothelium. Blood 2001;98(6):1955–62.

69. Johnson C, Telen MJ. Adhesion molecules and hydroxyurea in the pathophysiology of sickle cell disease 1. Haematologica 2008;93:481–6.

70. Telen MJ, Wun T, McCavit TL, et al. Randomized phase 2 study of GMI-1070 in SCD: reduction in time to resolution of vaso-occlusive events and decreased opioid use. #NCT01119833. Blood 2015;125(17):2656–64.

71. Ataga KI, Kutlar A, Kanter J, et al. Crizanlizumab for the prevention of pain crises in sickle cell disease. N Engl J Med 2017;376:429–39.

72. De Castro LM, Zennadi R, Jonassaint JC, et al. Effect of propranolol as antiadhesive therapy in sickle cell disease. Clin Transl Sci 2012;5:437–44.

73. Jasuja R, Hett SP, Kaila N, et al. Effect of PSI697, a small molecule inhibitor of P-selectin, in the Townes model of sickle cell disease. Blood 2015;126.

74. Chang J, Shi PA, Chiang EY, et al. Intravenous immunoglobulins reverse acute vaso-occlusive crises in sickle cell mice through rapid inhibition of neutrophil adhesion. Blood 2008;111:915–23.

75. Manwani D, Chen G, Carullo V, et al. Single-dose intravenous gammaglobulin can stabilize neutrophil Mac-1 activation in sickle cell pain crisis. Am J Hematol 2015; 90:381–5.

Genetic Therapies for Sickle Cell Disease

Rajeswari Jayavaradhan, MS[a,b], Punam Malik, MD[a,b],*

KEYWORDS

- Sickle cell anemia • Viral vectors • Gene therapy • HSC gene editing

KEY POINTS

- Gene therapy has the potential for curing hemoglobinopathies such as sickle cell anemia permanently.
- Lentivirus vectors have revolutionized genetic correction, with several patients with thalassemia and one with sickle cell anemia cured of their disease.
- The actual correction of the sickle mutation or permanent reactivation of fetal hemoglobin with gene editing may be possible in the near future.

INTRODUCTION

Historically, sickle shaped red blood cells (RBCs) were first described in a patient with sickle cell anemia (SCA) by James Herrick.[1] It was not until almost two decades later that the RBC sickling phenomenon was shown to be dependent on oxygen concentration.[2,3] In 1949, Linus Pauling was the first to show that the hemoglobin (Hb) in sickle RBC differed in structure from normal Hb.[4] That same year, Janet Watson predicted the importance of fetal Hb (HbF) by showing paucity of sickled RBC in newborns compared with adults with SCA.[5] By 1955, Ingram and Hunt showed that glutamic acid at position 6 of the beta-globin gene was replaced by a valine, which resulted in SCA,[6] which made SCA the first genetic disorder whose molecular basis was discovered. However, it took more than one-half of a century thereafter before the globin genes were cloned and sequenced, the organization of the globin gene clusters was characterized, and a great deal of insight was provided into the mechanisms of their regulated expression.[7]

Human Hb, the protein that carries oxygen from the lungs to the tissues, is a tetrameric molecule that consists of 2 pairs of identical polypeptide subunits (2 α-like globin peptides and 2 β-like globin peptides). The human α-like globin gene cluster (ζ, α_1, and

[a] Division of Experimental Hematology and Cancer Biology, Cancer and Blood Disease Institute (CBDI), Cincinnati Children's Hospital Medical Center (CCHMC), Mail Location 7013, 3333 Burnet Avenue, Cincinnati, OH 45229, USA; [b] Pathobiology and Molecular Medicine Graduate Program, Mail Location: 0529, 231 Albert Sabin Way, Cincinnati, OH 45267-0529, USA
* Corresponding author. Cincinnati Children's Hospital Medical Center (CCHMC), Mail Location 7013, 3333 Burnet Avenue, Cincinnati, OH 45229.
E-mail address: Punam.Malik@cchmc.org

Pediatr Clin N Am 65 (2018) 465–480
https://doi.org/10.1016/j.pcl.2018.01.008
0031-3955/18/© 2018 Elsevier Inc. All rights reserved.

α_2) is located on chromosome 16, and the β-like globin gene cluster (ϵ, Gγ, Aγ, δ, and β) is located on chromosome 11. Interestingly, the globin genes present on both these clusters are in the same order in which they are expressed during development.[8] During fetal life, the predominant Hb produced is HbF ($\alpha_2\gamma_2$), which is gradually replaced post-natally by HbA ($\alpha_2\beta_2$) when the γ-globin gene gets silenced. Upon this switch from HbF to HbA, β-globinopathies, such as sickle cell disease (SCD) and β-thalassemia manifest clinically.[5] This important observation, and natural mutations resulting in hereditary persistence of fetal hemoglobin with no clinical consequence led into an understanding of the process of switching from γ- to β-globin, and has formed the basis behind designing genetic therapies that reactivate γ-globin or similar antisickling globins.

SCA is caused by a homozygous point mutation (A-T) in the sixth codon of the β-globin/*HBB* gene. The dimerization of the mutant β-globin (β^S) chains with α-globin results in the formation of sickle Hb S (HbS, $\alpha_2\beta^S_2$). Various other β-globin mutations, like β-thalassemia, HbC, HbD, and HbE, when coinherited in compound heterozygosity with β^S mutations, also result in a sickle cell phenotype, and are grouped broadly as SCD, with patients that only make β^S-globin ($\beta^S\beta^S$ and $\beta^S/\beta^{0-thalassemia}$) termed as having SCA. SCD is among the most common monogenic diseases, with 330,000 affected births per year worldwide.[9] The sickle mutation was selected for in areas affected by malaria, because it conferred protection from severe forms of malaria in heterozygous individuals (HbAS), who are largely asymptomatic.[10,11]

MEDICAL MANAGEMENT OF SICKLE CELL DISEASE

The first breakthrough occurred when the use of pneumococcal vaccine with penicillin prophylaxis was found to be effective in preventing death from pneumococcal sepsis in children with SCD.[12] Next, hydroxyurea was shown to increase HbF and reduce the frequency of pain episodes,[13] and was approved by the US Food and Drug Administration in 1998 for adults with SCD. Chronic blood transfusions were also shown to reduce the risk of stroke by 90%.[14,15] Acute sickle events are managed with supportive care. Together, these are the cornerstones of preventive and symptomatic management in SCD that have prolonged survival in this disease. However, disease-modifying therapies, such as hydroxyurea, are not equally effective in all patients, often owing to poor compliance of life-long administration. Therefore, there remains significant morbidity and shortened life span in patients with SCD with the median age of death being 42 years for men and 48 years for women.[16] Current medical management of SCD are reviewed in Emily Riehm Meier's article, "Treatment Options for Sickle Cell Disease," and Ahmar U. Zaidi and Matthew M. Heeney's article, "A Scientific Renaissance: Novel Drugs in Sickle Cell Disease (SCD)," in this issue.

CURATIVE OPTIONS

The first cure of SCD occurred by serendipity in 1984, when a bone marrow transplant was performed to treat acute leukemia in a child with SCD and it eradicated both the leukemia and SCD,[11] setting the precedence for hematopoietic stem cell transplant (HSCT) as a curative modality. At present, allogeneic HSCT is the only definitive cure, with a disease-free survival of greater than 80% with HLA-matched sibling donor transplants.[17] However, most patients lack matched sibling donors. The use of unrelated donors increases the mortality and morbidity associated from transplant and its immune side effects, such as graft-versus-host disease and graft rejection/failure, thus limiting allogeneic HSCT as the major treatment option.[18] Only about 1200 HSCT have been performed so far for SCD, a disproportionately small number compared to the huge global burden of this disease.[19]

AUTOLOGOUS HEMATOPOIETIC STEM CELL TRANSPLANTATION WITH GENE TRANSFER

Transplantation of genetically modified autologous HSCs (gene therapy) is an attractive alternative to allogeneic HSCT. Gene therapy is accomplished in 3 steps (**Fig. 1**): (i) harvesting autologous hematopoietic stem and progenitor cells (HSPC) from either bone marrow, or peripheral blood, (ii) genetically modifying the sickle HSPC, and (iii) transplanting them back into the patient after chemotherapy conditioning. The gene-modified HSPC engraft and repopulate the hematopoietic compartment, producing genetically corrected RBC progeny.[20]

A variety of viral[21] and nonviral[22] vector-based gene delivery mechanisms have been developed, although viral vectors are currently the most efficient way to deliver genes into HSPC.[23] This review focuses on SCD gene therapy via an antisickling globin gene addition, a therapy that is in clinical trials. The article also reviews gene editing–mediated correction of the sickle mutation or activating HbF using site-directed nucleases, which can eventually become the next generation of genetic therapies.

VIRAL VECTORS

For HSC, vectors that can permanently integrate into the cellular genome are used so that all the HSC progeny carry the therapeutic gene for the life of the individual. Viral vectors used for transducing HSC are derived from the gamma-retrovirus (RV), lentivirus (LV), and foamy virus (FV) that belong to the Retroviridae family. These are RNA viruses that are capable of reverse transcribing their genome and integrating it into the host/cellular genome.[21] Viral vectors are bioengineered viral particles that are rendered replication-incompetent, and genetic elements needed for pathogenicity and replication are removed and replaced by the therapeutic transgene.

RETROVIRAL VECTORS

Initial attempts of *HBB* gene transfer were performed using RV vectors that had intact viral long terminal repeats (LTRs). LTRs of retroviruses contain strong viral promoters/enhancers at either end of the virus/vector. Initial RV vectors, that only encoded the beta-globin gene, resulted in little or negligible β-globin production after hematopoietic reconstitution in mice.[24] The discovery and characterization of the β-globin locus

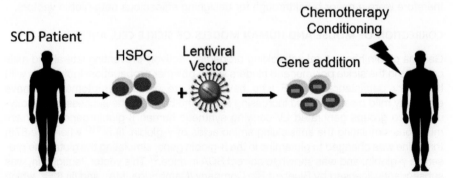

Fig. 1. Autologous gene-modified hematopoietic stem cell (HSC) transplant. Gene therapy is accomplished by first harvesting patient's hematopoietic stem and progenitor cells (HSPC) from either bone marrow or peripheral blood. Second, the harvested sickle HSPC are genetically modified. Finally, the gene-modified HSPC are transplanted back into the chemotherapy conditioned patient where they proliferate and repopulate the hematopoietic compartment with genetically corrected red blood cell progeny. SCD, sickle cell disease.

control region (LCR), a 16-kb regulatory element 40 to 60 kb upstream of the β-globin gene. The LCR was found to be necessary for high-level erythroid-specific globin gene expression,[25] and paved the way for incorporating sequences of the LCR into RV. However, owing to the limited packaging capacity of RV (4–5 kb), only small LCR core elements could be incorporated in beta-globin RV, which were insufficient for high-level β-globin expression. In addition, β-globin RV were unstable and together, this resulted in failure of RV vectors as effective vectors for the gene therapy for hemoglobinopathies despite a 15-year effort by numerous investigators.[26–33]

Moreover, although RV vectors led to clinical success in patients with X-linked severe combined immunodeficiency and Wiskott-Aldrich syndrome, the success in these trials was marred by insertional oncogenesis[20]: several patients developed leukemias from activation of protooncogenes in the vicinity of the integrated vector (provirus) by the LTR enhancers in the RV. Chromatin insulators that decrease *trans*-activation of genes from nearby enhancers (enhancer-blocking activity) and shield downstream sequences from repressive effects of neighboring chromatin (barrier activity) were incorporated into vectors to improve safety and efficiency. The chicken hypersensitive site-4 insulator was shown to promote the safety and efficacy of integrating vectors in experimental models.[34] Addition of insulators added to the size limitation of RV. However, insertional oncogenesis laid the last nail in the coffin of RV vectors for globin gene therapy, because RV vectors were already fraught with problems of efficacious expression of globin genes, and had inherent issues of only being able to transduce actively dividing HSC.

LENTIVIRAL VECTORS

A breakthrough in gene therapy occurred with the advent of human immunodeficiency virus-1–based LV vectors that offered several unique advantages over RV vectors.[34] LV vectors can transduce nondividing cells. HSC are primarily quiescent and enforcing them to divide in vitro results in a large loss in their "stemness" or long-term repopulating potential. In addition, LV were shown to be able to sustain a self-inactivating design without loss of potency. The SIN design deletes the LTR viral promoter/enhancers in the provirus (integrated vector), and hence allows transgenes expression to be driven by internal tissue-specific enhancer/promoters, minimizing the potential for insertional oncogenesis and resulting in tissue-specific expression.[35] LV vectors therefore were a major breakthrough for designing efficacious beta-globin vectors.

CORRECTION OF MOUSE AND HUMAN MODELS OF SICKLE CELL ANEMIA

Gamma globin has natural antisickling properties, actively preventing lateral and axial contacts in the sickle polymer and hinders sickle polymer propagation. Individuals with hereditary persistence of HbF who have SCA are either asymptomatic or have extremely mild disease[36]; and increasing HbF is the basis for the success of hydroxyurea. Two groups generated LV-carrying synthetic human β-globin genes that have mutations simulating the antisickling amino acids of γ-globin: (i) β^{T87Q} where the 87th threonine was changed to glutamine in the β-globin gene, simulating the glutamine present in γ-globin, and was shown to correct SCA in mice.[37] This vector, lentiglobin, was subsequently licensed by Bluebird Bio Company (Cambridge, MA), and (ii) β^{AS3}, which incorporated 3 amino acid substitutions in β-globin (T87Q, E22A, and G16D),[38] which would render β-globin with the same antisickling properties and potency as γ-globin and this also corrected the sickle phenotype in mice.[39] Romero and colleagues[40] used β^{AS3} in an LV that also carried a small insulator element in sickle HSPC and showed the reversal of sickle phenotype in RBCs differentiated from HSPC in vitro.

Although conferring antisickling properties to β-globin, a gene that naturally expresses in postnatal RBC, was 1 way to express an antisickling globin, 2 groups made LV that were able to express γ-globin itself in postnatal RBC. The rationale was that expressing γ-globin, a naturally present globin, will not be immunogenic; further, it is the most potent antisickling globin. Hanawa and colleagues[41] showed that the γ-globin gene could be driven by the β-globin promoter and LCR, and resulted in postnatal HbF expression that corrected SCD in mice. Our group substituted the exons of the β-globin gene for γ-globin exons, and this γ-globin vector, which contained the noncoding β-globin sequences and β-promoter, showed high HbF expression and corrected SCD in mice,[42] even after reduced intensity conditioning.[42]

HUMAN CLINICAL TRIALS

The success in preclinical studies in SCD mouse models, supported by safety studies on β-globin LV vectors by our group,[43] prompted the initiation of human clinical trials (summarized in **Table 1**). BB305 LentiGlobin[44] was used to treat patients with SCD in France (HGB-205 study) and in the United States (HGB-206 study) following myeloablative conditioning. The child with SCA treated in France exhibited substantial clinical benefit over the first year of treatment, with nearly one-half of the globin chains composed of β^{T87Q}, and remains completely free of SCD symptoms.[45] However, the data reported on 7 adult patients so far, who were treated in the United States, showed only modest increases in β^{T87Q}, and did not have a significant clinical benefit, possibly owing to lower numbers of HSC obtained from adults, and poor engraftment of the gene-modified cells.[46] These patients are all within 12 months of transplant, and there may yet be a positive selection of gene-modified cells. Important differences exist between the 2 studies. The French patient received a high dose of 5.6 million $CD34^+$ cells/kg that exhibited approximately 1 vector copy per cell in vitro that was sustained in vivo, whereas in the adult patients, the HSPC dose was lower and the vector copy number could not be sustained in vivo, suggesting loss or failure of the gene-modified HSC to engraft. Furthermore, this child treated in France had a high degree of myeloablation with a markedly prolonged duration of neutropenia of approximately 40 days before neutrophil recovery, which may have led to engraftment of only ex vivo treated HSC.[47]

Two other clinical trials of gene therapy for SCD have been initiated in the United States: the NCT02247843 trial led by Kohn and colleagues is investigating the efficacy of Lenti-βAS3-FB vector[40] using full myeloablative conditioning with busulfan. The NCT02186418 trial led by our group is testing the efficacy of sG^{b}GM γ-globin LV vector using reduced intensity conditioning with another chemotherapy agent, melphalan.[42] Both trials are enrolling patients and the results are eagerly awaited.

FOAMY VIRUS VECTORS

Even though the safety of gene therapy has been clinically observed in patients treated thus far with the advent of self-inactivating LV vectors, and the erythroid-specific promoter/enhancers (LCR) in self-inactivating LV carrying globin genes further limits inadvertent activation of cellular oncogenes, another potentially favorable vector may be the FV vector. FV is a nonpathogenic RV that offers several unique benefits; it is nonpathogenic, it has large packaging capacity (12 kb), and it has a safer integration profile with a higher preference for nongenic integrations than RV and LV vectors. We have recently shown that FV vectors are far less genotoxic owing to natural insulator sequences in their LTR.[48] FV vectors have been shown to be efficient vehicles for β-globin gene expression in HSPC[49] and may become an alternative in the future.

Table 1
Current human clinical trials for sickle cell gene therapy

Identifier/Study ID Number	Sponsor	Chemotherapy Conditioning	Lentiviral Vector	Phase	Estimated Enrollment	Location	Study Start Date	Estimated Study Completion Date
NCT02151526/HGB-205	Bluebird Bio (France)	Myeloablative busulfan (3.2/kg/d × 4 d)	LentiGlobin BB305 drug (Lentiviral Beta-A-T87Q Globin Vector)	II	7	France	July 2013	2019
NCT02140554/HGB-206	Bluebird Bio (Multicenter, USA)	Myeloablative Busulfan (3.2/kg/d × 4 d)	LentiGlobin BB305 Drug	I	29	United States	August 2014	2020
NCT02186418/2010–2588	Cincinnati Children's Hospital Medical Center	Reduced intensity melphalan (140 mg/m^2 × 1 dose)	Gamma Globin Vector	I/II	10	United States	December 2014	2019
NCT02247843/Lenti/βAS3-FB	University of California, Los Angeles	Myeloablative Busulfan (3.2/kg/d × 4 d)	βAS3-FB Vector	I	6	United States	July 2014	2018

GENE EDITING USING NUCLEASES

Recent advances in gene editing have revolutionized the field of gene therapy. The ability to make targeted double-stranded DNA breaks (DSB) by using different site-directed nucleases have been used to correct the disease causing mutations. Zinc finger nucleases (ZFNs),[50] transcription activator–like effector nucleases (TALENs),[51] and clustered regulatory interspaced short palindromic repeat and associated Cas9 (CRISPR/Cas9)[52] have been developed to make site-specific DSB.

After the induction of DSB, the cell repairs the DSBs generally by 3 major repair mechanisms: nonhomologous end joining (NHEJ), microhomology-mediated end joining, and homologous recombination (HR)[53] (**Fig. 2**). The NHEJ and microhomology-mediated end joining are error-prone repair processes that result in the insertions or deletions (indels) of base pairs at the DSB, thereby knocking out the gene.[53] In contrast, if a homologous DNA template is present, HR results precise repair. This DNA template can, within the homologous regions, carry the corrected gene and a selectable marker.[53] Nucleases with or without homology templates are transiently expressed, because they are not needed after the cellular repair of the DSB occurs. This avoids non-specific integration of the gene editing tools, and thereby eliminating the potential of insertional mutagenesis. However, off-target DSB can occur, and these can have deleterious genotoxic effects.

ZINC FINGER PROTEINS

A zinc finger is a small, zinc-dependent protein structural motif that is naturally present in numerous transcription factors, and confers the transcription factor the ability to

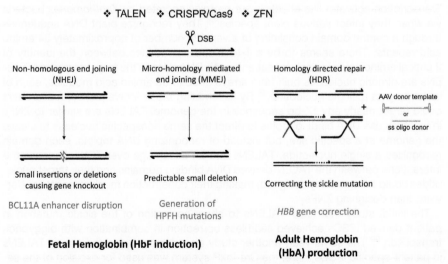

Fig. 2. Genome-editing strategies for correction of sickle mutation or reactivation of endogenous γ-globin expression. TALEN, CRISPR/Cas9 or ZFN induced DNA double strand breaks (DSB) can be repaired primarily by the three cell's DSB repair mechanisms. The non-homologous end joining (NHEJ) repair mechanism is exploited to cause BCL11A enhancer disruption or microhomology-mediated end joining (MMEJ) to generate mutations that cause hereditary persistence of fetal hemoglobin (HPFH). Both BCL11A enhancer disruption and HPFH mutations induce HbF. Gene correction utilizes homology directed repair (HDR) to replace the mutation causing SCD to the normal sequence, producing normal adult hemoglobin.

bind specific sequences in gene promoters. Researchers have made designer zinc finger proteins (ZFNs), such that they have zinc fingers that target a desired sequence in the genome and are fused to nucleases that create a DSB at the site zinc fingers bind DNA. To reduce off-target DSB, ZFNs were designed by designing 2 sets of zinc finger proteins, each recognizing a contiguous 9-bp DNA sequence; and each fused with the Fok1 endonuclease monomer. Together, only when binding of the 2 ZFNs occurred adjacent to each other, recognizing a contiguous 18-bp DNA sequence, only then Fok1 endonuclease would dimerize and cause a DSB at binding site.[54] Hence, ZFNs combine the ability to bind specific cellular DNA sequences (via designer zinc fingers) and cleave them (via Fok1 endonuclease).

The first indication of the therapeutic potential of ZFNs in SCD came from the studies in which ZFNs were used to correct the sickle mutation in patient-derived induced pluripotent stem cells (iPSCs).[55,56] In 2015, ZFNs were shown to correct approximately 18% of sickle alleles to wild-type alleles in HSPC derived from the patients with SCD in vitro.[57] The corrected sickle HSPC maintained their differentiation ability in vitro, leading to the formation of myeloid and erythroid clones and produced wild-type Hb tetramers. Despite the promising in vitro results of 10% to 20% gene modification in the HSPCs, when transplanted into immune-deficient mice, gene edited HSPC had less than 1% engraftment in vivo, suggesting a large loss of long-term repopulating potential with editing. The major disadvantage of ZFNs is the complexities of designing them and their limited modularity. Hence, more user-friendly modular platforms, such as TALENs, have largely replaced ZFN technology.

TRANSCRIPTION ACTIVATOR–LIKE EFFECTOR NUCLEASES

Transcription activator like effectors are proteins secreted by *Xanthomonas* bacteria via when they infect various plant species.[58] They recognize plant DNA sequences through a central domain consisting of a variable number of approximately 34 amino acid repeats. There seems to be a 1-to-1 correspondence between the identity of 2 critical amino acids in each repeat and each DNA base in the target sequence. TALENs are dimeric nucleases built from arrays of 33 to 35 amino acid modules, each of which targets a single nucleotide.[58] By assembling those arrays just so, researchers could target nearly any 17-bp sequence in the genome. TALENs are similar to ZNFs in that they use DNA binding motifs to direct the same nonspecific nuclease to cleave the genome at a specific site, but instead of recognizing DNA triplets, each domain recognizes a single nucleotide. TALENs had an advantage over ZFNs, because the interactions between the TALEN-derived DNA binding domains and their target nucleotides could be modularly designed, making their construction much more straightforward than designing ZNFs.

The initial study that used TALENs to show correction of the sickle mutation in patient-derived iPSCs achieved seamless correction in combination with piggyback transposon.[59] The same year, another study also demonstrated the use of TALENs in patient-specific iPSCs; here, the Cre-loxP system was used for excision of the selection marker,[60] and corrected iPSC-derived erythroid cells expressed 30% to 40% of the normal allele. These studies necessitate using a selectable marker to select for edited cells. Selection is only feasible when working with cell lines or iPSCs (which can be maintained in culture without the loss of the self-renewing potential). However, the culture time needed to select HSC, and to later remove the marker, would not allow for the retention of long-term repopulating HSC. Voit and colleagues[61] inserted the entire β-globin complementary DNA (cDNA) followed by a polyadenylation signal via TALEN upstream of the native *HBB* gene and downstream of the *HBB* promoter, as an alternative to correct different *HBB* mutations with 19% targeting efficiency without drug selection in the K562 erythroleukemia cell line. The use of TALENs to correct the sickle mutation in primary HSPC has not been demonstrated.

CLUSTERED REGULATORY INTERSPACED SHORT PALINDROMIC REPEAT/CAS9 SYSTEM

The CRISPR/Cas9 system is the latest and most popular genome editing tool owing to its ease of use.[52] Here, the Cas9 nuclease is guided to a specific site in the genome by a single guide RNA (sgRNA), the latter carrying a 20-bp homology to the targeted sequence. Hence, one only needs to change the 20-bp sgRNA recognition sequence to the desired targeted gene sequence, making this technology simple to use. A side-by-side comparison of ZFNs, TALENs, and CRISPR/Cas9 to target *HBB* locus near the β^s mutation in patient-derived iPSCs reported the CRISPR/Cas9 system to have better cutting efficiency at the *HBB* locus compared with ZFNs or TALENs.[62]

In an effort to rationally design CRISPR to target the sickle mutation, a detailed bioinformatics analysis of the *HBB* locus for suitable CRISPR target sites showed that targeting introns could have fewer off-target effects compared with exons[63] and because introns contained less single nucleotide polymorphisms, making a CRISPR design applicable to more people.[63]

Liang and colleagues[64] demonstrated the usefulness of CRISPR/Cas9–based gene editing in nonviable human zygotes, although this study raises serious ethical concerns. Nevertheless, HR efficiency at *HBB* locus of zygotes was low (4 in 54 embryos) and off-target mutations occurred. Although the CRISPR/Cas9 tool for gene editing has superseded all prior technologies, a number of CRISPRs designed to target *HBB* locus have been shown to have substantial off-target mutations,[65] highlighting the need to eliminate this CRISPR-associated genotoxicity before human applications.

Scientists have been working on first improving the efficacy/potency with improved design/delivery of CRISPR/Cas9 to correct the sickle mutation in clinically relevant HSPCs (summarized in **Table 2**). Hoban and colleagues[57] first showed ZFN-mediated correction of the sickle mutation and then demonstrated similar in vitro correction rates of approximately 20% using CRISPR/Cas9 in bone marrow–derived $CD34^+$ from patients with SCD. However, it is pertinent to note that there was a 100-fold decrease in the proportion of edited cells that engrafted in mice (0.2%).

HR-mediated gene correction using CRISPR requires presence of a protein (Cas9 nuclease), RNA (sgRNA), and DNA (homology donor template) to be available at the same time and location in the cell. Hence, to improve HR efficiency, when Cas9/sgRNA was delivered as a ribonucleoprotein complex along with a DNA homology template,[66,67] it met these requirements and improved both the overall DSB frequency and gene targeting efficiency. When this approach of ribonucleoprotein plus a single-strand oligonucleotide (as the DNA homology template) was transfected into sickle HSPC, DeWitt and colleagues[67] observed that approximately 25% of the alleles were corrected and produced approximately 29% HbA in vitro. However, when the HSPC were transplanted into immune-deficient mice, only 2% to 3% of edited cells engrafted animals. Dever and colleagues[66] improved on this by delivering the DNA homology template in adeno-associated virus type 6 vector. They used 3 different homology templates: (1) one that carried sequence homology to normal β-globin (with β^{T6A}), (2) one that carried antisickling *HBB* cDNA (HbAS3) along with a selectable marker green fluorescent protein, and (3) one that carried antisickling *HBB* cDNA (HbAS3) along with the truncated nerve growth factor receptor as a selectable marker. Ribonucleoprotein and

Table 2
Proof-of-concept studies showing gene correction of the sickle mutation

Gene Editing Nuclease	Study	Type of Gene Editing Components Delivered	CD34+ HSPC Source	In Vitro HR Efficiency in SS-CD34+	In Vivo Engraftment of HR + CD34+ in NSG Mice
ZFN	Hoban et al,[57] 2015	*Nuclease:* ZFN mRNA *HR Template:* IDLV/ssDNA	In vitro: SS-BM CD34+ In vivo: normal MPB CD34+	18 ± 7%	IDLV: 0.2 ± 0.4% in BM ssDNA: 0.9 ± 0.8% in BM
CRISPR/Cas9	Hoban et al,[78] 2016	*Nuclease:* Cas9 mRNA *HR template:* IDLV *sgRNA:* IDLV	In vitro: SS-BM CD34+	21%	Not performed
CRISPR/Cas9	DeWitt et al,[67] 2016	Nuclease + sgRNA: RNP *HR template:* ssDNA	In Vitro: SS-UMPB CD34+ In vivo: normal MPB CD34+	25%	2.3 ± 1.8% in BM 3.7 ± 1.4% in spleen
CRISPR/Cas9	Denver et al,[66] 2016	Nuclease + sgRNA: RNP *HR Templates:* in AAV6 with i. SNP (A→T) ii. HbAS3 with GFP iii. HbAS3 with tNGFR	In vitro: SS-UMPB CD34+ In vivo: normal MPB CD34+	SNP: 50% HbAS3/tNGFR: 11%	HbAS3 tNGFR: 7.5% in BM HbAS3 GFP: 1.9% in BM

Abbreviations: AAV6, adeno-associated virus type 6; GFP, green fluorescent protein; MPB, mobilized peripheral blood; mRNA, messenger RNA; RNP, ribonucleoprotein; SNP, single nucleotide polymorphism; SS-BM CD34+, sickle CD34+ HSPCs; ssDNA, single-stranded DNA; tNGFR, truncated nerve growth factor receptor; UMPB, unmobilized peripheral blood; ZFNs, zinc finger nucleases.

adeno-associated virus type 6 homology templates were delivered into sickle CD34$^+$ HSPC which resulted in 11% to 50% correction of the sickle alleles. Comparisons of the proportion of in vitro edited cells with those that engrafted in vivo showed that the *HBB*-truncated nerve growth factor receptor mice had 12% editing in vitro versus 7.5% editing in vivo, but the *HBB*-green fluorescent protein mice had 10% editing in vitro versus 1.9% editing in vivo. Furthermore, mice transplanted with truncated nerve growth factor receptor–selected edited HSPCs retained high in vivo engraftment of 10% to 75%, the highest in vivo editing in the beta-globin locus reported thus far.

FETAL HEMOGLOBIN REACTIVATION USING GENE EDITING

Therapeutic strategies aimed at reducing expression of factors silent the γ-globin gene have been tried. Several factors shown to be involved (KLF1, MYB, and LRF, to name a few) in HbF induction also have an essential role in erythroid development and thus not good targets for treating SCD.[68] However, BCL11A is a critical factor required to maintain repression of HbF in postnatal cells, and does not affect the process of erythropoiesis[69]; its knockdown has shown correction of SCD by increasing HbF.[70] However, BCL11A is essential in B-lymphopoiesis, dendritic cell development, and in HSCs,[71] and its knockout/knockdown in HSC is, therefore, not a feasible. However, Chang and colleagues[72] have identified an erythroid enhancer of BCL11A, which when knocked out using gene editing, does not affect any other hematopoietic lineage, and BCL11A enhancer ZFN–edited HSPCs can stably engraft in immunodeficient mice. Guda and colleagues[73] reported an alternative approach such as LCR-driven erythroid-specific expression of a short hairpin RNA for BCL11A overcomes the toxicity associated with polymerase III–dependent short hairpin RNAs and with knockdown of BCL11A in erythroid cells, which reverses the sickle phenotype. This approach was associated with a 90% decrease in BCL11A levels in RBCs derived from normal and SCD HSCs, and HbF represented up to 70% of the total Hb content.[71]

MANIPULATING THE CHROMATIN LOOPING IN THE β-GLOBIN LOCUS TO REACTIVATE γ-GLOBIN

Researchers have also been able to create synthetic transcription factors such as ZFN-binding domain recognizing the γ-globin promoter fused to an activation domain (VP64)[74] or LDB1, a factor involved in chromatin looping of the LCR[75] to increase HbF expression at the expense of β-globin. Interestingly, a low level of expression of the ZF-LDB1 was enough to force the formation of a loop between the LCR and the γ-globin promoter, which reduced sickling in RBCs from human SCD HSPCs in vitro.[75] Preclinical in vivo studies addressing the safety, potency, and specificity of this strategy and its translation to a clinical trial is awaited.

GENE EDITING TO INDUCE A HEREDITARY PERSISTENCE OF FETAL HEMOGLOBIN MUTATION

Hereditary persistence of HbF is a benign condition in which naturally occurring mutations in the regions that regulate expression of HBG1 and HBG2 genes result in increased HbF expression. Recently, Traxler and colleagues[76] used the CRISPR/Cas9 system to generate a 13bp hereditary persistence of HbF deletion in the γ-globin promoter via microhomology-mediated end-joining repair. In this study, HbF reactivation was associated with reduced levels of HbS and amelioration of the SCD phenotype in vitro.[77] The efficiency of genome editing in vivo and the potential off target effects of this approach need to be studied carefully in HSCs.

DISCUSSION

LV-based gene addition strategies have proven to be effective and safe in at least 1 child with SCD who is free of disease symptoms. However these results need to be reproduced in adults and in larger cohorts of patients, because other patients treated with the same vector, protocol, and gene transfer methodology showed only modest clinical benefit. Further improvements in gene transfer into HSC, retention of HSC long-term repopulating potential in vivo, the adequacy of myeloablative conditioning, number of transduced HSC, and/or protocol design are needed for clear clinical benefit and are being actively explored. Several groups have proposed alternative lentiviral vectors carrying chromatin loop proteins or small hairpins against BCL11A that await translation. These LV vectors, owing to smaller size and a lower bar for expression, and their ability to increase HbF at the expense of HbS, may be more potent.

Genome-editing strategies for correction of sickle mutation or reactivation of endogenous γ-globin expression (see **Fig. 2**) are likely the next future of gene therapy, although several issues of delivery, toxicity, and off-target effects with this approach need resolution before effective and safe translation to patients. Several obstacles face the field of gene editing for it to become clinically relevant. Although the proof-of-concept sickle correction in SCD patient derived HSPCs has been established, currently there is a large loss of the long-term repopulating ability of edited HSPC. Another obstacle is the need to increase the desired precise HR outcomes over NHEJ for correction of the mutation. HR and NHEJ are competitive processes, with NHEJ typically being the dominant process with most gene editing systems. The frequency of successful HR is still low and requires a selectable marker to sort gene targeted HSPC, that may not be practical at a clinical scale. Recent development of rapid hematopoietic stem and progenitor reporter systems will allow manipulation and optimization of the desired DNA double strand break repair outcomes, to achieve the optimal gene editing.[79,80] Simultaneous advances in iPSC to generate engraftable HSC could help to realize the potential of gene editing approaches in curing SCD. Further, there are limited tools available to measure the off-target effects of the endonuclease-induced DSB and nonspecific integration of homology template sequence. Ultimately, many different strategies may work and ameliorate the SCD phenotype, but the ease of translation and, most importantly, their transportability and affordability to resource-poor countries, where the greatest burden of SCD is present, will determine their usefulness for patients suffering from SCD.

REFERENCES

1. Herrick JB. Peculiar elongated and sickle-shaped red blood corpuscles in a case of severe anemia. 1910. Yale J Biol Med 2001;74:179–84.
2. Hahn E, Gillespie E. Sickle cell anemia: report of a case greatly improved by splenectomy. experimental study of sickle cell formation. Arch Intern Med 1927;39: 233–54.
3. Scriver JB, Waugh TR. Studies on a case of sickle-cell anaemia. Can Med Assoc J 1930;23:375–80.
4. Pauling L, Itano HA, Singer SJ, et al. Sickle cell anemia a molecular disease. Science 1949;110:543–8.
5. Watson J. The significance of the paucity of sickle cells in newborn Negro infants. Am J Med Sci 1948;215:419–23.
6. Ingram VM. Abnormal human haemoglobins. I. The comparison of normal human and sickle-cell haemoglobins by fingerprinting. Biochim Biophys Acta 1958;28: 539–45.

7. Stamatoyannopoulos G. Control of globin gene expression during development and erythroid differentiation. Exp Hematol 2005;33:259–71.
8. Frenette PS, Atweh GF. Sickle cell disease: old discoveries, new concepts, and future promise. J Clin Invest 2007;117:850–8.
9. Williams TN, Weatherall DJ. World distribution, population genetics, and health burden of the hemoglobinopathies. Cold Spring Harb Perspect Med 2012;2: a011692.
10. Eridani S. Sickle cell protection from malaria. Hematol Rep 2011;3:e24.
11. Johnson FL, Look AT, Gockerman J, et al. Bone-marrow transplantation in a patient with sickle-cell anemia. N Engl J Med 1984;311:780–3.
12. Babiker MA. Prophylaxis of pneumococcal infection in sickle-cell disease by the combined use of vaccination and penicillin. Ann Trop Paediatr 1986;6:179–81.
13. Charache S, Terrin ML, Moore RD, et al. Effect of hydroxyurea on the frequency of painful crises in sickle cell anemia. N Engl J Med 1995;332:1317–22.
14. Adams RJ, McKie VC, Hsu L, et al. Prevention of a first stroke by transfusions in children with sickle cell anemia and abnormal results on transcranial doppler ultrasonography. N Engl J Med 1998;339:5–11.
15. Bender MA. Sickle cell disease. GeneReviews® [Internet] 2003 Sep 15 [Updated 2017 Aug 17]. In: Adam MP, Ardinger HH, Pagon RA, et al, editors. GeneReviews®. Seattle (WA): University of Washington, Seattle; 1993-2018. Available from: https://www.ncbi.nlm.nih.gov/books/NBK1377/.
16. Platt OS, Brambilla DJ, Rosse WF, et al. Mortality in sickle cell disease. Life expectancy and risk factors for early death. N Engl J Med 1994;330:1639–44.
17. Walters MC, Patience M, Leisenring W, et al. Stable mixed hematopoietic chimerism after bone marrow transplantation for sickle cell anemia. Biol Blood Marrow Transplant 2001;7:665–73.
18. La Nasa G, Argiolu F, Giardini C, et al. Unrelated bone marrow transplantation for beta-thalassemia patients: the experience of the Italian Bone Marrow Transplant Group. Ann N Y Acad Sci 2005;1054:186–95.
19. Bhatia M, Sheth S. Hematopoietic stem cell transplantation in sickle cell disease: patient selection and special considerations. J Blood Med 2015;6:229–38.
20. Chandrakasan S, Malik P. Gene therapy for hemoglobinopathies: the state of the field and the future. Hematol Oncol Clin North Am 2014;28:199–216.
21. Finer M, Glorioso J. A brief account of viral vectors and their promise for gene therapy. Gene Ther 2017;24:1–2.
22. Hardee CL, Arévalo-Soliz LM, Hornstein BD, et al. Advances in non-viral DNA vectors for gene therapy. Genes 2017;8:65.
23. Katzourakis A, Gifford RJ, Tristem M, et al. Macroevolution of complex retroviruses. Science 2009;325:1512.
24. Karlsson S, Bodine DM, Perry L, et al. Expression of the human beta-globin gene following retroviral-mediated transfer into multipotential hematopoietic progenitors of mice. Proc Natl Acad Sci U S A 1988;85:6062–6.
25. Hardison RC. Evolution of hemoglobin and its genes. Cold Spring Harb Perspect Med 2012;2:a011627.
26. Chang JC, Liu D, Kan YWA. 36-base-pair core sequence of locus control region enhances retrovirally transferred human beta-globin gene expression. Proc Natl Acad Sci U S A 1992;89:3107–10.
27. Collis P, Antoniou M, Grosveld F. Definition of the minimal requirements within the human beta-globin gene and the dominant control region for high level expression. EMBO J 1990;9:233–40.

28. Cone RD, Weber-Benarous A, Baorto D, et al. Regulated expression of a complete human beta-globin gene encoded by a transmissible retrovirus vector. Mol Cell Biol 1987;7:887–97.
29. Dzierzak EA, Papayannopoulou T, Mulligan RC. Lineage-specific expression of a human [beta]-globin gene in murine bone marrow transplant recipients reconstituted with retrovirus-transduced stem cells. Nature 1988;331:35–41.
30. Ellis J, Tan-Un KC, Harper A, et al. A dominant chromatin-opening activity in 5' hypersensitive site 3 of the human beta-globin locus control region. EMBO J 1996;15:562–8.
31. Leboulch P, Huang GM, Humphries RK, et al. Mutagenesis of retroviral vectors transducing human beta-globin gene and beta-globin locus control region derivatives results in stable transmission of an active transcriptional structure. EMBO J 1994;13:3065–76.
32. Novak U, Harris EA, Forrester W, et al. High-level beta-globin expression after retroviral transfer of locus activation region-containing human beta-globin gene derivatives into murine erythroleukemia cells. Proc Natl Acad Sci U S A 1990; 87:3386–90.
33. Sadelain M, Wang CH, Antoniou M, et al. Generation of a high-titer retroviral vector capable of expressing high levels of the human beta-globin gene. Proc Natl Acad Sci U S A 1995;92:6728–32.
34. Goodman MA, Malik P. The potential of gene therapy approaches for the treatment of hemoglobinopathies: achievements and challenges. Ther Adv Hematol 2016;7:302–15.
35. Miyoshi H, Blomer U, Takahashi M, et al. Development of a self-inactivating lentivirus vector. J Virol 1998;72:8150–7.
36. Akinsheye I, Alsultan A, Solovieff N, et al. Fetal hemoglobin in sickle cell anemia. Blood 2011;118:19–27.
37. Pawliuk R, Westerman KA, Fabry ME, et al. Correction of sickle cell disease in transgenic mouse models by gene therapy. Science 2001;294:2368–71.
38. Levasseur DN, Ryan TM, Pawlik KM, et al. Correction of a mouse model of sickle cell disease: lentiviral/antisickling beta-globin gene transduction of unmobilized, purified hematopoietic stem cells. Blood 2003;102:4312–9.
39. Levasseur DN, Ryan TM, Reilly MP, et al. A recombinant human hemoglobin with anti-sickling properties greater than fetal hemoglobin. J Biol Chem 2004; 279:27518–24.
40. Romero Z, Urbinati F, Geiger S, et al. beta-globin gene transfer to human bone marrow for sickle cell disease. J Clin Invest 2013. https://doi.org/10.1172/jci67930.
41. Hanawa H, Hargrove PW, Kepes S, et al. Extended beta-globin locus control region elements promote consistent therapeutic expression of a gamma-globin lentiviral vector in murine beta-thalassemia. Blood 2004;104:2281.
42. Perumbeti A, Higashimoto T, Urbinati F, et al. A novel human gamma-globin gene vector for genetic correction of sickle cell anemia in a humanized sickle mouse model: critical determinants for successful correction. Blood 2009;114:1174.
43. Arumugam PI, Higashimoto T, Urbinati F, et al. Genotoxic potential of lineage-specific lentivirus vectors carrying the beta-globin locus control region. Mol Ther 2009;17:1929–37.
44. Negre O, Bartholomae C, Beuzard Y, et al. Preclinical evaluation of efficacy and safety of an improved lentiviral vector for the treatment of beta-thalassemia and sickle cell disease. Curr Gene Ther 2015;15:64–81.

45. Ribeil J-A, Hacein-Bey-Abina S, Payen E, et al. Gene therapy in a patient with sickle cell disease. N Engl J Med 2017;376:848–55.

46. Kanter J, Walters MC, Hsieh MM, et al. Interim results from a phase 1/2 clinical study of lentiglobin gene therapy for severe sickle cell disease. Blood 2016; 128:1176.

47. Malik P. Gene therapy for hemoglobinopathies: tremendous successes and remaining caveats. Mol Ther 2016;24:668–70.

48. Goodman MA, Arumugam P, Pillis DM, et al. Foamy virus vector carries a strong insulator in its long terminal repeat which reduces its genotoxic potential. Journal of Virology 2018;92(1):e01639–17.

49. Morianos I, Siapati EK, Pongas G, et al. Comparative analysis of FV vectors with human [alpha]- or [beta]-globin gene regulatory elements for the correction of [beta]-thalassemia. Gene Ther 2012;19:303–11.

50. Choo Y, Klug A. Selection of DNA binding sites for zinc fingers using rationally randomized DNA reveals coded interactions. Proc Natl Acad Sci U S A 1994; 91:11168–72.

51. Bogdanove AJ, Schornack S, Lahaye T. TAL effectors: finding plant genes for disease and defense. Curr Opin Plant Biol 2010;13:394–401.

52. Jinek M, Chylinski K, Fonfara I, et al. A programmable dual-RNA-guided DNA endonuclease in adaptive bacterial immunity. Science 2012;337:816–21. https://doi.org/10.1126/science.1225829.

53. Shrivastav M, De Haro LP, Nickoloff JA. Regulation of DNA double-strand break repair pathway choice. Cell Res 2008;18:134–47.

54. Durai S, Mani M, Kandavelou K, et al. Zinc finger nucleases: custom-designed molecular scissors for genome engineering of plant and mammalian cells. Nucleic Acids Res 2005;33:5978–90.

55. Sebastiano V, Maeder ML, Angstman JF, et al. In situ genetic correction of the sickle cell anemia mutation in human induced pluripotent stem cells using engineered zinc finger nucleases. Stem Cells 2011;29:1717–26.

56. Zou J, Mali P, Huang X, et al. Site-specific gene correction of a point mutation in human iPS cells derived from an adult patient with sickle cell disease. Blood 2011;118:4599–608.

57. Hoban MD, Cost GJ, Mendel MC, et al. Correction of the sickle cell disease mutation in human hematopoietic stem/progenitor cells. Blood 2015;125:2597–604.

58. Joung JK, Sander JD. TALENs: a widely applicable technology for targeted genome editing. Nat Rev Mol Cell Biol 2013;14:49–55.

59. Xie F, Ye L, Chang JC, et al. Seamless gene correction of β-thalassemia mutations in patient-specific iPSCs using CRISPR/Cas9 and piggyBac. Genome Res 2014; 24:1526–33.

60. Ramalingam S, Annaluru N, Kandavelou K, et al. TALEN-mediated generation and genetic correction of disease-specific human induced pluripotent stem cells. Curr Gene Ther 2014;14:461–72.

61. Voit RA, Hendel A, Pruett-Miller SM, et al. Nuclease-mediated gene editing by homologous recombination of the human globin locus. Nucleic Acids Res 2014;42: 1365–78.

62. Xu P, Tong Y, Liu XZ, et al. Both TALENs and CRISPR/Cas9 directly target the HBB IVS2-654 (C > T) mutation in beta-thalassemia-derived iPSCs. Sci Rep 2015;5: 12065.

63. Luo Y, Zhu D, Zhang Z, et al. Integrative analysis of CRISPR/Cas9 target sites in the human HBB gene. Biomed Res Int 2015;2015:514709.

64. Liang P, Xu Y, Zhang X, et al. CRISPR/Cas9-mediated gene editing in human tri-pronuclear zygotes. Protein Cell 2015;6:363–72.
65. Cradick TJ, Fine EJ, Antico CJ, et al. CRISPR/Cas9 systems targeting β-globin and CCR5 genes have substantial off-target activity. Nucleic Acids Res 2013; 41:9584–92.
66. Dever DP, Bak RO, Reinisch A, et al. CRISPR/Cas9 β-globin gene targeting in human haematopoietic stem cells. Nature 2016;539:384–9.
67. DeWitt MA, Magis W, Bray NL, et al. Selection-free genome editing of the sickle mutation in human adult hematopoietic stem/progenitor cells. Sci Transl Med 2016;8:360ra134.
68. Bauer DE, Orkin SH. Update on fetal hemoglobin gene regulation in hemoglobin-opathies. Curr Opin Pediatr 2011;23:1–8.
69. Sankaran VG, Menne TF, Xu J, et al. Human fetal hemoglobin expression is regu-lated by the developmental stage-specific repressor BCL11A. Science 2008; 322:1839.
70. Xu J, Peng C, Sankaran VG, et al. Correction of sickle cell disease in adult mice by interference with fetal hemoglobin silencing. Science 2011;334:993.
71. Brendel C, Guda S, Renella R, et al. Lineage-specific BCL11A knockdown cir-cumvents toxicities and reverses sickle phenotype. J Clin Invest 2016;126: 3868–78.
72. Chang KH, Smith SE, Sullivan T, et al. Long-term engraftment and fetal globin in-duction upon BCL11A gene editing in bone-marrow-derived CD34(+) hemato-poietic stem and progenitor cells. Mol Ther Methods Clin Dev 2017;4:137–48.
73. Guda S, Brendel C, Renella R, et al. miRNA-embedded shRNAs for lineage-specific BCL11A knockdown and hemoglobin F induction. Mol Ther 2015;23: 1465–74.
74. Wilber A, Tschulena U, Hargrove PW, et al. A zinc-finger transcriptional activator designed to interact with the gamma-globin gene promoters enhances fetal he-moglobin production in primary human adult erythroblasts. Blood 2010;115: 3033–41.
75. Deng W, Rupon JW, Krivega I, et al. Reactivation of developmentally silenced globin genes by forced chromatin looping. Cell 2014;158:849–60.
76. Traxler EA, Yao Y, Wang YD, et al. A genome-editing strategy to treat [beta]-hemoglobinopathies that recapitulates a mutation associated with a benign ge-netic condition. Nat Med 2016;22:987–90.
77. Ye L, Wang J, Tan Y, et al. Genome editing using CRISPR-Cas9 to create the HPFH genotype in HSPCs: an approach for treating sickle cell disease and β-thalassemia. Proc Natl Acad Sci U S A 2016;113:10661–5.
78. Hoban MD, Lumaquin D, Kuo CY, et al. CRISPR/Cas9-Mediated correction of the sickle mutation in human CD34+ cells. Mol Ther 2016;24(9):1561–9.
79. Jayavaradhan R, Pillis D, Malik P. A versatile tool for the quantification of CRISPR/Cas9-induced genome editing events in human hematopoietic cell lines and hematopoietic stem/progenitor cells. J Mol Biol 2018. [Epub ahead of print].
80. Gundry MC, Brunetti L, Lin A, et al. Highly efficient genome editing of murine and human hematopoietic progenitor cells by CRISPR/Cas9. Cell reports 2016;17(5): 1453–61.

The Epidemiology and Management of Lung Diseases in Sickle Cell Disease

Lessons Learned from Acute and Chronic Lung Disease in Cystic Fibrosis

Shaina M. Willen, MD, Michael R. DeBaun, MD, MPH*

KEYWORDS

• Sickle cell disease • Cystic fibrosis • Lung disease

KEY POINTS

• Both sickle cell disease and cystic fibrosis are common monogenic disorders with significant improvements seen in survival across the lifespan but with vast differences in collaboration and funding efforts.

• There is much to be learned by the sickle cell community from the advances made in cystic fibrosis.

INTRODUCTION

Sickle cell disease (SCD) and cystic fibrosis (CF) are two of the most common monogenic diseases presenting in childhood worldwide. SCD affects approximately 100,000 individuals in the United States and is more common in individuals of African-American descent, occurring in 1 out of every 365 black births.[1] Worldwide, estimates suggest 300,000 babies with SCD are born every year.[2] Approximately 30,000 individuals are living with CF in the United States, and 70,000 worldwide. CF is most common in individuals of European ancestry, occurring in 1 out of every 3200 white births in the United States.[3] Significant advances in medical management of CF and SCD over the past two decades have transformed what were once a near fatal childhood diseases into chronic conditions with survival into the fifth or sixth decade of life.[4,5] This success creates new challenges, as more is learned about

The authors have no disclosures.
Department of Pediatrics, Division of Hematology/Oncology, Vanderbilt-Meharry Center for Excellence in Sickle Cell Disease, Vanderbilt University Medical Center, Nashville, TN, USA
* Corresponding author. Vanderbilt-Meharry Center of Excellence in Sickle Cell Disease, Vanderbilt University School of Medicine, 2200 Children's Way, 11206 DOT, Nashville, TN 37232-9000.
E-mail address: m.debaun@vanderbilt.edu

Pediatr Clin N Am 65 (2018) 481–493
https://doi.org/10.1016/j.pcl.2018.01.007
0031-3955/18/© 2018 Elsevier Inc. All rights reserved.

how both diseases develop across the lifespan, with disease-specific manifestations that change with age.

Despite these commonalities, CF and SCD enjoy vastly different funding and collaborative research efforts.[6] Currently the CF registry has more than 20,000 registrants providing key information regarding the clinical history and comparativeness of various interventions. A similar registry has not been established for SCD, limiting the broader understanding changing disease phenotype as affected individuals age. Additionally, disease-specific funding for CF as compared with SCD from the National Institutes of Health and national foundations is approximately 3.5-fold and 440-fold higher, respectively.[6] In 2011, funding per affected individual was 11.4-fold greater for CF than SCD, and there were nearly twice as many publications in the field of CF when compared with SCD.[6] Clearly, there are likely opportunities for the SCD research community to learn from the work being done in CF.

Both SCD and CF are multisystem diseases and require multidisciplinary care. However, CF has primarily been considered a disease of the lungs, with inflammation, recurrent infections, and lung pathology known to be present as early as the first few months of life.[4] Defining, monitoring, and treating lung disease is considered central to the clinical management of CF, but in SCD pulmonary complications have been considered one of many separate morbidities. To the extent that the lung in SCD has been studied, attention has mainly focused on acute life-threatening complications, such as acute chest syndrome (ACS). The following review compares and contrasts significant knowledge about acute and chronic lung disease and optimal management in CF with the dearth of knowledge regarding acute and chronic lung disease in SCD.

ACUTE LUNG DISEASE EXACERBATIONS ARE COMMON IN BOTH SICKLE CELL DISEASE AND CYSTIC FIBROSIS

Periodic flares of lung disease in CF and SCD are associated with significant morbidity and mortality. The accepted definition of these flares is not universally accepted in either disease, making understanding of the triggers, mechanism, and pathophysiologic consequences challenging.

"Pulmonary exacerbation" describes periodic episodes of acute worsening of pulmonary status, commonly seen in CF. More than a third of individuals with CF experience at least one pulmonary exacerbation requiring intravenous antibiotics per year.[7] A universally accepted definition of what constitutes an exacerbation is not currently in use. However, symptoms include decreased exercise tolerance, increased cough, increased sputum production, abnormal respiratory examination, decreased appetite, and school or work absenteeism.[8] Severe pulmonary exacerbations have well-established long-term effects including a decline in lung function[9] and decreased 5-year survivorship.[10] A retrospective cohort study of 851 individuals with CF demonstrated that half of the decline seen in forced expiratory volume in 1 second (FEV_1) was associated with pulmonary exacerbations, and for a given number of exacerbations, the annual rate of FEV_1 decline was greatest in individuals with less than 6 months between exacerbations.[11] These associations motivated the development of clear guidelines for recommended management and targeted therapy for pulmonary exacerbations in CF.[7]

An acute flare in respiratory disease in individual with SCD is termed ACS. ACS is also a common complication with a reported rate of 12.8 hospitalizations per 100-patient years.[12] As in CF, there is no universally accepted definition of ACS. Common criteria used for research include a new infiltrate seen on chest radiograph and one of the following symptoms: cough, chest pain, fever, tachypnea, abnormal respiratory examination, or decrease in oxygen saturation.[13] This definition of ACS is so broad that other common ailments, such as community-acquired pneumonia, bronchiolitis, and acute asthma exacerbations, would all be termed an episode of ACS.[13] ACS is the most common cause of death in individuals with SCD,[14] with a reported death rate of 1.8% in children and 4.3% in adults.[13] As in CF, recurrent episodes of ACS seem to impact lung function parameters in adults with SCD.[15] However, because routine pulmonary function testing is not a part of standard of care in SCD, the connection is less clear, particularly in children.[16] The unclear pathophysiology, definition, and long-term consequences of ACS have prevented the development of specific therapies to treat or prevent ACS events.

ASTHMA IS A COMMON COMORBID DISEASE FOR CHILDREN WITH CYSTIC FIBROSIS AND SICKLE CELL DISEASE

Asthma has proven to be a common comorbidity in CF and SCD. Similar to what has been observed in acute flares of lung disease, there have been inherent challenges in accurately and uniformly defining asthma in CF and SCD.

Asthma is a common chronic illness in the general population, affecting more than 6 million children and 18.4 million adults in the United States.[17] Pulmonologists have recognized that many children and adults with CF also carry a diagnosis of asthma, which confers an increased odds of pulmonary exacerbations requiring antibiotics.[18] The concomitant diagnosis of asthma and CF poses many treatment and diagnostic challenges because individuals with CF and asthma may be using medications with good evidence for their use in asthma but of uncertain benefit in the CF population and vice versa.[19]

Asthma is a clear comorbidity in children and adults with SCD. The prevalence of asthma is highest among children in low-income families (13.5%) and non-Hispanic black children (17.0%),[20] and studies have suggested that asthma may be more common in children with SCD compared with those without SCD.[21,22] Those with a diagnosis of both SCD and asthma have demonstrated higher rates of pain and ACS episodes[21,23,24] and earlier mortality.[25,26]

The definition of asthma in individuals with CF and SCD poses a challenge. For the general population, an expert panel assembled by the National Heart, Lung, and Blood Institute defined asthma as "a chronic inflammatory disorder of the airways in which many cells and cellular elements play a role, in particular, mast cells, eosinophils, T lymphocytes, macrophages, neutrophils, and epithelial cells. In susceptible individuals, this inflammation causes recurrent episodes of wheezing, breathlessness, chest tightness, and coughing, particularly at night or in the early morning. These episodes are usually associated with widespread but variable airflow obstruction that is often reversible either spontaneously or with treatment."[27] Part of the inherent challenge is that these characteristics of asthma are common in SCD and CF and can occur without other features consistent with a diagnosis of asthma.

Despite the challenging clinical diagnosis of asthma in individuals with CF, multiple studies have demonstrated the benefit of asthma therapies in the CF population. Several randomized controlled trials have been performed to examine the impact of inhaled bronchodilators,[28,29] montelukast,[30] inhaled glucocorticoids,[31–33] and systemic glucocorticoids[34,35] on individuals with CF without a focus on distinguishing those with a concomitant asthma diagnosis or not.

The definition of asthma in SCD often relies on whether asthma medication has been prescribed. In a multicenter, prospective cohort study, Strunk and colleagues[23] defined asthma as a physician diagnosis plus prescription of an asthma medication (albuterol, inhaled corticosteroid, or both). Having a parent with asthma and wheezing further strengthened this definition and had a clear association with future ACS episodes. A retrospective study in France demonstrating asthma is associated with increased rates of ACS episodes defined asthma as three or more episodes of bronchiolitis younger than 2 years of age or wheezing heard at clinic visit or hospitalization.[36] An analysis from the Cooperative Study for Sickle Cell Disease defined asthma as a physician diagnosis recorded in the medical history or use of prescribed asthma medications, such as short-acting β-agonists, inhaled corticosteroids, or both.[24] A study performed in Jamaica defined asthma based on parental completion of a modified International Study of Asthma and Allergies in Childhood questionnaire.[21] These various definitions of asthma raise the possibility that the associations identified in these studies may reflect nonoverlapping subsets of SCD-associated asthma. A more formal uniform definition of asthma must be applied to improve clinical care and define future clinical trials for this subgroup of children with both morbidities.

Unfortunately, no SCD-specific asthma randomized controlled trial has been undertaken. Little is known about the benefit of acute asthma therapy in children or adults with SCD. In the absence of evidence specific to managing asthma in individuals with SCD, with few exceptions, we recommend managing asthma in those with SCD as we would manage asthma in those without SCD according to the National Heart, Lung, and Blood Institute guidelines.[22] However, unlike CF, in which treating this population with standard asthma algorithms has proven beneficial, treatment of acute asthma exacerbations in SCD with oral steroids, the standard therapy for acute asthma exacerbation, is associated with an increased risk for adverse events. In individuals with SCD, oral corticosteroids given for an acute asthma exacerbation may result in acute vaso-occlusive pain temporally associated with the steroids. This treated group is also at increased risk for 30-day readmission.[37,38] A similar risk has not been observed with inhaled corticosteroids. In fact, a single-center trial in participants without asthma with SCD receiving daily inhaled mometasone furoate for 16 weeks demonstrated a significant decrease in daily pain scores over time.[39] Further studies are needed to understand the pathophysiology and ideal interventions for asthma-related complications for children and adults with SCD.

CYSTIC FIBROSIS AND SICKLE CELL DISEASE DIFFER IN THE ROUTINE ASSESSMENT OF PULMONARY DISEASE

Clear parameters exist for the timing and technique for surveillance of lung disease and function in CF. However, the most recent guidelines in SCD recommendation against serial monitoring of lung function,[27] which is in need of further exploration.

Spirometry has been deemed the most important tool to assess lung function in CF, assisting clinicians in monitoring disease status and response to inpatient and outpatient treatments. Both the European Cystic Fibrosis Society and the Cystic Fibrosis Foundation recommend yearly spirometry measurements starting at 3 years of age, even in the absence of significant symptom development.[40,41] FEV_1 is typically monitored as the main indicator of disease progression[42] and risk for exacerbation.[43] FEV_1 has even been used as a surrogate marker for defining a clinically significant pulmonary exacerbation[44] and to assist in decision to pursue lung transplantation.[45] Decreased $FEV_1\%$ predicted has been associated with an increased risk for earlier death in individuals with CF.[46,47]

Unlike CF where pulmonary function surveillance is considered standard care with several assessments per year, pulmonary function surveillance is not yet considered routine in SCD.[48] However, we believe that these recommendations are out of date, and do not reflect the current body of literature demonstrating that approximately one in four children with SCD will have a diagnosis of asthma.[21] Furthermore, as is the case in CF and the older general population, spirometry can be used to identify a group at high risk for earlier death. In a prospective cohort study, young adults with SCD with a decreased FEV_1% predicted had a higher rate of death over the course of 5 years.[49] Routine pulmonary imaging is also not recommended in standard SCD clinical care[48] and few studies have examined the clinical utility of serial lung imaging. Two small studies in adults with SCD have shown that computed tomography scan findings correlate to pulmonary function changes. In a single-center, prospective study of 35 adults with SCD, 30 were noted to have abnormalities on high-resolution computed tomography scan. Lobar volume loss and central vessel prominence were negatively associated with FEV_1 and FVC.[50] In a follow-up study of 20 of the participants, pulmonary vasculature deteriorated over time in correlation with a decrease in lung function parameters.[51] Overall, further studies are needed in SCD to understand the utility of screening with regular spirometry or routine imaging and to assess the longitudinal change in these measurements over time to improve outcomes in sickle cell lung disease.

BOTH CYSTIC FIBROSIS AND SICKLE CELL DISEASE ARE ASSOCIATED WITH INCREASED SUSCEPTIBILITY TO SELECT INFECTIONS

Individuals with CF and with SCD are at increased risk for the development of pathogenic infections. However, the mechanisms for predispositions are completely different. Individuals with CF are known to have infections localized to the lung, frequently with chronic colonization of these pathogens because of increased inflammation and decreased mucociliary clearance. Individuals with SCD are at increased risk for systemic infections because of functional hyposplenism secondary to splenic infarction. Infections in SCD are episodic in nature and not associated with chronic colonization. However, pulmonary infection is a known trigger for an ACS episode.

Symptomatic lung disease in CF is typically correlated with the recognition of bacterial infection in the lung, such as *Staphylococcus aureus*, nontypeable *Haemophilus influenzae*, and *Pseudomonas aeruginosa*.[52] Viral infections are also commonly identified in the airways, and have been implicated in pulmonary exacerbations.[53] Of the organisms commonly causing infection in individuals with CF, only *S aureus* is generally pathogenic in immunocompetent individuals. *P aeruginosa*, *Burkhholderia cepacia*, nontypeable *H influenzae*, *Stenotrophomonas maltophilia*, and *Achromobacter xylosoxidans* are all considered opportunistic pathogens. Aspergillus and nontuberculous mycobacteria are other organisms seen in CF that are generally nonpathogenic in the healthy host.[54] Collectively, the predisposition to infections that are rare in an immunocompetent host suggests an alteration in the immune response of individuals with CF. The prevalence of chronic bacterial infections in children and adults with CF has led to improved use of antibiotics in this population and is thought to have contributed to an increase in survival over the years.[55]

Regardless of the microbiologic profile in children with CF, oral azithromycin prophylaxis is recommended as standard care for children older than 6 years of age with clinical evidence of chronic inflammation, such as cough or reduced FEV_1.[56] Although the exact mechanism of action is unclear, its clinical effectiveness has been well-established. Azithromycin is thought to have antibacterial and immunomodulatory effects against the marked neutrophilic inflammation characteristic of CF[57] and may change the microbiome flora of the airway and gut, altering immune response and colonization in a favorable fashion.

Individuals with SCD also have a propensity for airway-specific pathogens. In the largest study done to date to examine the causes of ACS in SCD, a specific cause was only identified in 38% of all episodes.[14] When bronchoscopic or sputum samples were obtained, frequently the samples were uninterpretable because of a large quantity of inflammatory cells making it impossible to identify pulmonary macrophages. When a pathogen was identified, *Chlamydia pneumoniae* was the most frequent, followed by *Mycoplasma pneumoniae* and respiratory syncytial virus. Treatment of ACS episodes includes the use of a third-generation cephalosporin plus a macrolide to cover the most common pathogens. These pathogens are found at an increased rate in individuals with SCD when compared with the general population.[58] However, similar to CF, select bacterial airway pathogens have a more severe course in SCD than in the general population, specifically *M pneumoniae* and *C pneumoniae*.[59–61] Population studies have not been done to identify the incidence or prevalence of these two organisms in children with SCD; however, published case series, before the routine use of a macrolide for ACS treatment, demonstrated a more virulent than expected clinical course when compared with the general pediatric population.[62]

Unlike CF, in SCD, no studies have investigated the effect of a chronic anti-inflammatory regimen, such as oral azithromycin, for individuals with SCD. This antibiotic has been shown to have anti-inflammatory and immunomodulatory effects in the lungs and inhibition of neutrophil activation suggesting a clinical benefit in SCD, similar to what has been observed in CF.[63] Additional studies with the use of azithromycin or other anti-inflammatory agents are also needed to understand the potential pulmonary benefit in SCD.

NUTRITIONAL DEFICIENCIES ARE COMMON IN CYSTIC FIBROSIS AND SICKLE CELL DISEASE

Growth failure and malnutrition is a common problem in CF and SCD. For both diseases, this is caused by an energy imbalance from an increase in metabolic demand and reduced protein-calorie intake. Individuals with CF also have malabsorption secondary to pancreatic insufficiency and are at increased risk for micronutrient deficiencies. Malnutrition also has a clear connection to decreased lung function in CF,[64] but this area has not been fully explored in SCD. The Cystic Fibrosis Foundation has established clear guidelines for monitoring nutritional status and interventions to prevent progression and its sequelae.[40] The evidence is not as well-established in guiding nutritional care for individuals with SCD.

Malnutrition has been identified as a critical feature in children with SCD for more than 30 years.[65,66] Similar to what has been observed in CF, malnutrition is caused by elevated protein turnover and an increase in resting energy expenditure[67,68] in conjunction with decreased intake because of frequent acute disease flares.[69] Also in parallel to studies in CF, SCD complications seem to be related to growth and nutritional status. In a study of 1618 children and adults with SCD in Tanzania, body mass index and weight for age z score was associated with hospitalizations (hazard ratio, 0.90; $P = .04$; and hazard ratio, 0.88; $P = .02$).[70] Both lung function[71] and cognitive function[72] have been suggested to have a relationship to somatic growth in children with SCD. However, no uniform strategy in high- and low-resource settings has been undertaken to monitor, prevent, and treat acute malnutrition in children with SCD.

Similar to children with CF, children with SCD have a significant risk for micronutrient deficiencies, such as folic acid, vitamin D, zinc, and iron. In high-income countries, folic acid deficiency is far less common now than in the prior era because of folic acid supplementation.[73] A recent Cochrane review of the evidence for folic acid supplementation in SCD stated an unclear impact of folic acid supplementation on clinical outcomes in SCD.[74] Based on the conclusions from this Cochrane review and folic acid fortification of US food, we do not emphasize daily folic acid administration. However, in settings where folic acid fortification is not routine, potential benefit may still exist for prophylactic treatment.

Vitamin D deficiency has also been reported in SCD and has been suggested to relate to osteopenia and chronic pain.[59–61] Small studies have suggested a benefit in supplementing vitamin D and calcium to adults with SCD to improve bone mineral density.[62] The challenge of keeping the vitamin D levels higher than nondeficient threshold levels is challenging; hence, we have resulted in simply providing 2000 IU daily of vitamin D to all children with SCD.

Zinc deficiency has also been consistently reported in children with SCD. The cause of zinc deficiency is most likely multifactorial, depending on adequate nutritional intake, along with increased hemolysis causing an increase in plasma zinc that cannot be reabsorbed by the renal tubules.[75,76] Pooled analysis demonstrated mixed evidence regarding the benefit of zinc supplementation in individuals with SCD. Although supplementation seems to increase serum zinc levels, no improvement is seen in hemoglobin or height and weight parameters. However, zinc supplementation does seem to lead to a decrease in hospitalizations for infection and vaso-occlusive pain episodes.[77] Further prospective high-quality studies are needed to understand the impact of nutritional interventions on lung function and acute and chronic complications of SCD, ultimately leading to formal guidelines to improve nutritional interventions and monitoring in this population.

DISEASE-SPECIFIC THERAPY HAS MADE SIGNIFICANT ADVANCEMENT IN CYSTIC FIBROSIS BUT NOT SICKLE CELL DISEASE

The primary treatment for CF and SCD has generally focused on supportive care. However, new disease-specific therapies are rapidly being researched and approved for CF without the same rapid development seen in SCD. From 2010 to 2013, five new drugs have received Food and Drug Administration (FDA) approval for CF, which is not the case for SCD.[6] Supportive care for CF has been focused on optimizing nutrition, airway clearance, reducing inflammation, and treating airway infections. Disease-specific supportive therapies are currently in use including inhalations with hypertonic saline or recombinant human deoxyribonuclease (dornase alfa) to improve mucociliary clearance. However, with the discovery of the CFTR gene, therapies are now focusing on either reversing the consequences of the gene defect on protein function[78] or on replacing the abnormal gene itself.[79]

Treatment of SCD is largely supportive and focuses on routine screening, prevention, and treatment of complications. In contrast to CF, only one new FDA-approved medication has been introduced since hydroxyurea was approved in 1998. Hydroxyurea is used to reduce SCD-related complications in adults,[80] children,[81] and infants[82] with SCD; improve quality of life[83]; and is also thought to improve survival.[84] Use is uniformly recommended for all infants 9 months of age or older with HgbSS or HgbSβ[0] genotypes, regardless of disease-severity.[27] The use of hydroxyurea in other genotypes, such as HgbSC or HgbSβ[+], is individualized based on disease severity. Data are more limited in this context, because no randomized controlled trials have taken place.[85] For decades, hydroxyurea was the only FDA-approved therapy for SCD. In July 2017, Endari (L-glutamine) was approved for the reduction of acute complications in individuals with SCD greater than 4 years of age. In a small study of 27 children and adolescents, oral glutamine was shown to decrease resting energy expenditure and improve nutritional parameters.[86] Regular blood transfusion therapy is another disease-modifying therapy to limit disease-related morbidity in prevention of primary and secondary stroke,[87] silent cerebral infarcts,[88] and other recurrent disease-related complications refractory to hydroxyurea. Current standards of care are reviewed elsewhere in this issue (See Emily Riehm Meier's article, "Treatment Options for Sickle Cell Disease," in this issue). However, regular blood transfusion therapy is associated with difficulties related to venous access, alloimmunization, chronic iron overload, and family/patient burden, urging researchers in the field to develop better therapeutic options. Preclinical data and clinical trials have offered some promise in other therapies, such as antipolymerizing agents (eg, GBT440),[89] hypomethylating agents,[90] and inhibitors of selectin binding (eg, crizanlizumab).[91] A review of the SCD pipeline is found elsewhere in this issue (See Ahmar U. Zaidi and Matthew M. Heeney's article, "A Scientific Renaissance: Novel Drugs in Sickle Cell Disease (SCD)," in this issue) and gene therapy for SCD is reviewed elsewhere in this issue (See Rajeswari Jayavaradhan and Punam Malik's article, "Genetic Therapies for Sickle Cell Disease," in this issue). Overall, targeted therapeutic options remain limited for individuals with SCD.

DEVELOPMENTS IN CYSTIC FIBROSIS CAN PAVE THE WAY FOR COLLABORATIVE RESEARCH, GUIDELINE-FOCUSED MONITORING, AND TARGETED THERAPY DEVELOPMENT IN SICKLE CELL DISEASE

The CF community, with the start of the Cystic Fibrosis Foundation, patient registry, and evidence-based guidelines for assessment of standards of care tied to funding, has changed the landscape for children and adults with CF. The focus on understanding, monitoring, and treating lung disease, even before the development of disease-specific treatment, provided a foundation for standardizing patient care supportive measures, including routine surveillance spirometry and optimizing nutritional support.

With clear evidence that lung disease is a major cause of morbidity and mortality in children and adults with SCD, and lessons learned from the CF community, we are at a point where pulmonologists can significantly contribute to the care of individuals with SCD. Given the high prevalence of asthma and recurrent wheezing in children with SCD, asthma-specific therapy for SCD and anti-inflammatory therapies are a reasonable next step. A more central focus on nutritional monitoring and intervention may improve secondary complications of the disease, as has been demonstrated in CF. The use of routine pulmonary function testing, such as spirometry or novel pulmonary imaging studies, can assist in understanding the longitudinal course of sickle cell lung disease from pediatrics to adulthood. Finally, collaborative efforts between hematologist and pulmonologists are needed to better define, categorize, and treat lung disease in individuals with SCD.

REFERENCES

1. Hassell KL. Population estimates of sickle cell disease in the U.S. Am J Prev Med 2010;38:S512–21.
2. Diallo D, Tchernia G. Sickle cell disease in Africa. Curr Opin Hematol 2002;9: 111–6.
3. Hamosh A, FitzSimmons SC, Macek M, et al. Comparison of the clinical manifestations of cystic fibrosis in black and white patients. J Pediatr 1998;132:255–9.
4. Elborn JS. Cystic fibrosis. Lancet 2016;388:2519–31.

5. Chaturvedi S, DeBaun MR. Evolution of sickle cell disease from a life-threatening disease of children to a chronic disease of adults: the last 40 years. Am J Hematol 2016;91:5–14.
6. Strouse JJ, Lobner K, Lanzkron S, et al. NIH and national foundation expenditures for sickle cell disease and cystic fibrosis are associated with pubmed publications and FDA approvals. Blood 2013.
7. Flume PA, Mogayzel PJ, Robinson KA, et al. Cystic fibrosis pulmonary guidelines: treatment of pulmonary exacerbations. Am J Respir Crit Care Med 2009;180: 802–8.
8. Rosenfeld M, Emerson J, Williams-Warren J, et al. Defining a pulmonary exacerbation in cystic fibrosis. J Pediatr 2001;139:359–65.
9. Sanders DB, Bittner RCL, Rosenfeld M, et al. Failure to recover to baseline pulmonary function after cystic fibrosis pulmonary exacerbation. Am J Respir Crit Care Med 2010;182:627–32.
10. Liou TG, Adler FR, Fitzsimmons SC, et al. Predictive 5-year survivorship model of cystic fibrosis. Am J Epidemiol 2001;153:345–52.
11. Waters V, Stanojevic S, Atenafu EG, et al. Effect of pulmonary exacerbations on long-term lung function decline in cystic fibrosis. Eur Respir J 2012;40:61–6.
12. Castro O, Brambilla DJ, Thorington B, et al. The acute chest syndrome in sickle cell disease: incidence and risk factors. The cooperative study of sickle cell disease. Blood 1994;84:643–9.
13. Vichinsky EP, Styles LA, Colangelo LH, et al. Acute chest syndrome in sickle cell disease: clinical presentation and course. Blood 1997;89:1787–92.
14. Vichinsky E, Neumayr L, Earles A. Causes and outcomes of acute chest syndrome in sickle cell disease. N Engl J Med 2000;342:1855–66.
15. Knight-Madden JM, Forrester TS, Lewis NA, et al. The impact of recurrent acute chest syndrome on the lung function of young adults with sickle cell disease. Lung 2010;188:499–504.
16. Cohen R, Strunk RC, Rodeghier M, et al. Pattern of lung function is not associated with prior or future morbidity in children with sickle cell anemia. Ann Am Thorac Soc 2016;13:1314–23.
17. National Center for Health Statistics. Age adjusted percentages of ever having asthma for children under age 18 years, by selected characteristics: United States, 2015. Summ Heal Stat Natl Heal Interview Surv 2015. Available at: https://ftp.cdc.gov/pub/Health_Statistics/NCHS/NHIS/SHS/2015_SHS_Table_C-1.pdf. Accessed August 30, 2017.
18. Rabin HR, Butler SM, Wohl MEB, et al. Pulmonary exacerbations in cystic fibrosis. Pediatr Pulmonol 2004;37:400–6.
19. Balfour-Lynn IM, Elborn JS. "CF asthma": what is it and what do we do about it? Thorax 2002;57:742–8.
20. Centers for Disease Control and Prevention (CDC). Vital signs: asthma prevalence, disease characteristics, and self-management education: United States, 2001–2009. MMWR Morb Mortal Wkly Rep 2011;60:547–52.
21. Knight-Madden JM, Forrester TS, Lewis NA, et al. Asthma in children with sickle cell disease and its association with acute chest syndrome. Thorax 2005;60: 206–10.
22. Morris CR. Asthma management: reinventing the wheel in sickle cell disease. Am J Hematol 2009;84:234–41.
23. Strunk RC, Cohen RT, Cooper BP, et al. Wheezing symptoms and parental asthma are associated with a physician diagnosis of asthma in children with sickle cell anemia. J Pediatr 2014;164:821–6.e1.

24. Boyd JH, Macklin EA, Strunk RC, et al. Asthma is associated with acute chest syndrome and pain in children with sickle cell anemia. Blood 2006;108: 2923–7.

25. Knight-Madden JM, Barton-Gooden A, Weaver SR, et al. Mortality, asthma, smoking and acute chest syndrome in young adults with sickle cell disease. Lung 2013;191:95–100.

26. Boyd JH, Macklin EA, Strunk RC, et al. Asthma is associated with increased mortality in individuals with sickle cell anemia. Haematologica 2007;92:1115–8.

27. National Asthma Education and Prevention Program. Expert Panel Report 3 (EPR-3): Guidelines for the Diagnosis and Management of Asthma-Summary Report. J Allergy Clin Immunol 2007;120(5 Suppl):S94–138.

28. Eggleston PA, Rosenstein BJ, Stackhouse CM, et al. A controlled trial of long-term bronchodilator therapy in cystic fibrosis. Chest 1991;99:1088–92.

29. Salvatore D, D'Andria M. Effects of salmeterol on arterial oxyhemoglobin saturations in patients with cystic fibrosis. Pediatr Pulmonol 2002;34:11–5.

30. Stelmach I, Korzeniewska A, Stelmach W, et al. Effects of montelukast treatment on clinical and inflammatory variables in patients with cystic fibrosis. Ann Allergy Asthma Immunol 2005;95:372–80.

31. Bisgaard H, Pedersen SS, Nielsen KG, et al. Controlled trial of inhaled budesonide in patients with cystic fibrosis and chronic bronchopulmonary *Pseudomonas aeruginosa* infection. Am J Respir Crit Care Med 1997;156:1190–6.

32. Nikolaizik WH, Schöni MH. Pilot study to assess the effect of inhaled corticosteroids on lung function in patients with cystic fibrosis. J Pediatr 1996;128:271–4.

33. Balfour-Lynn IM, Lees B, Hall P, et al. Multicenter randomized controlled trial of withdrawal of inhaled corticosteroids in cystic fibrosis. Am J Respir Crit Care Med 2006;173:1356–62.

34. Tepper RS, Eigen H, Stevens J, et al. Lower respiratory illness in infants and young children with cystic fibrosis: evaluation of treatment with intravenous hydrocortisone. Pediatr Pulmonol 1997;24:48–51.

35. Eigen H, Rosenstein BJ, FitzSimmons S, et al. A multicenter study of alternate-day prednisone therapy in patients with cystic fibrosis. Cystic Fibrosis Foundation Prednisone Trial Group. J Pediatr 1995;126:515–23.

36. Bernaudin F, Strunk RC, Kamdem A, et al. Asthma is associated with acute chest syndrome, but not with an increased rate of hospitalization for pain among children in France with sickle cell anemia: a retrospective cohort study. Haematologica 2008;93(12):1917–8.

37. Darbari DS, Castro O, Taylor JG, et al. Severe vaso-occlusive episodes associated with use of systemic corticosteroids in patients with sickle cell disease. J Natl Med Assoc 2008;100:948–51.

38. Strouse JJ, Takemoto CM, Keefer JR, et al. Corticosteroids and increased risk of readmission after acute chest syndrome in children with sickle cell disease. Pediatr Blood Cancer 2008;50:1006–12.

39. Glassberg J, Minnitti C, Cromwell C, et al. Inhaled steroids reduce pain and sVCAM levels in individuals with sickle cell disease: a triple-blind, randomized trial. Am J Hematol 2017. https://doi.org/10.1002/ajh.24742.

40. Lahiri T, Hempstead SE, Brady C, et al. Clinical practice guidelines from the cystic fibrosis foundation for preschoolers with cystic fibrosis. Pediatrics 2016; 137 [pii:e20151784].

41. Kerem E, Conway S, Elborn S, et al. Standards of care for patients with cystic fibrosis: a European consensus. J Cyst Fibros 2005;4:7–26.

42. Stanojevic S, Bilton D, McDonald A, et al. Global lung function Initiative equations improve interpretation of FEV1 decline among patients with cystic fibrosis. Eur Respir J 2015;46(1):262–4.
43. Block JK, Vandemheen KL, Tullis E, et al. Predictors of pulmonary exacerbations in patients with cystic fibrosis infected with multi-resistant bacteria. Thorax 2006; 61:969–74.
44. Fuchs HJ, Borowitz DS, Christiansen DH, et al. Effect of aerosolized recombinant human DNase on exacerbations of respiratory symptoms and on pulmonary function in patients with cystic fibrosis. N Engl J Med 1994;331:637–42.
45. Orens JB, Estenne M, Arcasoy S, et al. International guidelines for the selection of lung transplant candidates: 2006 update-a consensus report from the pulmonary scientific council of the International Society for Heart and Lung Transplantation. J Heart Lung Transplant 2006;25:745–55.
46. Kerem E, Reisman J, Corey M, et al. Prediction of mortality in patients with cystic fibrosis. N Engl J Med 1992;326:1187–91.
47. Kerem E, Viviani L, Zolin A, et al. Factors associated with FEV1 decline in cystic fibrosis: analysis of the ECFS patient registry. Eur Respir J 2013;43:125–33.
48. Melorose J, Perroy R, Careas S. Evidence-based management of sickle cell disease. Expert panel report, 2014. Bethesda (MD): US Dep Heal Humand Serv NIH; 2015. p. 1.
49. Kassim AA, Payne AB, Rodeghier M, et al. Low forced expiratory volume is associated with earlier death in sickle cell anemia. Blood 2015;126:1544–50.
50. Sylvester KP, Desai SR, Wells AU, et al. Computed tomography and pulmonary function abnormalities in sickle cell disease. Eur Respir J 2006;28:832–8.
51. Lunt A, Desai SR, Wells AU, et al. Pulmonary function, CT and echocardiographic abnormalities in sickle cell disease. Thorax 2014;3:1–6.
52. Balough K, McCubbin M, Weinberger M, et al. The relationship between infection and inflammation in the early stages of lung disease from cystic fibrosis. Pediatr Pulmonol 1995;20:63–70.
53. Wark PAB, Tooze M, Cheese L, et al. Viral infections trigger exacerbations of cystic fibrosis in adults and children. Eur Respir J 2012;40(2):510–2.
54. Gibson RL, Burns JL, Ramsey BW. Pathophysiology and management of pulmonary infections in cystic fibrosis. Am J Respir Crit Care Med 2003;168(8):918–51.
55. Goss CH, Rosenfeld M. Update on cystic fibrosis epidemiology. Curr Opin Pulm Med 2004;10:510–4.
56. Flume PA, O'Sullivan BP, Robinson KA, et al. Cystic fibrosis pulmonary guidelines: chronic medications for maintenance of lung health. Am J Respir Crit Care Med 2007;176:957–69.
57. Yousef AA, Jaffe A. The role of azithromycin in patients with cystic fibrosis. Paediatr Respir Rev 2010;11(2):108–14.
58. Bates JH, Campbell GD, Barron AL, et al. Microbial etiology of acute pneumonia in hospitalized patients. Chest 1992;101:1005–12.
59. Chapelon E, Garabedian M, Brousse V, et al. Osteopenia and vitamin D deficiency in children with sickle cell disease. Eur J Haematol 2009;83:572–8.
60. Buison AM, Kawchak DA, Schall J, et al. Low vitamin D status in children with sickle cell disease. J Pediatr 2004;145:622–7.
61. Osunkwo I, Hodgman EI, Cherry K, et al. Vitamin D deficiency and chronic pain in sickle cell disease. Br J Haematol 2011;153:538–40.
62. Adewoye AH, Chen TC, Ma Q, et al. Sickle cell bone disease: response to vitamin D and calcium. Am J Hematol 2008;83:271–4.

63. Zarogoulidis P, Papanas N, Kioumis I, et al. Macrolides: from in vitro anti-inflammatory and immunomodulatory properties to clinical practice in respiratory diseases. Eur J Clin Pharmacol 2012;68(5):479–503.
64. Solomon M, Bozic M, Mascarenhas MR. Nutritional issues in cystic fibrosis. Clin Chest Med 2016;37(1):97–107.
65. Reed JD, Redding-Lallinger R, Orringer EP. Nutrition and sickle cell disease. Am J Hematol 1987;24:441–55.
66. Prasad AS. Malnutrition in sickle cell disease patients. Am J Clin Nutr 1997;66(2): 423–4.
67. Hibbert JM, Hsu LL, Bhathena SJ, et al. Proinflammatory cytokines and the hyper-metabolism of children with sickle cell disease. Exp Biol Med (Maywood) 2005; 230:68–74.
68. Barden EM, Zemel BS, Kawchak DA, et al. Total and resting energy expenditure in children with sickle cell disease. J Pediatr 2000;136:73–9.
69. Gray NT, Bartlett JM, Kolasa KM, et al. Nutritional status and dietary intake of children with sickle cell anemia. Am J Pediatr Hematol Oncol 1992;14:57–61.
70. Cox SE, Makani J, Fulford AJ, et al. Nutritional status, hospitalization and mortality among patients with sickle cell anemia in Tanzania. Haematologica 2011;96: 948–53.
71. Catanzaro T, Koumbourlis AC. Somatic growth and lung function in sickle cell disease. Paediatr Respir Rev 2014;15:28–32.
72. Puffer ES, Schatz JC, Roberts CW. Relationships between somatic growth and cognitive functioning in young children with sickle cell disease. J Pediatr Psychol 2010;35:892–904.
73. Honein MA, Paulozzi LJ, Mathews TJ, et al. Impact of folic acid fortification of the US food supply on the occurrence of neural tube defects. JAMA 2001;285:2981.
74. Dixit R, Nettem S, Madan SS, et al. Folate supplementation in people with sickle cell disease. Cochrane Database Syst Rev 2016;(2):CD011130.
75. Prasad AS, Schoomaker EB, Ortega J, et al. Zinc deficiency in sickle cell disease. Clin Chem 1975;21:582–7.
76. Karayalcin G, Lanzkowsky P, Kazi AB. Zinc deficiency in children with sickle cell disease. Am J Pediatr Hematol Oncol 1979;1:283–4.
77. Swe KMM, Abas ABL, Bhardwaj A, et al. Zinc supplements for treating thalas-saemia and sickle cell disease. Cochrane Database Syst Rev 2013;(6):CD009415.
78. Davies JC, Wainwright CE, Canny GJ, et al. Efficacy and safety of ivacaftor in patients aged 6 to 11 years with cystic fibrosis with a G551D mutation. Am J Respir Crit Care Med 2013;187:1219–25.
79. Kuk K, Taylor-Cousar JL. Lumacaftor and ivacaftor in the management of patients with cystic fibrosis: current evidence and future prospects. Ther Adv Respir Dis 2015;9:313–26.
80. Charache S, Terrin ML, Moore RD, et al. Effect of hydroxyurea on the frequency of painful crises in sickle cell anemia. N Engl J Med 1995;332:1317–22.
81. Kinney TR, Helms RW, O'Branski EE, et al. Safety of hydroxyurea in children with sickle cell anemia: results of the HUG-KIDS study, a phase I/II trial. Blood 1999; 94:1550–4.
82. Wang WC, Ware RE, Miller ST, et al. Hydroxycarbamide in very young children with sickle-cell anaemia: a multicentre, randomised, controlled trial (BABY HUG). Lancet 2011;377:1663–72.
83. Ballas SK, Barton FB, Waclawiw MA, et al. Hydroxyurea and sickle cell anemia: effect on quality of life. Health Qual Life Outcomes 2006;4:59.

84. Lê PQ, Gulbis B, Dedeken L, et al. Survival among children and adults with sickle cell disease in Belgium: benefit from hydroxyurea treatment. Pediatr Blood Cancer 2015;62:1956–61.

85. Luchtman-Jones L, Pressel S, Hilliard L, et al. Effects of hydroxyurea treatment for patients with hemoglobin SC disease. Am J Hematol 2016;91:238–42.

86. Williams R, Olivi S, Li CS, et al. Oral glutamine supplementation decreases resting energy expenditure in children and adolescents with sickle cell anemia. J Pediatr Hematol Oncol 2004;26:619–25.

87. Estcourt LJ, Fortin PM, Hopewell S, et al. Blood transfusion for preventing primary and secondary stroke in people with sickle cell disease. Cochrane Database Syst Rev 2017;(1):CD003146.

88. Estcourt LJ, Fortin PM, Hopewell S, et al. Interventions for preventing silent cerebral infarcts in people with sickle cell disease. Cochrane Database Syst Rev 2017;(5):CD012389.

89. Oksenberg D, Dufu K, Patel MP, et al. GBT440 increases haemoglobin oxygen affinity, reduces sickling and prolongs RBC half-life in a murine model of sickle cell disease. Br J Haematol 2016;175:141–53.

90. Saunthararajah Y, Hillery CA, Lavelle D, et al. Effects of 5-aza-2'-deoxycytidine on fetal hemoglobin levels, red cell adhesion, and hematopoietic differentiation in patients with sickle cell disease. Blood 2003;102:3865–70.

91. Ataga KI, Kutlar A, Kanter J, et al. Crizanlizumab for the prevention of pain crises in sickle cell disease. N Engl J Med 2017;376:429–39.

Pulmonary Embolism in Children

Sarah Ramiz, MD, Madhvi Rajpurkar, MD*

KEYWORDS

- Children • Pediatric • Pulmonary embolism • Pulmonary artery thrombosis
- Venous thromboembolism • Deep vein thrombosis

KEY POINTS

- Compared to adults, pulmonary embolism (PE) in children is vastly different in terms of incidence, predisposition, pathophysiology, presenting symptoms, and management strategies.
- Pediatric treatment guidelines for PE are extrapolated from adult data, thus there is a critical need for clinical trials in childhood PE.
- This article reviews the incidence, presentation, diagnostic workup, management, and long-term outcome of PE in children. It also highlights recent advances in imaging technology and anticoagulation therapy.

INTRODUCTION

Venous thromboembolic (VTE) disease encompasses pulmonary embolism (PE) and deep vein thrombosis (DVT). PE is believed to be a rare event in children.[1,2] However, the incidence of PE in children has been steadily increasing, which can be attributed to numerous factors, including increased awareness and recognition, increased survival of children with underlying predisposing conditions, increased use of central venous catheters (CVCs) in infants and neonates, hormonal supplementation in female adolescents, and the availability of noninvasive diagnostic modalities.[3,4]

In comparison with the adult population, PE in children is vastly different in terms of incidence, predisposition, pathophysiology, presenting symptoms, and management strategies. However, to date, pediatric treatment guidelines for PE are extrapolated from adult data, thus there is a critical need for clinical trials in childhood PE.

This article reviews the incidence, presentation, diagnostic workup, management, and long-term outcome of PE in children. It also highlights recent advances in imaging technology and anticoagulation therapy.

The authors have no financial interest or other potential conflict of interest to disclose.
Division of Pediatric Hematology Oncology, Carman and Ann Adams Department of Pediatrics, Wayne State University School of Medicine, Children's Hospital of Michigan, 3901 Beaubien Street, Detroit, MI 48201, USA
* Corresponding author.
E-mail address: mrajpurk@med.wayne.edu

EPIDEMIOLOGY

The early incidence estimates of PE stem from autopsy studies and report an incidence of 0.05% to 4.2%.[5–8] Buck and colleagues[7] reported a higher prevalence of pediatric PE at 4.2% on autopsy reports, of which 30% were clinically relevant. In clinically relevant cases, 50% of cases presented with signs and symptoms suggestive of PE but in only 15% of cases the diagnosis of PE had been considered. These findings highlight the underdiagnosis and need for a high index of suspicion for detection of PE in children.

Subsequent registry reports have yielded variable incidence estimates. The Canadian and Dutch registries report VTE disease incidence rates of 0.07 per 10,000 to 0.14 per 10,000 children, respectively.[1,2] The National Hospital Discharge survey data from 1979 to 2001 show comparable incidence of VTE disease (DVT and/or PE) of 0.49 per 100,000 children per year and PE of 0.09 per 100,000 children per year.[9] However, VTE disease incidence is found to be dramatically higher in the Pediatric Health Information System administrative data from 2001 to 2007, which demonstrates a 70% higher VTE disease incidence of 34 to 58 cases per 10,000 hospital admissions. PE accounts for 11% of VTE disease admissions.[3]

The variability in the incidence of various registries may again reflect the limitations of diagnosing PE in an effective manner. Besides reporting the incidence, registry reports highlight important characteristics of PE in children. Because PE is often diagnosed in children with underlying serious medical disorders, the incidence is significantly lower in the community compared with hospitalized children. Studies report an incidence of 8.6 to 57 per 100,000 in hospitalized children,[1,10] whereas the incidence in all children in the community is estimated to be 0.14 to 0.9 per 100,000.[2,9]

PE shows a bimodal distribution in children; a higher incidence is reported in infants (younger than the age of 1 year) and in teenagers.[1–4,9] Neonates account for most PEs in the first year of life, as demonstrated by the Dutch study, which shows that 47% of PE cases in infancy are in the neonatal group.[2] This bimodal pattern of distribution can be attributed to increased utilization of CVCs in the neonate and infant age group, whereas pregnancy and use of hormonal contraceptive methods account for the higher incidence among female adolescents.[9] No gender predilection has been demonstrated, although in adolescents a slightly higher incidence may be seen in female patients.[1–4,9] Black children are found to have 2.38-fold higher risk compared with white children.[9]

RISK FACTORS

As previously described, registry studies show that more than 95% of children with VTE disease have at least 1 underlying clinical condition[1,2]; this is in contrast to the adult population in which up to 30% of PE is idiopathic.[11] A recent systematic review of literature on pediatric PE describes 2 distinct variants of PE in children: in situ pulmonary artery thrombosis (ISPAT) and classic thromboembolic PE. Each category differs in underlying etiologic factors, long-term management, and outcomes.[4] ISPAT usually occurs in younger children with congenital heart disease or anomalies of pulmonary arteries.

Similarly, classic thromboembolic PE is correlated with underlying risk factors. Among hospitalized children, the most important predisposing factor for PE is the presence of CVCs, which are increasingly being used in pediatric care for drug administration, parenteral nutrition, and chemotherapy.[3,9,12] On the other hand, the use of oral contraceptive pills or hormonal supplementation is considered to be the most significant risk factor for PE in community-based children.[13,14]

Other risk factors include cancer, immobility, infection, nephrotic syndrome, inflammatory conditions (eg, systemic lupus erythematosus and inflammatory bowel disease), surgery, ventriculoatrial shunts, and congenital stenosing vascular anomaly (May-Thurner anomaly or Paget-Schroetter syndrome).[3,4,9,10,12,14,15]

The association between sickle cell disease and increased VTE disease risk has been established in the adult literature[16–18]; this has not been shown to be clinically significant in children. As reported by Boechat Tde and colleagues,[19] in a cohort of 1063 children younger than 12 years of age with sickle cell disease, only 2 DVT cases are reported and both are associated with CVCs.

Acquired or congenital thrombophilia states are common among children presenting with PE, especially in adolescents and non-CVC–related PE.[10,15] Biss and colleagues[10] have demonstrated positive thrombophilia screening in 14 out of 40 patients in their case series. Comparable rates have been reported by Rajpurkar and colleagues.[15] Overall, anticardiolipin antibody, antithrombin deficiency, and heterozygous F2 G20210A mutation are the most frequently reported risk factors. Antiphospholipid antibody syndrome is present with PE in 31% of cases in a pediatric cohort in which a substantial number of patients showed a delayed onset of diagnostic antibodies.[14]

PE is associated with DVT in 30% to 60% of cases.[20] Rajpurkar and colleagues,[4] in their recent systematic review, demonstrated the prevalence of thromboembolic PE associated with upper extremity DVT in 12%, with lower extremity DVT in 34%, and with nonextremity DVT in 47% of cases.

PRESENTATION

The classic triad of PE symptoms consists of pleuritic chest pain, shortness of breath and hemoptysis, and is common to both adults and children. However, the diagnosis of PE can be missed in children, as seen in autopsy studies, or delayed, as reported by Rajpurkar and colleagues,[15] when the time to PE diagnosis is made at an average of 7 days (range 1–21 days) after the onset of symptoms.[7]

Numerous factors contribute to this delay. Symptoms of PE are nonspecific and can mimic other childhood conditions such as pneumonia, atelectasis, and thoracic tumors.[12] It is also difficult to assess symptoms such as pain in young children.[12,21,22] Additionally, PE in children can be asymptomatic in up to 16% of cases.[10] Thus, the diagnosis of PE in children requires a high index of suspicion.

In a retrospective review of 54 patients diagnosed radiologically with PE, the most frequent symptoms of PE are shortness of breath (57%) and pleuritic chest pain (32%), with 16 patients (28%) demonstrating symptoms of DVT at presentation.[10] Furthermore, unexplained persistent tachypnea can be an important indication of PE in pediatric patients of all age categories.[23] Additional signs and symptoms include cough, fever, hemoptysis, tachycardia, and hypoxemia.[1,2,9,10,12,24] Massive PE as defined by an embolus sufficient to cause obstruction of the pulmonary flow, resulting in hemodynamic instability, is considered a rare event in children and is associated with a high mortality of greater than 50%.[25,26] Presenting symptoms include hypotension, dyspnea, hypoxemia, syncope, right-sided ventricular failure, and it can occasionally present with sudden death.[2,12,25–27]

In adults, the combination of validated clinical probability scores, with Well's Simplified Score being the most commonly used, and D-dimer results provide an effective tool to safely exclude PE.[28,29] Unfortunately, it has low diagnostic utility when adapted in children.[30] A more useful method is the assessment of risk factors, as demonstrated by Lee and colleagues[31] in a retrospective review of 227 patients who underwent multidetector computed tomography (CT) and pulmonary angiography (PA) (CT-PA) for suspected PE, of whom 36 (16%) had confirmed PE. Five independent risk factors for PE were identified, including the presence of immobilization, hypercoagulable state (defined as presence of factor V Leiden, protein C or S deficiency, or antiphospholipid antibodies), a CVC, associated estrogen use, and a prior PE or DVT. Using 2 or more risk factors as the clinical threshold for obtaining a diagnostic CT scan, the sensitivity for PE detection reaches 89% (32 of 36 patients), and the specificity is 94% (180 of 191 patients).

DIAGNOSIS

Diagnostic workup can be categorized into the following groups: investigations for PE diagnosis, severity assessment, management-related, and underlying factors (**Table 1**).

Investigations for Pulmonary Embolism Diagnosis

Laboratory evaluation: D-dimer, a fibrin degradation product, has been demonstrated to be a sensitive test to screen for PE in adults.[32] It is, however, nondiscriminatory in the diagnosis of PE in children. Normal D-dimer has been reported in 15% to 40% of children diagnosed with PE.[10,15,27]

Cardiac evaluation: Electrocardiogram (ECG) changes consistent with right heart strain and atrial enlargement patterns can occur in the setting of acute PE, as a result of mechanical PA flow obstruction, subsequent elevation in pulmonary artery and right heart pressures, and right atrial and ventricular dilatation. ECG findings include sinus tachycardia, right axis deviation, right bundle branch block, and ST-T segment changes, as well as the classic S1-Q3-T3 pattern.[14,33] Hancock and colleagues[14] report the classic pattern in 12% of children within 72 hours of presentation. Notably,

Table 1	
Categories of diagnostic workup	
Investigations for diagnosis of PE	• Laboratory: D-dimer • Imaging: PA, V/Q scan, CT-PA, MRA
Investigations for severity assessment	• Clinical examinations: signs of respiratory distress, sweating etc. • POC: pulse oximetry, ABG, ECG • Laboratory: troponin, BNP • Imaging: echocardiogram
Investigations to guide management	• Laboratory: pregnancy test, CBC, CMP, PT/INR, PTT, fibrinogen, plasminogen

Investigations of underlying cause	• Laboratory: thrombophilia screening
	  ○ Congenital: protein C, protein S, ATIII, prothrombin, factor VIII, vWF, homocysteine, lipoprotein (a), factor V R506Q, prothrombin G20210A,MTHFR C677T
	  ○ Acquired: ANA, ACLA IgG or IgM, Circulating anticoagulant
	• Imaging: ultrasound of extremities

Abbreviations: ABG, arterial blood gas; ACLA, anticardiolipin antibody test; ANA, antinuclear antibody; ATIII, antithrombin III; BNP, brain natriuretic peptide; CBC, complete blood count; CMP, comprehensive metabolic panel; ECG, electrocardiogram; IgG, immunoglobulin G; IgM, immunoglobulin M; MRA, magnetic resonance arteriography; POC, point of care; PT/INR, prothrombin time/international normalized ratio; PTT, partial thromboplastin time; V/Q scan, ventilation to perfusion scan; vWF, von Willebrand factor.

a normal ECG does not rule out PE.[14,33] An echocardiogram (ECHO) can aid in the diagnosis of PE either directly via the visualization of the thrombus in the heart or central pulmonary vessels, or indirectly by evaluating right ventricular dysfunction.

Imaging evaluation: The chest radiograph is frequently normal in the setting of PE.[34] However, it can be helpful to exclude other conditions such as pneumonia or pneumothorax. Nonspecific signs seen in patients with PE include parenchymal infiltrates, atelectasis, and an ipsilateral pleural effusion. More specific signs, which are difficult to define, include the Westermark sign (hypovascularity in parts of the lung affected by the emboli), the Hampton hump (a peripheral wedge-shaped density with the peak directed to the hilum), and the Fleischner sign (a prominent central pulmonary artery).[12,20,24,34]

PA is considered the gold standard for diagnosing PE. Contrast is injected into a pulmonary artery branch after percutaneous catheterization, usually via the femoral or jugular vein. Filling defects or an abrupt ending of a vessel suggests an embolus. Although highly reliable, it is an invasive procedure and associated with risk of sedation or contrast medium reaction, arrhythmia, bleeding, infection, and death.[35] It has been replaced in both adults and children by less invasive methods.

Historically, the ventilation to perfusion (V/Q) scan has been considered the test of choice for the diagnosis of PE in adults and children.[1,36] It is safe, sensitive, reproducible, and uses relatively low radiation without the need for iodinated contrast media. However, the V/Q scan requires the cooperation of the child, which is usually attained at the age of 5 or 6 years.[12,20,24] Additionally, V/Q mismatch is not specific to PE and can also be seen in several other conditions, including congenital and acquired arterial stenosis, tuberculosis, air, fat and foreign body embolism, pneumonia, and sickle cell disease.[37] Interpretation can also be difficult in the setting of congenital heart disease, especially those with right-to-left shunts and high hematocrits.

In the adult population, the Prospective Investigation of Pulmonary Embolism Diagnosis (PIOPED) study demonstrates that high probability scans are highly specific for the diagnosis of PE (97%) but lack sensitivity because they fail to identify 59% of patients with PE.[36] Furthermore, V/Q scans are frequently nondiagnostic (28%–46% of cases), necessitating further investigation. Also, the PIOPED criteria used to interpret V/Q scans in children are extrapolated from adults, with no studies evaluating their specificity or sensitivity in children.[12,20,24]

The multidetector CT-PA is now the primary imaging modality for evaluation of PE in adults and children, due to its high sensitivity and specificity, wide availability, short imaging time, high spatial resolution, 2-dimensional (D) and 3D imaging reconstruction capabilities, and evaluation of parenchymal and mediastinal structures.[34,38–40] The main disadvantage with CT is the radiation exposure.[41] Other concerns in the pediatric population include a sedation requirement for infants and children younger than 5 years old, whereas older children can follow breathing instructions and sedation is not required. Also, a large intravenous bore cannula is necessary for rapid pump injection of iodinated contrast.[34,42]

In this modality, acute PE is defined by the presence of a sharply marginated complete or partial pulmonary arterial filling defect present on at least 2 consecutive images. Acute PE is usually located centrally within the vessel wall or has an acute margin within the vessel wall. On the other hand, chronic PE is generally eccentric and adherent to the vessel wall.[34]

The adult-based PIOPED II study shows a CT-PA sensitivity of 83%, which increases to 95% when CT venography is included. The specificity is reported to be 95%, which remains unchanged with the addition of CT venography (96%). The sensitivity, however, is found to be lower when evaluating the subsegmental branches (positive predictive value of 25%).[43] Comparable results are demonstrated by Victoria and colleagues,[39] and Kritsaneepaiboon and colleagues,[41] emphasizing the high diagnostic value of CT-PA for PE in children.

Recent advances in CT techniques aim to increase diagnostic accuracy of PE. Dual-energy CT is an innovative technique, providing both anatomic and functional information in a single contrast-enhanced CT scan.[42,44] The addition of ventilation imaging allows the demonstration of V/Q mismatch, thus increasing the accuracy of the diagnosis of PE. Studies have demonstrated the feasibility of this technique in adults but the experience in children remains limited. Other advancements include 3D reconstruction algorithms, such as model-based iterative reconstruction (MBIR) and adaptive statistical iterative reconstruction (ASIR). These reconstruction techniques provide the same anatomic detail as conventional scans at lower radiation doses.[34]

Magnetic resonance PA (MRPA) is a promising diagnostic modality when CT-PA is contraindicated, allowing evaluation of the pulmonary arteries without radiation exposure. Furthermore, the MRPA provides visualization of the upper body and central venous systems, and the pulmonary arteries, in the same investigation. When combined with magnetic resonance venography (MRV), it shows comparative sensitivity and specificity to CT-PA in adult studies but is limited by technical difficulty.[45,46]

Investigations for Assessment of Severity

Arterial blood gas measurement and saturation of peripheral oxygen (spO2) can demonstrate hypoxemia, hypocapnia, and respiratory alkalosis. In adults, markers of cardiac injury (eg, troponins) and natriuretic peptides have been incorporated in prognostic risk categorization and therapy choices.[47]

An ECHO may demonstrate signs of right ventricular dysfunction including right ventricular enlargement and hypokinesis as measured by myocardial doppler tissue imaging, and evidence of pulmonary hypertension as indicated by tricuspid regurgitation velocity.[14]

Additionally, the ECHO is particularly important in the setting of massive PE and hemodynamic instability, when more invasive diagnostic studies are not feasible and urgent intervention is warranted.

Evidence of right ventricular dysfunction detected by ECG, ECHO, or biomarkers are correlated with higher mortality.[48,49] Early mortality rates for PE range from 5% in patients who are clinically stable to 58% in patients with cardiogenic shock.[50] Accordingly, PE can be stratified into risk groups, which affects intervention and care. High-risk PE refers to symptoms consistent with cardiovascular collapse, whereas intermediate-risk PE indicates findings of myocardial injury based on ECG or ECHO, or elevated cardiac biomarkers. Low-risk PE refers to the presence of PE in the absence of these findings.[51]

Investigations to Guide Management

Baseline laboratory workup required before initiation of anticoagulation includes full blood count with a differential count, partial thromboplastin time, prothrombin time, international normalized ratio, fibrinogen level, and plasminogen. Pregnancy tests are necessary in female patients.

Investigations of Underlying Etiologic Factors

Comprehensive evaluation of underlying inherited and acquired thrombophilia states is necessary. Congenital thrombophilia testing includes the evaluation of protein C deficiency, protein S deficiency, antithrombin deficiency, factor V variants, factor II variant, factor VIII, lipoprotein(a), and homocysteine level. Acquired thrombophilia testing includes evaluation of ANA, anticardiolipin antibody and lupus anticoagulants.

Ultrasonography of all 4 extremities is required to evaluate for a possible PE source. Doppler ultrasound is also sensitive for evaluation of thrombosis in jugular veins, which is the most common site for CVC-associated thrombosis.[44] However, CT or MRV might be required for evaluation of pelvic, intraabdominal, or central upper venous system.[52]

TREATMENT

Treatment of PE in children is adapted from the adult clinical trials and small pediatric studies. However, neonates and children differ from adults in physiology, pharmacologic responses to drugs, and long-term consequences of thrombosis.[53] Thus, large pediatric clinical trials are urgently needed to provide stronger evidence-based guidelines.

Pharmacologic Treatment

Anticoagulation should be initiated with a rapid-acting agent, either unfractionated heparin (UH) or low-molecular-weight heparin (LMWH), followed by continued anticoagulation with LMWH or vitamin K antagonist (VKA). UH is the optimal choice in the presence of high bleeding risk, given its short half-life and easy reversibility. However, LMWH is now the preferred agent in children. It has several advantages, including easy subcutaneous administration, minimal laboratory monitoring, predictable anticoagulant effect, and longer half-life.[53,54] The use of VKA in children is limited by variability of dietary intake of vitamin K, difficult and frequent monitoring, unavailability of a liquid formulation, and numerous medication interactions. Additionally, it has well-established teratogenicity, imposing an added consideration for adolescent female patients.[54]

Bleeding is the main risk associated with anticoagulation. Variable risks of bleeding are reported in the literature with UH, ranging from 1.5% to 24%.[53–55] LMWH and warfarin are associated with lower risks of bleeding, estimated at 3% and 5%, respectively.[55]

There is no consensus regarding duration of therapy, with American College of Chest Physicians (CHEST) guidelines recommending anticoagulation for 3 months or until resolution of the precipitating risk factor for secondary PE, and longer anticoagulation of 6 to 12 months for idiopathic PE.[53] Currently, there is an on-going trial evaluating the optimal duration of anticoagulation for children with provoked DVT. This study, however, excludes children with PE.[56] Furthermore, there is insufficient pediatric data evaluating the use of alternative anticoagulants, such as direct thrombin inhibitors (lepirudin, argatroban, and bivalirudin) and selective Xa inhibitors (fondaparinux and idraparinux).

Few studies evaluating pharmacokinetic and pharmacodynamic effects of the oral anti-Xa inhibitor rivaroxaban in children are completed,[57,58] and there are ongoing trials evaluating rivaroxaban and other direct oral anticoagulants in children. Their use in children remains restricted to clinical trials because there is insufficient pediatric safety and dosing data. A clear exception would be in adult-size older adolescents.

Management of ISPAT differs from classic thromboembolic PE, in which most patients undergo surgical intervention, with surgical thrombectomy or stent placement as the initial intervention. Patients are subsequently kept on anticoagulation in the acute phase, then maintained on antiplatelet agents for subacute or chronic phases.[4]

Mechanical Treatment

Thrombolysis, thrombectomy, or embolectomy are indicated in the setting of massive PE and associated hemodynamic instability. In pediatric PE, thrombolysis is reported as the initial treatment in approximately one-third of children. It should be kept in mind that this could reflect a reporting bias in which patients with more dramatic presentation may have received thrombolysis and may have been reported in the literature.[4]

Catheter-directed thrombolysis (CDT) has shown similar efficacy rates compared with systemic thrombolysis with reduced bleeding risks in adults.[59,60] In a pediatric series of 6 cases, CDT achieved complete resolution of PE in 4 out of 6 instances and partial resolution in the remaining 2 cases. Ultrasound agitation is used in combination with CDT in 5 out of 6 cases. There has been no reported mortality or complications.[61]

There is a paucity of pediatric data to guide indications, route, dosing, or duration of pharmacologic thrombolysis. Among various thrombolytic agents, tissue plasminogen activator (tPA) has become the preferred agent of choice, which can be administered either systematically or locally.[53,62] One consideration regarding the use of tPA in neonates is that supplementation of plasminogen using fresh frozen plasma may be required due to physiologically decreased levels in newborns.

Surgical or transvenous catheter thrombectomy is reserved for massive PE when thrombolysis is contraindicated and there is insufficient time for anticoagulation to be effective. A review of the literature shows that surgical pulmonary embolectomy is successful in 80% of pediatric cases.[26] It is associated with high mortality and significant risks, such as vessel perforation and distal migration of embolus. Additionally, incomplete embolectomy may result in other complications, such as chronic thromboembolic pulmonary hypertension (CTEPH).[26]

PROPHYLAXIS

There are few studies to guide thromboprophylaxis in older hospitalized children (>14 years) based on their VTE disease risks, with early ambulation and adequate hydration being the preventive strategies of choice in low-risk patients. In moderate-risk to high-risk patients, mechanical and pharmacologic prophylaxis can be used but there is little evidence to inform these strategies.[63–68]

Inferior vena cava (IVC) filters are used to prevent PE. In adults, use of IVC filters has significantly increased with the availability of retrievable filters, and the expansion of indications to include PE prophylaxis.[69] On the other hand, use of IVC filters in children is rare and has remained stable over time.[70] Pediatric CHEST guidelines recommend considering the placement of a retrievable IVC filter only in children greater than 10 kg with a lower extremity DVT and a contraindication to anticoagulation.[53] Additionally, the American Heart Association recommended IVC filter use in case of recurrent DVT despite anticoagulation.[71] A retrospective multicenter study has evaluated the use of IVC filters in children, demonstrating that IVC filters are mostly used in adolescents aged 13 to 18 years, and most cases have an isolated diagnosis of DVT. Prophylaxis is the reported indication in 24% of cases, mainly in the setting of orthopedic surgery.[70] There are significant complications associated with IVC filters, including migration, thrombosis, and hemorrhage, which are directly related to longer duration of placement.[70]

OUTCOME

Overall mortality with PE is reported at about 10%,[2,10] with the cause of death usually related to underlying disease. Reported recurrence rates for PE range from 7% to

18%. It is important to identify patients at the highest risk of recurrence because these patients will benefit the most from long-term anticoagulation.

Hancock and colleagues[14] have evaluated long-term cardiac outcome with pediatric acute PE. They demonstrated that, although right ventricular strain is common in the setting of acute PE, chronic ventricular strain is rare provided aggressive treatment occurs.

CTEPH is a major long-term complication of acute PE, with considerable morbidity and mortality. Incidence is reported in a wide range of 0.4% to 8.8% in the adult literature but no pediatric estimates are available.[72]

FUTURE DIRECTION

Currently, there are few clinical trials underway evaluating the use of direct oral anticoagulants in the prevention and treatment of venous thromboembolism in children, including neonates.[73–75] Such trials are essential for formulating precise pediatric guidelines for the management of PE.

REFERENCES

1. Andrew M, David M, Adams M, et al. Venous thromboembolic complications (VTE) in children: first analyses of the Canadian Registry of VTE. Blood 1994; 83(5):1251–7.
2. Van Ommen CH, Heijboer H, Büller HR, et al. Venous thromboembolism in childhood: a prospective two-year registry in The Netherlands. J Pediatr 2001. https://doi.org/10.1067/mpd.2001.118192.
3. Raffini L, Huang Y-S, Witmer C, et al. Dramatic increase in venous thromboembolism in children's hospitals in the United States from 2001 to 2007. Pediatrics 2009;124(4):1001–8.
4. Rajpurkar M, Biss TT, Amankwah EK, et al. Pulmonary embolism and in situ pulmonary artery thrombosis in paediatrics. A systematic review. Thromb Haemost 2017;117:1199–207.
5. Jones RH, Sabiston DC. Pulmonary embolism in childhood. Monogr Surg Sci 1966;3(1):35–51. Available at: http://www.ncbi.nlm.nih.gov/pubmed/5937913. Accessed August 4, 2017.
6. Emery JL. Pulmonary embolism in children. Arch Dis Child 1962;37(196):591–5. Available at: http://www.ncbi.nlm.nih.gov/pubmed/21032397. Accessed August 4, 2017.
7. Buck JR, Connors RH, Coon WW, et al. Pulmonary embolism in children. J Pediatr Surg 1981;16(3):385–91. Available at: http://www.ncbi.nlm.nih.gov/pubmed/7252746. Accessed August 4, 2017.
8. Byard RW, Cutz E. Sudden and unexpected death in infancy and childhood due to pulmonary thromboembolism. An autopsy study. Arch Pathol Lab Med 1990; 114(2):142–4. Available at: http://www.ncbi.nlm.nih.gov/pubmed/2302030. Accessed August 4, 2017.
9. Stein PD, Kayali F, Olson RE. Incidence of venous thromboembolism in infants and children: data from the National Hospital Discharge Survey. J Pediatr 2004;145(4):563–5.
10. Biss TT, Brandão LR, Kahr WH, et al. Clinical features and outcome of pulmonary embolism in children. Br J Haematol 2008;142(5). https://doi.org/10.1111/j.1365-2141.2008.07243.x.
11. Torbicki A, Perrier A, Konstantinides S, et al. Guidelines on the diagnosis and management of acute pulmonary embolism: the task force for the diagnosis

and management of acute pulmonary embolism of the European Society of Cardiology (ESC). Eur Heart J 2008;29(18):2276–315.

12. Dijk FN, Curtin J, Lord D, et al. Pulmonary embolism in children. Paediatr Respir Rev 2012;13(2):112–22.

13. Wang CY, Ignjatovic V, Francis P, et al. Risk factors and clinical features of acute pulmonary embolism in children from the community. Thromb Res 2016;138: 86–90.

14. Hancock HS, Wang M, Gist KM, et al. Cardiac findings and long-term thromboembolic outcomes following pulmonary embolism in children: a combined retrospective-prospective inception cohort study. Cardiol Young 2013;23(3): 344–52.

15. Rajpurkar M, Warrier I, Chitlur M, et al. Pulmonary embolism-experience at a single children's hospital. Thromb Res 2007;119(6). https://doi.org/10.1016/j.thromres.2006.05.016.

16. Brunson A, Lei A, Rosenberg AS, et al. Increased incidence of VTE in sickle cell disease patients: risk factors, recurrence and impact on mortality. Br J Haematol 2017;178(2):319–26.

17. Little I, Vinogradova Y, Orton E, et al. Venous thromboembolism in adults screened for sickle cell trait: a population-based cohort study with nested case-control analysis. BMJ Open 2017;7(3):e012665.

18. Wun T, Brunson A. Sickle cell disease: an inherited thrombophilia. Hematology 2016;2016(1):640–7.

19. Boechat Tde O, do Nascimento EM, de Castro Lobo CL, et al. Deep venous thrombosis in children with sickle cell disease. Pediatr Blood Cancer 2015; 62(5):838–41.

20. Babyn PS, Gahunia HK, Massicotte P. Pulmonary thromboembolism in children. Pediatr Radiol 2005;35(3):258–74.

21. Van Ommen CH, Peters M. Acute pulmonary embolism in childhood. Thromb Res 2006;118(1):13–25.

22. Patocka C, Nemeth J. Pulmonary embolism in pediatrics. J Emerg Med 2012. https://doi.org/10.1016/j.jemermed.2011.03.006.

23. van Ommen CH, Heyboer H, Groothoff JW, et al. Persistent tachypnea in children: keep pulmonary embolism in mind. J Pediatr Hematol Oncol 1998;20(6):570–3. Available at: http://www.ncbi.nlm.nih.gov/pubmed/9856682. Accessed July 24, 2017.

24. Brandao LR, Labarque V, Diab Y, et al. Pulmonary embolism in children. Semin Thromb Hemost 2011. https://doi.org/10.1055/s-0031-1297168.

25. Baird JS, Killinger JS, Kalkbrenner KJ, et al. Massive pulmonary embolism in children. J Pediatr 2010;156(1):148–51.

26. Motti Eini Z, Houri S, Cohen I, et al. Massive pulmonary emboli in children does fiber-optic-guided embolectomy have a role? Review of the literature and report of two cases. Chest 2013;143(2):544–9.

27. Biss TT, Brandão LR, Kahr WHA, et al. Clinical probability score and D-dimer estimation lack utility in the diagnosis of childhood pulmonary embolism. J Thromb Haemost 2009;7(10):1633–8.

28. Philip S, Anderson DR, Rodger M, et al. Derivation of a simple clinical model to categorize patients probability of pulmonary embolism: increasing the models utility with the SimpliRED D-dimer. Thromb Haemost 2000;83(3):416–20. Available at: https://th.schattauer.de/en/contents/archive/issue/882/manuscript/2372/show.html. Accessed August 7, 2017.

29. Gibson NS, Sohne M, Kruip MJHA, et al. Further validation and simplification of the Wells clinical decision rule in pulmonary embolism. Thromb Haemost 2007; 99(1):229–34.
30. Hennelly KE, Baskin MN, Monuteuax MC, et al. Detection of pulmonary embolism in high-risk children. J Pediatr 2016. https://doi.org/10.1016/j.jpeds.2016.07.046.
31. Lee EY, Tse SKS, Zurakowski D, et al. Children suspected of having pulmonary embolism: multidetector CT pulmonary angiography—thromboembolic risk factors and implications for appropriate use. Radiology 2012;262(1):242–51.
32. Perrier A, Desmarais S, Miron M-J, et al. Non-invasive diagnosis of venous thromboembolism in outpatients. Lancet 1999;353(9148):190–5.
33. Chan TC, Vilke GM, Pollack M, et al. Electrocardiographic manifestations: pulmonary embolism. J Emerg Med 2001;21(3):263–70.
34. Thacker PG, Lee EY. Pulmonary embolism in children. Am J Roentgenol 2015; 204(6):1278–88.
35. Zuckerman DA, Sterling KM, Oser RF. Safety of pulmonary angiography in the 1990s. J Vasc Interv Radiol 1996;7(2):199–205. Available at: http://www.ncbi. nlm.nih.gov/pubmed/9007798. Accessed August 17, 2017.
36. PIOPED Investigators. Value of the ventilation/perfusion scan in acute pulmonary embolism. Results of the prospective investigation of pulmonary embolism diagnosis (PIOPED). JAMA 1990;263(20):2753–9. Available at: http://www.ncbi.nlm. nih.gov/pubmed/2332918. Accessed August 17, 2017.
37. Evander E, Holst H, Jarund A, et al. Role of ventilation scintigraphy in diagnosis of acute pulmonary embolism: an evaluation using artificial neural networks. Eur J Nucl Med Mol Imaging 2003;30(7):961–5.
38. Lee EY, Zurakowski D, Boiselle PM. Pulmonary embolism in pediatric patients. Acad Radiol 2010;17(12):1543–9.
39. Victoria T, Mong A, Altes T, et al. Evaluation of pulmonary embolism in a pediatric population with high clinical suspicion. Pediatr Radiol 2009;39(1):35–41.
40. Remy-Jardin M, Pistolesi M, Goodman LR, et al. Management of suspected acute pulmonary embolism in the era of CT angiography: a statement from the fleischner society. Radiology 2007;245(2):315–29.
41. Kritsaneepaiboon S, Lee EY, Zurakowski D, et al. MDCT pulmonary angiography evaluation of pulmonary embolism in children. Am J Roentgenol 2009;192(5): 1246–52.
42. Tang CX, Schoepf UJ, Chowdhury SM, et al. Multidetector computed tomography pulmonary angiography in childhood acute pulmonary embolism. Pediatr Radiol 2015;45(10):1431–9.
43. Stein PD, Fowler SE, Goodman LR, et al. Multidetector computed tomography for acute pulmonary embolism. N Engl J Med 2006;354(22):2317–27.
44. Thacker PG, Lee EY. Advances in multidetector CT diagnosis of pediatric pulmonary thromboembolism. Korean J Radiol 2016;17(2):198–208.
45. Meaney JFM, Weg JG, Chenevert TL, et al. Diagnosis of pulmonary embolism with magnetic resonance angiography. N Engl J Med 1997;336(20):1422–7.
46. Stein PD, Chenevert TL, Fowler SE, et al. Gadolinium-enhanced magnetic resonance angiography for pulmonary embolism. Ann Intern Med 2010;152(7):434.
47. Kucher N, Goldhaber SZ. Cardiac biomarkers for risk stratification of patients with acute pulmonary embolism. Circulation 2003;108(18):2191–4.
48. Sanchez O, Trinquart L, Caille V, et al. Prognostic factors for pulmonary embolism. Am J Respir Crit Care Med 2010;181(2):168–73.
49. Donadini MP, Dentali F, Castellaneta M, et al. Pulmonary embolism prognostic factors and length of hospital stay: a cohort study. Thromb Res 2017;156:155–9.

50. White RH. The epidemiology of venous thromboembolism. Circulation 2003;107: I-4–8. Available at: http://circ.ahajournals.org/content/107/23_suppl_1/I-4. Accessed August 11, 2017.
51. Jiménez D, Lobo JL, Barrios D, et al. Risk stratification of patients with acute symptomatic pulmonary embolism. Intern Emerg Med 2016;11(1):11–8.
52. Monagle P. Diagnosis and management of deep venous thrombosis and pulmonary embolism in neonates and children. Semin Thromb Hemost 2012;38(07):683–90.
53. Monagle P, Chan AKC, Goldenberg NA, et al. Antithrombotic therapy in neonates and children: antithrombotic therapy and prevention of thrombosis, 9th ed: American College of Chest physicians evidence-based clinical practice guidelines. Chest 2012;141(2 Suppl):e737S–801S.
54. Radulescu V. Anticoagulation therapy in children. Semin Thromb Hemost 2017. https://doi.org/10.1055/s-0036-1598004.
55. Kuhle S, Eulmesekian P, Kavanagh B, et al. A clinically significant incidence of bleeding in critically ill children receiving therapeutic doses of unfractionated heparin: a prospective cohort study. Haematologica 2007;92(2):244–7. Available at: http://www.ncbi.nlm.nih.gov/pubmed/17296576. Accessed August 18, 2017.
56. Goldenberg NA, Abshire T, Blatchford PJ, et al. Multicenter randomized controlled trial on duration of therapy for thrombosis in children and young adults (the Kids-DOTT trial): pilot/feasibility phase findings. J Thromb Haemost 2015; 13(9):1597–605.
57. Attard C, Monagle P, Kubitza D, et al. The in vitro anticoagulant effect of rivaroxaban in children. Thromb Res 2012;130(5):804–7.
58. Willmann S, Becker C, Burghaus R, et al. Development of a paediatric population-based model of the pharmacokinetics of rivaroxaban. Clin Pharmacokinet 2014; 53(1):89–102.
59. Todoran TM, Sobieszczyk P. Catheter-based therapies for massive pulmonary embolism. Prog Cardiovasc Dis 2010;52(5):429–37.
60. Engelberger RP, Kucher N, Müller OJ, et al. Catheter-based reperfusion treatment of pulmonary embolism. Circulation 2011;124(19):2139–44.
61. Bavare AC, Naik SX, Lin PH, et al. Catheter-directed thrombolysis for severe pulmonary embolism in pediatric patients. Ann Vasc Surg 2014;28(7):1794.e1-7.
62. Albisetti M. Thrombolytic therapy in children. Thromb Res 2006;118(1):95–105.
63. Braga AJ, Young AER. Preventing venous thrombosis in critically ill children: what is the right approach? Paediatr Anaesth 2011;21(4):435–40.
64. Mahajerin A, Branchford BR, Amankwah EK, et al. Hospital-associated venous thromboembolism in pediatrics: a systematic review and meta-analysis of risk factors and risk-assessment models. Haematologica 2015. https://doi.org/10. 3324/haematol.2015.123455.
65. Raffini L, Trimarchi T, Beliveau J, et al. Thromboprophylaxis in a pediatric hospital: a patient-safety and quality-improvement initiative. Pediatrics 2011;127(5):e1326–32.
66. Meier KA, Clark E, Tarango C, et al. Venous thromboembolism in hospitalized adolescents: an approach to risk assessment and prophylaxis. Hosp Pediatr 2015; 5(1):44–51.
67. Hanson SJ, Punzalan RC, Arca MJ, et al. Effectiveness of clinical guidelines for deep vein thrombosis prophylaxis in reducing the incidence of venous thromboembolism in critically ill children after trauma. J Trauma Acute Care Surg 2012; 72(5):1292–7.
68. Jaffray J, Buckner T, Vincent E, et al. Prevention of hospital-acquired venous thromboembolism in children: a review of published guidelines. Front Pediatr 2017;5.

69. Prasad V, Rho J, Cifu A. The inferior vena cava filter. JAMA Intern Med 2013; 173(7):493.
70. Blevins EM, Glanz K, Huang YSV, et al. A multicenter cohort study of inferior vena cava filter use in children. Pediatr Blood Cancer 2015;62(12):2089–93.
71. Jaff MR, McMurtry MS, Archer SL, et al. Management of massive and submassive pulmonary embolism, iliofemoral deep vein thrombosis, and chronic thromboembolic pulmonary hypertension: a scientific statement from the American Heart Association. Circulation 2011;123(16):1788–830.
72. Yang S, Yang Y, Zhai Z, et al. Incidence and risk factors of chronic thromboembolic pulmonary hypertension in patients after acute pulmonary embolism. J Thorac Dis 2015;7(11):1927–38.
73. Catheter-related early thromboprophylaxis with enoxaparin (crete) trial - full text view - ClinicalTrials.gov. Available at: https://clinicaltrials.gov/ct2/show/NCT03003390?term=pediatric&cond=Venous+Thromboembolism&draw=3&rank=18. Accessed October 23, 2017.
74. Rivaroxaban for treatment in venous or arterial thrombosis in neonates - full text view - ClinicalTrials.gov. Available at: https://clinicaltrials.gov/ct2/show/NCT02564718?term=pediatric&cond=Venous+Thromboembolism&draw=3&rank=17. Accessed October 23, 2017.
75. Apixaban for the acute treatment of venous thromboembolism in children - full text view - ClinicalTrials.gov. Available at: https://clinicaltrials.gov/ct2/show/NCT02464969?term=pediatric&cond=Venous+Thromboembolism&draw=4&rank=5. Accessed October 23, 2017.

Atypical Hemolytic Uremic Syndrome

Bradley P. Dixon, MD[a], Ralph A. Gruppo, MD[b],*

KEYWORDS

- Atypical hemolytic uremic syndrome • Thrombotic microangiopathies
- Complement activation • Eculizumab

KEY POINTS

- Atypical hemolytic uremic syndrome is a rare form of thrombotic microangiopathy resulting from chronic uncontrolled activation of the alternative pathway of complement.
- Untreated, it carries a high degree of morbidity and mortality.
- Atypical hemolytic uremic syndrome is associated with nonimmune hemolytic anemia, thrombocytopenia, and renal involvement; it is distinguished from thrombotic thrombocytopenic purpura and Shigatoxin-positive *Escherichia coli* hemolytic uremic syndrome.
- Atypical hemolytic uremic syndrome is a systemic microangiopathy with extrarenal manifestations that involve the heart, brain, lungs, gastrointestinal tract, pancreas, and skin.
- Acquired and genetic abnormalities in the complement regulatory system can be demonstrated in up to 70% of patients with atypical hemolytic uremic syndrome.

INTRODUCTION

The term thrombotic microangiopathy (TMA) refers to a spectrum of disorders characterized by widespread thrombosis of the arterioles and capillaries of the microvasculature affecting multiple organs including the kidneys, brain, heart, lungs, and gastrointestinal tract.[1] The pathologic features are vascular damage manifested by arteriolar occlusion with endothelial cell detachment, widening of the subendothelial space, and the presence of intraluminal fibrin and platelet thrombi (**Fig. 1**).[2] Hemolytic uremic syndrome (HUS) and thrombotic thrombocytopenic purpura (TTP) comprise the primary TMA syndromes, but with different pathophysiology (**Fig. 2**). TMA is also associated with a number of miscellaneous conditions (see **Fig. 2**). The pathophysiology of

Conflict of Interest: Dr R.A. Gruppo has received honoraria for speaking engagements from Alexion Pharmaceuticals. Dr B. Dixon has received honoraria for speaking engagements from Alexion Pharmaceuticals, and has served as a consultant for Alexion Pharmaceuticals and Achillion Pharmaceuticals.

[a] Renal Section, Department of Pediatrics, University of Colorado School of Medicine, 13123 East 16th Avenue, Aurora, CO 80045, USA; [b] Division of Hematology, Cancer and Blood Diseases Institute, Cincinnati Children's Hospital Medical Center, 3333 Burnet Avenue, Cincinnati, OH 45229, USA
* Corresponding author.
E-mail address: ralph.gruppo@cchmc.org

Pediatr Clin N Am 65 (2018) 509–525
https://doi.org/10.1016/j.pcl.2018.02.003
0031-3955/18/© 2018 Elsevier Inc. All rights reserved.

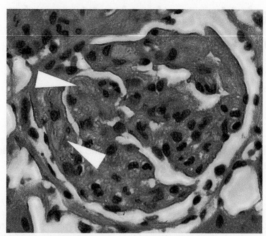

Fig. 1. Thrombotic microangiopathy evident on a renal biopsy from a patient with atypical hemolytic uremic syndrome (aHUS). Note the fibrin thrombi and red blood cell fragments present in the capillary loops (*white arrowheads*). (Hematoxylin and eosin stain, 40× magnification.)

TMA associated with these conditions is less well-understood. HUS is characterized by the triad of microangiopathic hemolytic anemia, thrombocytopenia and acute renal failure. In children, approximately 85% to 90% of cases of HUS are caused by Shigatoxin-positive *Escherichia coli* enteric infection (STEC-HUS).[3] The remaining cases, so-called atypical HUS, are due to genetic or acquired defects of the alternative pathway of

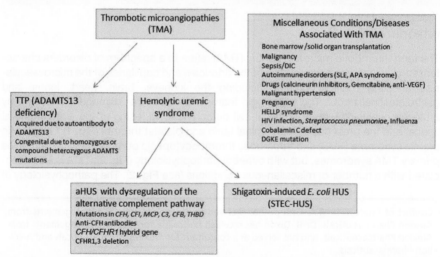

Fig. 2. Classification of the thrombotic microangiopathies based on etiology. ADAMTS13, A disintegrin and metalloproteinase with a thrombospondin type 1 motif, member 13; APA, antiphospholipid antibody syndrome; CFB, complement Factor B; CFH, complement Factor H; CFI, complement Factor I; DGKE, diacylglycerol kinase ε; DIC, disseminated intravascular coagulation; HELLP syndrome, hemolysis, elevated liver enzymes and low platelet count syndrome; HIV, human immunodeficiency virus; HUS, hemolytic uremic syndrome; MCP, Membrane Cofactor Protein (CD46); SLE, systemic lupus erythematosus; STEC, Shiga toxin-producing *Escherichia coli*; THBD, thrombomodulin gene; TMA, thrombotic microangiopathy; TTP, thrombotic thrombocytopenic purpura; VEGF, vascular endothelial growth factor.

complement leading to unregulated complement activation. TTP, in contrast, is a primary TMA syndrome caused by an acquired or congenital deficiency of the von Willebrand factor (vWF) cleaving protease, A disintegrin and metalloproteinase with a thrombospondin type 1 motif, member 13 (ADAMTS13). In the absence of ADAMTS13, ultralarge multimers of vWF promote the formation of microvascular platelet thrombi and endothelial damage.[4,5] Previously, the TMA syndromes were poorly differentiated, but advances in recent years have allowed their reclassification based on distinct molecular mechanisms. This knowledge has led to the development of targeted therapies, which have dramatically improved clinical outcomes. Therefore, it is incumbent on the physician to recognize and differentiate the TMA syndromes, because the early institution of appropriate therapy can prevent multiorgan damage and death. This review focuses on atypical HUS, a subtype of HUS, caused by a dysregulated activation of the alternative pathway of complement.

EPIDEMIOLOGY

The estimated annual incidence of atypical HUS in children less than 18 years of age is approximately 1.0 to 3.3 per million.[6–8] Atypical HUS occurs with equal frequency in boys and girls when onset occurs during childhood. In the global atypical HUS registry of 516 registered patients of all ages, 39% of patients developed the disease before 18 years of age.[9] Approximately 44% of children experienced their first episode before the age of 2 years. Atypical HUS may be sporadic or familial, with family members affected in 20% of childhood cases.[9]

CLINICAL PRESENTATION

In children, the onset of atypical HUS is usually abrupt, although up to 20% of patients may present with slowly progressive symptoms. In 191 patients registered on the International Registry of Recurrent and Familial HUS/TTP for whom data were available, underlying complement amplifying conditions/diseases were present in 69% of patients (**Fig. 3**).[10] Diarrhea/gastroenteritis and upper respiratory tract infections were associated with atypical HUS in 42% of patients, whereas a variety of other conditions, including malignant hypertension, pregnancy, solid organ and bone marrow transplant, glomerular diseases, autoimmune diseases, and malignancy, were present in 27%.

The clinical characteristics of atypical HUS are summarized in **Box 1**. Hemolytic anemia may present with pallor and fatigue. Thrombocytopenia is usually not severe enough to cause symptoms of bleeding. In a retrospective study of 43 patients by Sallee and coauthors,[11] 14% of patients presented with normal platelet counts. Renal involvement is usually predominant at the time of presentation, and is most commonly associated with proteinuria and hematuria, elevated creatinine level, hypertension, and a decreased glomerular filtration rate. However, up to 20% of children may present with only proteinuria and hematuria, with preserved renal function.[12] Extrarenal manifestations are prominent in up to 20% of patients, with neurologic involvement being the most common.[10,12] Gastrointestinal involvement may present with symptoms of abdominal pain, vomiting, or gastrointestinal bleeding. Cardiac involvement,[13] skin involvement,[14] and ischemia of the fingers and toes[15] have also been reported.

PATHOPHYSIOLOGY

The pathogenesis of atypical HUS stems from genetic or acquired defects in the regulation of the alternative complement pathway. This pathway (**Fig. 4**) is constitutively active in plasma by the hydrolysis of the reactive thioester bond of C3 to $C3(H_2O)$, a

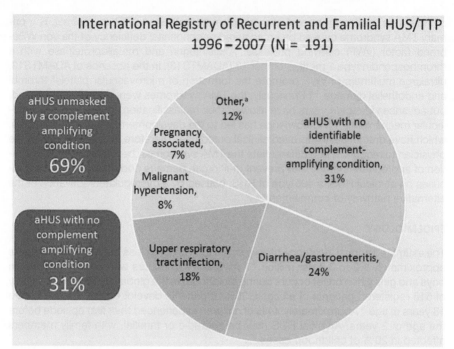

Fig. 3. Association of complement amplifying conditions in 191 patients with atypical hemolytic uremic syndrome (aHUS) entered on the International Registry of Recurrent and Familial HUS/thrombotic thrombocytopenic purpura (TTP) from 1996 to 2007.[10] [a] Other: post-transplant (5%), glomerulopathy (4%), autoimmune disease (2%), and malignancy (1%).

Box 1
Clinical characteristics of atypical hemolytic uremic syndrome in children

- Slightly greater frequency in adults (60%) than children under 18 years of age (40%).
- Equal frequency in boys and girls.
- Familial in 20% of cases.
- In children, more than 40% of cases occur under age 2 years and 25% under 6 months.
- Infections or inflammatory conditions trigger complement activation in 70% of patients. Upper respiratory tract infections or diarrhea are the most common triggering events.
- Usually sudden onset with fatigue, pallor, poor feeding, vomiting, shortness of breath, edema.
- Hypertension, renal failure, and oliguria.
- Extrarenal manifestations are present in up to 20% of patients:
  ○ Cardiac failure;
  ○ Neurologic involvement (10%) with irritability, drowsiness, seizures, diplopia, cortical blindness, hemiparesis or hemiplegia, stupor, or coma;
  ○ Myocardial infarction;
  ○ Distal gangrene of fingers and toes;
  ○ Pulmonary hemorrhage or edema;
  ○ Abdominal pain, nausea/vomiting, and intestinal bleeding; and
  ○ Pancreatitis.

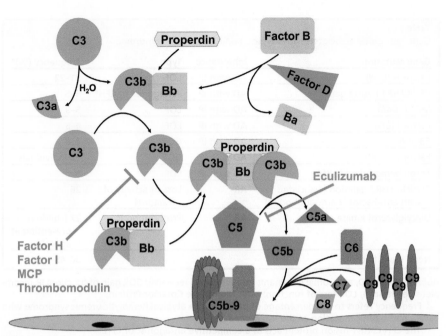

Fig. 4. Alternative pathway of the complement system. With ongoing activation of the alternative pathway C3 convertase C3bBb, a C5 convertase (C3Bb•C3b) is formed, leading to activation of the terminal pathway and formation of the membrane attack complex (C5b-9). Complement regulatory proteins that have been associated with atypical hemolytic uremic syndrome (aHUS) intervene at the level of inactivation of C3b, whereas eculizumab intervenes downstream at the level of the terminal pathway (C5). MCP, Membrane Cofactor Protein (CD46).

process known as the tickover mechanism, where it can bind to Factor B. Factor B when bound to $C3(H_2O)$ is a substrate for Factor D, and is cleaved to its fragments Bb, which remains a part of the molecular complex, and Ba. The complex $C3(H_2O)$ Bb functions as a C3 convertase, cleaving new molecules of C3 to C3a, a proinflammatory anaphylatoxin, and C3b, the latter of which can then bind to new molecules of Factor B, leading to the formation of additional C3 convertase complexes of C3bBb. This robust amplified formation of C3b, known as the amplification loop, leads to the decoration of cell surfaces with many molecules of C3b, opsonizing these cell surfaces for the recruitment of inflammatory and phagocytic cells. C3bBb, when complexed with a second C3b molecule as C3bBb•C3b, then functions as both a C3 convertase and a C5 convertase, cleaving C5 to its fragments C5a, an additional proinflammatory anaphylatoxin, and C5b, which initiates the formation of the lytic membrane attack complex C5b-9.

Because this process is constitutively active, is rapidly amplified, and does not easily distinguish between foreign microbial surfaces and self-surfaces, a series of membrane-bound and fluid phase regulatory proteins within the complement system serve to modulate its destructive power on self-surfaces. Factor H (encoded by the *CFH* gene) is a plasma glycoprotein produced by the liver that binds C3b and sialic acid on the cell surface and serves as a cofactor for the enzymatic inactivation of C3b by Factor I. Factor H was the first complement regulatory gene in which a loss-of-function mutation was identified in association with atypical HUS. Loss-of-function heterozygous mutations in *CFH* are the most frequently identified cause of complement dysregulation in patients with atypical HUS (**Table 1**).[8] Loss-of-function mutations in

Table 1
Gene mutations associated with atypical hemolytic uremic syndrome

Gene Mutation	Inheritance	Type	Frequency (%)[a]
Factor H (CFH)	AD with IP	LOF	21–22
CFH/CFHR1 hybrid gene	AD with IP	Antagonist to CFH[b]	3–5
MCP (CD46)	AD with IP	LOF	5–9
Factor I (CFI)	AD with IP	LOF	4–8
C3 (C3)	AD with IP	GOF	2–8
Factor B (CFB)	AD with IP	GOF	12 individuals
Thrombomodulin (THBD)	AD with IP	LOF	5
CFHR1/CFHR3 deletion (associated with anti-Factor H autoantibodies)	AR	Loss of activity of Factor H	26
Diacylglycerol kinase ε	AR	Prothrombotic	27 (children presenting at age <1 y)
None identified			30–48

Abbreviations: AD, autosomal dominant; AR, autosomal recessive; GOF, gain of function; IP, incomplete penetrance; LOF, loss of function; MCP, Membrane Cofactor Protein.
[a] Frequency refers to the percentage of patients with atypical hemolytic uremic syndrome who have a pathogenic mutation of the listed gene.
[b] The CFH/CFHR1 fusion protein acts as a competitive antagonist of CFH.
Adapted from Noris M, Breslin E, Mele C, Remuzzi G. Genetic atypical hemolytic-uremic syndrome. In: Pagon RA, Adam MP, Ardinger HH, et al., editors. GeneReviews. Seattle (WA): University of Washington, Seattle;1993–2017. Available at: https://www.ncbi.nlm.nih.gov/books/NBK1367/. ©University of Washington 1993–2017. GeneReviews (R) is a registered trademark of the University of Washington, Seattle. The content is used with permission. All rights reserved.

additional complement regulatory proteins such as Factor I (*CFI*), Membrane Cofactor Protein (*CD46*), and thrombomodulin (*THBD*), have also been described in association with atypical HUS, as well as gain-of-function mutations in pathway components C3 (*C3*) and Factor B (*CFB*).[8] These mutations are generally heterozygous, but exhibit incomplete penetrance. An acquired form of complement dysregulation has also been described, in which autoantibodies directed against Factor H may inhibit its function, although even this acquired form of complement dysregulation seems to have a genetic susceptibility through homozygous deletion of the Factor H-related gene *CFHR1*.[8]

If one or more of these regulatory proteins has an inherent defect in the ability to modulate complement activation, exuberant complement activity may occur if complement activation is stimulated by a variety of clinical conditions and disease states. This exaggerated and dysregulated complement activation may lead to endothelial cell injury and the final common pathway of TMA, with subsequent platelet and coagulation activation with thrombotic occlusion of the microvasculature leading to tissue ischemia and organ dysfunction.

In addition to mutations in the regulatory proteins of the alternative pathway of complement, atypical HUS has been identified in children with homozygous mutations of the diacylglycerol kinase ε (*DGKE*) gene,[16] an intracellular protein that seems to confer a prothrombotic state to the microvasculature when defective, but does not seem to interact with the complement system. Affected individuals usually present before 1 year of age with persistent hypertension, hematuria, and proteinuria. Mutations in the plasminogen gene *PLG* have also been noted in a cohort of patients with atypical HUS.[17]

LABORATORY DIAGNOSIS

Laboratory features of atypical HUS are listed in **Box 2**. Clinically, atypical HUS is characterized by hemolytic anemia and consumptive thrombocytopenia. Endothelial damage and thrombosis in the microvasculature result in abnormally high shear stress leading to platelet aggregation and mechanical (nonimmune) red cell destruction. Thrombocytopenia is modest with platelet counts uncommonly less than 30×10^9/L. Examination of the peripheral blood smear characteristically demonstrates fragmented red blood cells (schistocytes), a finding common to the TMA syndromes (**Fig. 5**). The direct antiglobulin test (Coombs test) is negative. Elevated levels of serum lactic dehydrogenase correspond with the degree of hemolysis and tissue damage from microvascular thrombosis, and can be useful diagnostically as well as in following disease progression and response to therapy. The serum haptoglobin level is typically decreased owing to intravascular hemolysis.

Atypical HUS is largely a clinical diagnosis, because no diagnostic test is currently available that can confirm or refute the diagnosis with a high degree of sensitivity and specificity. Distinguishing between atypical HUS and the microangiopathy associated with other miscellaneous conditions and diseases (see **Fig. 2**) can be challenging diagnostically. Treatment options, and the efficacy of these options, may vary depending on the specific form of TMA. Serious clinical sequelae may result if the correct diagnosis is not promptly recognized and treated, making an accurate diagnosis early in the patient's presentation critical.

DIFFERENTIAL DIAGNOSIS
Thrombotic Thrombocytopenic Purpura

Atypical HUS can usually be distinguished from TTP based on the clinical presentation and laboratory features. In general, more modest laboratory evidence of renal impairment would be most consistent with TTP, although great caution must be exercised in applying this paradigm because the severity of individual organ system involvement in atypical HUS can vary greatly from patient to patient. An analysis of multiple cohorts of adult patients has yielded the insight that if thrombocytopenia is not severe (ie, platelet count $>30 \times 10^9$/L) or if renal dysfunction is more prominent (serum creatinine >1.7–2.3), a diagnosis of TTP is almost entirely excluded.[18]

The laboratory hallmark of TTP is a severe deficiency (<5%–10%) of the vWF-cleaving protease ADAMTS13.[19] Currently, clinical assays of ADAMTS13 activity are relatively widely available and can provide results to the clinician with a rapid turnaround time, allowing for prompt decision making. The clinician should be aware of the

---

Box 2
Laboratory features of thrombotic microangiopathy

- Hemolytic anemia (with elevated reticulocyte percentage)
- Presence of fragmented red cells (schistocytes) on blood smear
- Thrombocytopenia
- Direct antiglobulin test (Coomb's test) negative
- Elevated lactic dehydrogenase level
- Decreased haptoglobin
- Elevated serum blood urea nitrogen and creatinine with renal involvement
- Hemoglobinuria and proteinuria with renal involvement

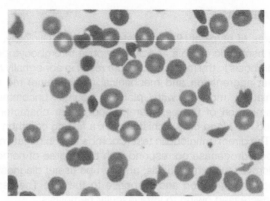

Fig. 5. Peripheral blood smear stained with hematoxylin and eosin (100× magnification) demonstrating fragmentation of red blood cells (schistocytes) associated with the thrombotic microangiopathy syndromes.

laboratory's lower cutoff for ADAMTS13 activity, which may vary, depending on the sensitivity of the assay used. The earliest methods of measuring ADAMTS13 activity were directly through the electrophoretic analysis of vWF multimers or vWF fragments, or indirectly by the measurement of the residual collagen binding capacity of vWF or ristocetin-induced platelet aggregation.[20] Newer methodologies using synthetic vWF-based peptides as ADAMTS13 substrates[21–23] have improved the reproducibility and assay performance time of this testing, which is of great benefit in facilitating an early distinction between TTP and other forms of TMA, including atypical HUS. Obtaining blood samples for this testing before the initiation of plasma therapy (plasma infusion or plasmapheresis) is critical, because such interventions may obscure a severe deficiency and make the diagnosis of TTP difficult.[24]

Shigatoxin-Positive Escherichia coli Hemolytic Uremic Syndrome

Distinguishing STEC-HUS from atypical HUS is facilitated by laboratory testing. Testing for the presence of Shigatoxin is appropriate in the setting of TMA with gastrointestinal symptoms such as watery or bloody diarrhea. Stool culture with selective and differential media such as sorbitol MacConkey agar effectively identifies the most common serotype of Shigatoxin-producing E coli in the United States, O157:H7. However, a number of non-O157 Shigatoxin-producing strains may also cause disease but not be identified by routine microbiological techniques, particularly outside of the United States. Therefore, molecular testing for Shigatoxin by either immunoassay for the toxin itself or by polymerase chain reaction to detect the toxin genes stx1 and stx2 is now uniformly recommended to accompany routine stool culture techniques.[25] Although a history of preceding bloody diarrhea should suggest the possibility of STEC-HUS, caution should be exercised because bloody diarrhea may be a symptom of gastrointestinal involvement in atypical HUS. Confirmatory tests are mandatory for a diagnosis of STEC-HUS.

Complement Assays in the Diagnosis of Atypical Hemolytic Uremic Syndrome

The diagnosis of atypical HUS can sometimes by aided by laboratory tests interrogating the complement system. This evaluation generally includes 3 aspects of testing: quantitative testing, functional testing, and genetic analysis. Quantitative measurement of serum levels of complement components, specifically C3, C4, and Factor B, may provide insight as to the pattern of complement activation present in a patient. A low level of C3 and/or Factor B, with a normal level of C4, suggests an isolated activation of the alternative pathway, fitting with the pathobiology of atypical HUS. However, normal levels of complement components are commonly seen in the majority of patients with atypical HUS[10]; therefore, these levels may only occasionally provide added diagnostic insight. Similarly, genetic defects in the complement regulators Factor H and Factor I may cause decreased levels of these proteins in the blood, but more commonly cause functional defects in the proteins without leading to a reduction in serum antigen levels[10,26]; thus, these measurements may also have limited diagnostic usefulness. One notable exception to the limited diagnostic role of quantitative complement testing is the measurement of Factor H autoantibodies. This testing, typically performed by enzyme linked immunosorbent assay, is vitally important in the initial diagnostic evaluation of suspected atypical HUS to detect the 5% to 10% of patients with atypical HUS associated with these autoantibodies,[8] and may not be directly detected by any other means. Furthermore, the identification of these antibodies may have therapeutic implications (ie, the use of plasmapheresis and immunosuppression to eliminate the autoantibodies), as well as implications for recurrence risk after kidney transplantation.

Biomarkers of Complement Activation

More recently, measurement of levels of complement split products in plasma or urine such as the soluble form of the membrane attack complex (sC5b-9) and the Factor B fragments Ba and Bb have shown promise as functional indicators of terminal pathway and alternative pathway activation, respectively.[27,28] However, these fragments may also be elevated in other complement activating conditions, including TTP.[27,29] Their lack of specificity may limit their diagnostic usefulness. Hemolytic assays such as CH50 and AH50 are also used as functional tests to indicate complement activation, although these may only be abnormal in the setting of complement factor depletion, and thus are also not specific or sensitive for detection of atypical HUS. Additional functional assay methods have also been recently described that provide greater specificity for the complement dysregulation associated with atypical HUS, but require highly specialized reagents and technical expertise,[30,31] currently limiting their widespread implementation in clinical diagnostic testing.

Genetic Mutation Analysis in Atypical Hemolytic Uremic Syndrome

The most comprehensive assessment of the complement system is by genetic analysis. The advent of next-generation sequencing and its application to molecular genetic diagnostic testing has greatly reduced both the cost and time needed for this testing. Presently, there is widespread consensus as to the minimum set of genes to be sequenced in the setting of atypical HUS: CFH, CFI, MCP, C3, CFB, THBD, CFHR5, and DGKE genes, as well as detection of complex rearrangements of the CFH gene with Factor H–related genes (CFHR1, CFHR3, CFHR4) and the common CFHR1-CFHR3 deletion that is present in the vast majority of patients with Factor H autoantibody-associated atypical HUS (see **Table 1**).[32] Genetic testing may identify either a type I mutation, in which reduced expression of the protein is noted, or a type II mutation, in which the expression of the protein product is normal but a functional defect is present. Despite its pivotal role in the diagnostic evaluation of atypical HUS, several challenges are associated with this aspect of the evaluation. Genetic testing is expensive, which may represent a barrier to access for patients. Test results typically require weeks for a thorough analysis of the sequencing data, and are therefore generally not practical for use in the acute setting. However, most important of all is that only approximately 60% of patients with a confirmed clinical diagnosis of atypical HUS will have an identified pathogenic variant by genetic testing. The absence of a mutation in one of the complement regulating genes does not rule out the diagnosis of atypical HUS, or the likelihood of response to anticomplement therapy.

The main usefulness of genetic testing in atypical HUS is for family counseling and, to some extent, the prediction of clinical severity and risk of relapse. Family counseling in cases where complement mutations are identified is also complicated by the incomplete penetrance of the disease, in that only approximately 50% of persons carrying an identified mutation in *C3*, *CD46*, *CFH*, *CFI*, *CFB*, *CFH/CFHR1* hybrid gene or *THBD* eventually develop disease, indicating that additional genetic and environmental factors contribute to disease development in affected individuals.[33] Also, the limitations of *in silico* methods for the prediction of variant pathogenicity (variants of uncertain significance) may leave the clinician to rely largely on a clinical diagnosis upon which to base therapeutic decisions and prognostic understanding. In the future, functional testing of the individual complement components paired with genetic testing may offer the most robust insight as to the pathogenicity of identified variants.

The Diagnosis of Atypical Hemolytic Uremic Syndrome in the Presence of Another Thrombotic Microangiopathy

A difficult diagnostic challenge arises when atypical HUS is suspected in the setting of TMA associated with another disease or condition, such as solid organ or stem cell transplantation, malignancy, sepsis, autoimmune disorders, drugs (including calcineurin inhibitors, gemcitabine, or anti-vascular endothelial growth factor), malignant hypertension, HELLP (hemolysis, elevated liver enzymes, and low platelet count) syndrome in pregnancy, and infections (human immunodeficiency virus, *Strep pneumoniae*, influenza). Unfortunately, the pathophysiology of TMA associated with these disorders is less well-understood, although complement activation as evidenced by elevated levels of sC5b-9 and C3a is common.[29] In this setting, complement activation may trigger or unmask atypical HUS in susceptible individuals with underlying abnormalities of complement regulation. In fact, more than one-quarter of atypical HUS cases are known to be associated with these miscellaneous disorders (see **Fig. 3**).[10] It is generally recommended in these cases that treatment consist of supportive care and treatment of the underlying condition, which often results in clinical improvement or resolution of the TMA. However, if after treatment of the underlying disorder, symptoms of TMA persist or worsen, as evidenced by the patient's clinical condition and laboratory findings, a diagnosis of atypical HUS should be seriously considered and treated accordingly.[24] An algorithm for the diagnosis of atypical HUS is presented (**Fig. 6**).

MANAGEMENT
Plasma Therapy

There is no evidence that plasma therapy (plasma infusion or plasmapheresis) affects the ultimate outcome of children or adults with atypical HUS. In a large study of more than 270 patients enrolled in an international registry of atypical HUS, plasma therapy was shown to induce hematologic remission in up to 78% of episodes in children and 53% in adults. Nevertheless, at 3 years of follow-up 48% of children and 67% of adults had end-stage renal disease or had died.[10] Similarly, in a French registry of more than 200 children and adults with atypical HUS, end-stage renal disease or death occurred in 56% of adults and 29% of children within 1 year of follow-up despite plasma therapy.[34] Although hematologic parameters may improve during plasma therapy, underlying complement activation remains unchanged, as demonstrated by the persistent elevation of biomarkers of complement activation, inflammation, renal injury, and endothelial damage.[28]

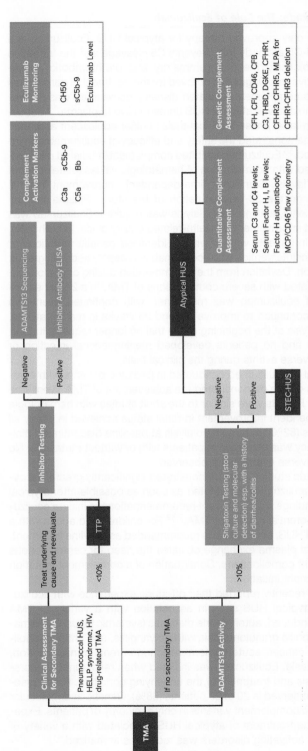

Fig. 6. Proposed diagnostic algorithm for the evaluation of a patient with thrombotic microangiopathy. After excluding TTP by investigation of ADAMTS13 activity, and excluding STEC-HUS by investigation for Shigatoxin, a comprehensive evaluation of the complement system is warranted in patients with suspected atypical HUS (aHUS). ADAMTS13, A disintegrin and metalloproteinase with a thrombospondin type 1 motif, member 13; CFB, complement Factor B; CFH, complement Factor H; CFI, complement Factor I; DGKE, diacylglycerol kinase ε; HELLP syndrome, hemolysis, elevated liver enzymes and low platelet count syndrome; HIV, human immunodeficiency virus; HUS, hemolytic uremic syndrome; MCP, Membrane Cofactor Protein (CD46); SLE, systemic lupus erythematosus; STEC, Shiga toxin-producing *Escherichia coli*; TMA, thrombotic microangiopathy; TTP, thrombotic thrombocytopenic purpura.

Terminal Complement Blockade: The Role of Eculizumab

Eculizumab currently is the only approved therapy for atypical HUS. Eculizumab is a monoclonal humanized anti-C5 antibody that prevents C5 cleavage and the formation of C5a and C5b-9, thus blocking the proinflammatory and prothrombotic consequences of complement activation. Originally approved for the treatment of paroxysmal nocturnal hemoglobinuria, a complement-mediated disease, eculizumab was first reported to be effective in an infant with atypical HUS unresponsive to plasma.[35] Subsequently, 2 prospective open-label phase II clinical trials in older adolescent and adult patients with atypical HUS demonstrated the safety and efficacy of eculizumab administered over a 26-week period.[36] Eculizumab inhibited complement-mediated microangiopathy and was associated with normalization of hematologic values (platelet count and lactic dehydrogenase levels). Significant time-dependent improvement in renal function was observed during the 26-week duration of the study. Plasma therapy was discontinued in all patients, and no new dialysis was required. Eculizumab was associated with a significant improvement of health-related quality of life. In both trials, positive results were seen in patients with or without identified genetic mutations or Factor H autoantibody. Earlier intervention with eculizumab was associated with greater improvement in renal function. Deviation from the recommended dosing or discontinuation of therapy was associated with severe complications of TMA. In a 2-year extension study, the efficacy of eculizumab was maintained with continued event-free survival.[37] Kidney function continued to improve beyond 26 weeks in many patients. Most patients receiving dialysis at the beginning of the trial no longer required it. Eculizumab was well-tolerated and no patients developed meningococcal infection or infection-related serious adverse events during the clinical trials.

A prospective clinical trial of eculizumab conducted in pediatric patients with atypical HUS less than 18 years of age demonstrated the achievement of TMA event-free status in 95% of patients.[38] Results were similar to the adult studies with hematologic normalization and time-dependent improvement in renal status achieved in nearly all patients. Nine of 11 patients (82%) undergoing dialysis at baseline discontinued dialysis during the study. Efficacy was observed in patients with or without mutations. No serious infection-related adverse events were observed.

Both the adult and pediatric studies have demonstrated significantly greater recovery of renal function when eculizumab is instituted as soon as possible after atypical HUS presentation. These findings support recent recommendations to initiate eculizumab after ruling out other potential causes of TMA.[7,39] For children and adults with a clinical suspicion of atypical HUS, eculizumab is recommended as first-line treatment. In children, the avoidance of plasma exchange obviates the need for central venous catheters with their attendant complications. Confirmation of a complement mutation is not required before treatment initiation.

Cavero and colleagues[40] recently reported their off-study experience with eculizumab in 29 patients with atypical HUS seen in association with a variety of TMA syndromes, including drug induced, autoimmune diseases (systemic lupus erythematosus, scleroderma, eosinophilic granulomatosis with polyangiitis, and antiphospholipid syndrome), pregnancy, cancer, acute humoral rejection in renal transplantation, and intestinal lymphangiectasia. Eculizumab was initiated when renal function worsened despite plasmapheresis and treatment of the underlying condition. Rapid resolution of atypical HUS was observed in 20 of 29 patients (68%). Genetic and molecular studies identified pathogenic complement variants in only a minority of patients. Experience with eculizumab in the treatment of atypical HUS associated with a variety of miscellaneous complement activating disorders was recently summarized.[41]

In the case of severe STEC-HUS, eculizumab has been reported to be effective in select patients. Evidence from both the bench and the bedside has demonstrated that complement may act as a secondary mediator of disease in STEC-HUS. Shigatoxin binds Factor H and can interfere with its complement regulatory functions,[42] and can thus promote deposition of C3b on the injured endothelial cell surface.[43] Furthermore, in an animal model of STEC-HUS, Factor B–deficient mice, which are unable to activate the alternative complement pathway, have an attenuated degree of thrombocytopenia and renal injury compared with wild-type mice.[43] Elevated levels of complement activation fragments sC5b-9 and Bb have been demonstrated in the plasma of patients with STEC-HUS that return to normal levels during convalescence.[44] These findings led to the successful use of complement-targeted therapy (eculizumab) in a small series of patients with STEC-HUS and severe neurologic involvement.[45] The use of eculizumab during the 2011 epidemic of STEC-HUS owing to *E coli* O104:H4 in Germany and other European countries seemed to be associated with a rapid recovery in selected patients with extrarenal complications,[46] including patients with early central nervous system involvement.[47] Overall, however, in a large group of patients with *E coli* O104:H4-induced HUS treated with eculizumab, no short-term[48,49] or intermediate-term benefit was apparent.[50]

Eculizumab was reported to be effective in a case of TTP with high titer anti-ADAMTS13 autoantibodies.[51] Subsequently, the patient was found to have a *CFH* mutation and anti-Factor H antibodies,[52] suggesting a link between the dysregulation of complement activation and refractory TTP. Eculizumab was also reported to be effective in a case of congenital TTP.[53] Experimental evidence suggests that vWF in the plasma from patients with congenital TTP interacts with C3b and initiates alternative pathway complement activation and formation of complement products C5a and C5b-9.[54] These investigators demonstrated in an ex vivo perfusion system that the vWF-mediated formation of terminal complement products could induce microvascular thrombosis.

Last, eculizumab has shown effectiveness in treating TMA associated with hematopoietic stem cell transplantation, a significant cause of morbidity and mortality in the posttransplant setting.[55] Surprisingly, posttransplant patients demonstrated significant variability in eculizumab clearance. Maintenance of therapeutic plasma levels of eculizumab required careful monitoring of drug serum concentrations, total hemolytic complement activity (which should be completely suppressed if therapeutic levels of eculizumab are maintained), and plasma C5b-9 levels.[56] A high prevalence of deletions in *CFH*-related genes 3 and 1 (*delCFHR3-CFHR1*) and CFH autoantibodies were identified in HSCT patients with TMA.[57]

Discontinuation of Therapy

After the resolution of the TMA in patients treated with eculizumab, the issue of whether to indefinitely continue or discontinue therapy is invariably raised. The risk of recurrence of atypical HUS after discontinuation of eculizumab has been reported to be 20% to 30%.[58–61] Relapse is more likely in patients with pathogenic variants in complement genes compared with patients without gene variants. No guidelines exist about which patients may be better candidates for stopping therapy. If the decision is made to discontinue therapy, careful monitoring should be done to closely monitor patients for signs and symptoms of TMA complications as well as progressive organ damage.

REFERENCES

1. Noris M, Remuzzi G. Atypical hemolytic-uremic syndrome. N Engl J Med 2009; 361:1676–87.

2. Tsai H-M. A mechanistic approach to the diagnosis and management of atypical hemolytic uremic syndrome. Transfus Med Rev 2014;28:187–97.

3. Fakhouri F, Zuber J, Fremeaux-Bacchi V, et al. Haemolytic uraemic syndrome. Lancet 2017;390:681–96.

4. Furlan M, Robles R, Galbusera M, et al. von Willebrand factor-cleaving protease in thrombotic thrombocytopenic purpura and the hemolytic-uremic syndrome. N Engl J Med 1998;339:1578–84.

5. Tsai HM, Lian EC. Antibodies to von Willebrand factor-cleaving protease in acute thrombotic thrombocytopenic purpura. N Engl J Med 1998;339: 1585–94.

6. Zimmerhackl LB, Besbas N, Jungraithmayr T, et al. Epidemiology, clinical presentation, and pathophysiology of atypical and recurrent hemolytic uremic syndrome. Semin Thromb Hemost 2006;32:113–20.

7. Campistol JM, Arias M, Ariceta G, et al. An update for atypical haemolytic uraemic syndrome: diagnosis and treatment. A consensus document. Nefrologia 2013;33:27–45.

8. Loirat C, Fremeaux-Bacchi V. Atypical hemolytic uremic syndrome. Orphanet J Rare Dis 2011;6:1150–72.

9. Licht C, Ardissino G, Ariceta G, et al. The global aHUS registry: methodology and initial patient characteristics. BMC Nephrol 2015;16:207.

10. Noris M, Caprioli J, Bresin E, et al. Relative role of genetic complement abnormalities in sporadic and familial aHUS and their impact on clinical phenotype. Clin J Am Soc Nephrol 2010;5:1844–59.

11. Sallee M, Ismail K, Fakhouri F, et al. Thromboctopenia is not mandatory to diagnose haemolytic and uremic syndrome. BMC Nephrol 2013;14:3–6.

12. Sellier-Lecleerc AL, Fremeaux-Bacchi V, Dragon-Durey MA, et al. Differential impact of complement mutations on clinical characteristics in atypical hemolytic uremic syndrome. J Am Soc Nephrol 2007;18:2392.

13. Hu H, Nagra A, Haq MR, et al. Eculizumab in atypical haemolytic uraemic syndrome with severe cardiac and neurological involvement. Pediatr Nephrol 2014;29:1103–6.

14. Ardissino G, Tel F, Testa S, et al. Skin involvement in atypical hemolytic uremic syndrome. Am J Kidney Dis 2014;63:652–5.

15. Malina M, Gulati A, Bagga A, et al. Peripheral gangrene in children with atypical hemolytic uremic syndrome. Pediatrics 2013;131:e331–5.

16. Lemaire M, Fremeaux-Bacchi V, Schaefer F, et al. Recessive mutations in DGKE cause atypical hemolytic-uremic syndrome. Nat Genet 2013;45:531–6.

17. Bu F, Maga T, Meyer NC, et al. Comprehensive genetic analysis of complement and coagulation genes in atypical hemolytic uremic syndrome. J Am Soc Nephrol 2014;25:55–64.

18. Cataland SR, Wu HM. How I treat: the clinical differentiation and initial treatment of adult patients with atypical hemolytic uremic syndrome. Blood 2014;123: 2478–84.

19. Bianchi V, Robles R, Alberio L, et al. von Willebrand factor-cleaving protease (ADAMTS13) in thrombocytopenic disorders: a severely deficient activity is specific for thrombotic thrombocytopenic purpura. Blood 2002;100:710–3.

20. Franchini M, Mannucci PM. Advantages and limits of ADAMTS13 testing in thrombotic thrombocytopenic purpura. Blood Transfus 2008;6:127–36.

21. Kokame K, Nobe Y, Kokubo Y, et al. FRETS-VWF73, a first fluorogenic substrate for ADAMTS13 assay. Br J Haematol 2005;129:93–100.

22. Kato S, Matsumoto M, Matsuyama T, et al. Novel monoclonal antibody-based enzyme immunoassay for determining plasma levels of ADAMTS13 activity. Transfusion 2006;46:1444–52.
23. Muia J, Gao W, Haberichter SL, et al. An optimized fluorogenic ADAMTS13 assay with increased sensitivity for the investigation of patients with thrombotic thrombocytopenic purpura. J Thromb Haemost 2013;11:1511–8.
24. Laurence J, Haller H, Mannucci PM, et al. Atypical hemolytic uremic syndrome (aHUS): essential aspects of an accurate diagnosis. Clin Adv Hematol Oncol 2016;14(Suppl 11):2–15.
25. Gould LH, Bopp C, Strockbine N, et al. Recommendations for diagnosis of Shiga toxin-producing *Escherichia coli* infections by clinical laboratories. MMWR Recomm Rep 2009;58(RR12):1–16.
26. Caprioli J, Noris M, Brioschi S, et al. Genetics of HUS: the impact of *MCP, CFH*, and *IF* mutations on clinical presentation, response to treatment, and outcome. Blood 2006;108:1267–79.
27. Cataland SR, Holers M, Geyer S, et al. Biomarkers of the alternative pathway and terminal complement activity at presentation confirms the clinical diagnosis of aHUS and differentiates aHUS from TTP. Blood 2014;123:3733–8.
28. Cofiell R, Kukreja A, Bedard K, et al. Eculizumab reduces complement activation, inflammation, endothelial damage, thrombosis, and renal injury markers in aHUS. Blood 2015;125:3253–62.
29. Farkas P, Csuka D, Mikes B, et al. Complement activation, inflammation and relative ADAMTS13 deficiency in secondary thrombotic microangiopathies. Immunobiology 2017;222:119–27.
30. Noris M, Galbusera M, Gastoldi S, et al. Dynamics of complement activation in aHUS and how to monitor eculizumab therapy. Blood 2014;124:1715–26.
31. Gavrilaki E, Yuan X, Ye Z, et al. Modified Ham test for atypical hemolytic uremic syndrome. Blood 2015;125:3637–46.
32. Zipfel PF, Mache C, Muller D, et al. DEAP-HUS: deficiency of CFHR plasma proteins and autoantibody-positive form of hemolytic uremic syndrome. Pediatr Nephrol 2010;25:2009–19.
33. Noris M, Breslin E, Mele C, et al. Genetic atypical hemolytic-uremic syndrome. In: Pagon RA, Adam MP, Ardinger HH, et al, editors. GeneReviews. Seattle (WA): University of Washington; 1993–2017. Available at: https://www.ncbi.nlm.nih.gov/books/NBK1367/.
34. Fremeaux-Bacchi V, Fakhouri F, Garnier A, et al. Genetics and outcome of atypical hemolytic uremic syndrome: a nationwide French series comparing children and adults. Clin J Am Soc Nephrol 2013;8:554–62.
35. Gruppo R, Rother RP. Eculizumab for congenital atypical hemolytic-uremic syndrome. N Engl J Med 2009;360:544–6.
36. Legendre CM, Licht C, Muus P, et al. Terminal complement inhibitor eculizumab in atypical hemolytic-uremic syndrome. N Engl J Med 2013;368:2169–81.
37. Licht C, Greenbaum LA, Muus P, et al. Efficacy and safety of eculizumab in atypical hemolytic uremic syndrome from 2-year extensions of phase 2 studies. Kidney Int 2015;87:1061–73.
38. Greenbaum LA, Fila M, Ardissino G, et al. Eculizumab is a safe and effective treatment in pediatric patients with atypical hemolytic uremic syndrome. Kidney Int 2016;89:701–11.
39. Loirat C, Fakhouri F, Ariceta G, et al. An international consensus approach to the management of atypical hemolytic uremic syndrome in children. Pediatr Nephrol 2016;31:15–39.

40. Cavero T, Rabasco C, Lopez A, et al. Eculizumab in secondary atypical haemolytic uraemic syndrome. Nephrol Dial Transplant 2017;32:466–74.
41. Asif A, Nayer A, Haas CS. Atypical hemolytic uremic syndrome in the setting of complement-amplifying conditions: case reports and a review of the evidence for treatment with eculizumab. J Nephrol 2017;30:347–62.
42. Orth D, Khan AB, Naim A, et al. Shiga toxin activates complement and binds factor H: evidence for an active role of complement in hemolytic uremic syndrome. J Immunol 2009;182:6394–400.
43. Morigi M, Galbusera M, Gastoldi S, et al. Alternative pathway activation of complement by shiga toxin promotes exuberant C3a formation that triggers microvascular thrombosis. J Immunol 2011;187:172–80.
44. Thurman JM, Marians R, Emlen W, et al. Alternative pathway of complement in children with diarrhea-associated hemolytic uremic syndrome. Clin J Am Soc Nephrol 2009;4:1920–4.
45. Lapeyraque A-L, Malina M, Fremeaux-Bacchi V, et al. Eculizumab in severe shiga-toxin-associated HUS. N Engl J Med 2011;364:2561–3.
46. Delmas Y, Vendrely B, Clouzeau B, et al. Outbreak of Escherichia coli O104:H4 haemolytic uraemic syndrome in France: outcome with eculizumab. Nephrol Dial Transplant 2014;29:565–72.
47. Pape L, Hartmann H, Bange FC, et al. Eculizumab in typical hemolytic uremic syndrome (HUS) with neurological involvement. Medicine 2015;94:e1000.
48. Menne J, Nitschke M, Stingele R, et al. Validation of treatment strategies for enterohaemorrhagic Escherichia coli O104:H4 induced haemolytic uraemic syndrome: case-control study. BMJ 2012;345:e4565.
49. Kielstein JT, Beutel G, Fleig S, et al. Best supportive care and therapeutic plasma exchange with or without eculizumab in Shiga-toxin-producing E. Coli O104:h4 induced haemolytic-uraemic syndrome: an analysis of the German STE C-HUS registry. Nephrol Dial Transplant 2012;27:3807–15.
50. Loos S, Aulbert W, Hoppe B, et al. Intermediate follow-up of pediatric patients with hemolytic uremic syndrome during the 2011 outbreak caused by E. coli O104:H4. Clin Infect Dis 2017;64:1637–43.
51. Chapin J, Weksler B, Magro C, et al. Eculizumab in the treatment of refractory idiopathic thrombotic thrombocytopenic purpura. Br J Haematol 2012;157:772–4.
52. Tsai E, Zhou W, Chapin J, et al. Use of eculizumab in the treatment of a case of refractory, ADAMTS13-deficient thrombotic thrombocytopenic purpura: additional data and clinical follow-up. Br J Haematol 2013;162:558–9.
53. Pecoraro C, Ferretti AV, Rurali E, et al. Treatment of congenital thrombotic thrombocytopenic purpura with eculizumab. Am J Kidney Dis 2015;66:1067–70.
54. Bettoni S, Galbusera M, Gastoldi S, et al. Interaction between multimeric von Willebrand factor and complement: a fresh look to the pathophysiology of microvascular thrombosis. J Immunol 2017;199:1021–40.
55. Jodele A, Fukuda T, Vinks A, et al. Eculizumab therapy in children with severe hematopoietic stem cell transplantation-associated thrombotic microangiopathy. Biol Blood Marrow Transplant 2014;20:518–25.
56. Jodele A, Fukuda T, Mizuno K, et al. Variable eculizumab clearance requires pharmacodynamics monitoring to optimize therapy for thrombotic microangiopathy after hematopoietic stem cell transplantation. Biol Blood Marrow Transplant 2016;22:307–15.
57. Jodele S, Licht C, Goebel J, et al. Abnormalities in the alternative pathway of complement in children with hematopoietic stem cell transplant-associated thrombotic microangiopathy. Blood 2013;122:2003–7.

58. Ardissino G, Testa S, Possenti I, et al. Discontinuation of eculizumab maintenance treatment for atypical hemolytic uremic syndrome: a report of 10 cases. Am J Kidney Dis 2014;64:633–7.
59. Macia M, de Alvaro Moreno F, Dutt T, et al. Current evidence on the discontinuation of eculizumab in patients with atypical haemolytic uraemic syndrome. Clin Kidney J 2017;10:310–9.
60. Merrill SA, Brittingham ZD, Yuan X, et al. Eculizumab cessation in atypical hemolytic uremic syndrome. Blood 2017;130:368–72.
61. Fakhouri F, Fila M, Provot F, et al. Pathogenic variants in complement genes and risk of atypical hemolytic uremic syndrome relapse after eculizumab discontinuation. Clin J Am Soc Nephrol 2017;12:50–9.

von Willebrand Disease
Diagnostic Strategies and Treatment Options

Christopher J. Ng, MD, Jorge Di Paola, MD*

KEYWORDS

- von Willebrand disease • von Willebrand factor • Mucocutaneous bleeding

KEY POINTS

- von Willebrand disease (VWD) is one of the most common inherited bleeding disorders.
- The clinical diagnosis of von Willebrand disease is usually made through the combination of clinical symptoms of mucocutaneous bleeding and laboratory-based evidence of von Willebrand factor (VWF) deficiency or dysfunction.
- Clinical subtypes of VWD are important to distinguish because they may have therapeutic implications.
- Treatment of VWD is designed to increase or replace circulating VWF, along with adjunctive therapies.

INTRODUCTION

First described by Erik von Willebrand[1] in a Scandinavian family in 1926, von Willebrand disease (VWD) is an inherited bleeding disorder with a reported symptomatic prevalence of 1 in 10,000. VWD affects individuals of all races and can have clinical implications from childhood, when it is usually first discovered, to adulthood, when management of comorbid conditions is complicated by the bleeding tendency. VWD is classically manifested by a predisposition to mucocutaneous bleeding (MCB); this leads to increased risks of postoperative blood loss; significant epistaxis; oral bleeding; and, in women, menorrhagia. Although rare, life-threatening bleeding can occur. VWD is characterized by a deficiency, either quantitative (type 1, type 3) or qualitative (type 2), of von Willebrand factor (VWF).[2] The diagnosis and treatment of VWD requires the understanding of the necessary functions of VWF in promoting

Department of Pediatrics, University of Colorado, Children's Hospital Colorado, 12800 East 19th Avenue, Research Center 1 North, MS 8302, Aurora, CO 80111, USA
* Corresponding author. Department of Pediatrics, University of Colorado, Children's Hospital Colorado, MS 8302, 12800 East 19th Avenue, Aurora, CO 80045.
E-mail address: jorge.dipaola@ucdenver.edu

Pediatr Clin N Am 65 (2018) 527–541
https://doi.org/10.1016/j.pcl.2018.02.004
0031-3955/18/© 2018 Elsevier Inc. All rights reserved.

hemostasis and a familiarity with the clinical assays and treatments necessary to correct the bleeding diathesis seen in VWD.

STRUCTURE AND FUNCTION OF VON WILLEBRAND FACTOR

VWF is a plasma glycoprotein that plays critical roles in promoting hemostasis by mediating the binding of platelets to collagen, mostly through its interaction with platelet glycoprotein (GPI)-1bα at sites of vessel injury and by stabilizing factor VIII (FVIII) from clearance in the circulation. VWF is the product of the *VWF* gene located in the short arm of chromosome 22. VWF contains a 22 amino acid signal peptide, followed by a 741 amino acid propeptide (commonly referred to as the D1-D2 domains) to ultimately generate a 2050 amino acid mature protein. The propeptide is critical for protein maturation and assembly; it is cleaved and released in equimolar amounts to the mature protein.[3] VWF is primarily synthesized in endothelial cells and megakaryocytes, and is stored in platelet alpha granules and Weibel-Palade bodies in endothelial cells. In terms of protein structure, the classic domain structure of the mature protein is D′-D3-A1-A2-A3-D4-B1-B2-B3-C1-C2-CK, although recent revisions have further segmented the protein into far more domains based on recent findings and correlation to function.[4] The different domains of VWF equip it with its varied functions in vivo. Collagen binding is primarily mediated by the A1 and A3 domains; platelet-binding function is primarily mediated by the A1 and C1-C2 domains, and FVIII binding is primarily mediated by the D′D3 domain.[4]

VWF has a unique ability to multimerize, in which individual VWF monomers undergo tail-to-tail dimerization in the C-terminus in the endoplasmic reticulum before N-terminal linkage via disulfide bonds at cysteine residues in the Golgi network.[5] This remarkable capability allows VWF to form a range of complexes, from individual monomers to large multimeric structures. This concept is critically important to the understanding of VWD because its multimeric structure is correlated with function, whereby increased large multimeric structure of VWD correspond with increased hemostatic ability. Abnormalities in multimer structure can lead to a qualitative defect in VWF (see later discussion). The primary modulator of VWF is ADAMTS13 (a disintegrin and metalloproteinase with a thrombospondin type-1 motif, member 13), which cleaves VWF at the A2 domain when VWF is unraveled under flow conditions. This can result in a change in multimeric distribution and may lead to an increased risk of bleeding with increased ADAMTS13 activity or conversely a predisposition to thrombosis if there is inhibition of ADAMTS13 function via autoantibodies, as seen in thrombotic thrombocytopenia purpura.[6,7]

CLINICAL DIAGNOSTIC CRITERIA FOR VON WILLEBRAND DISEASE

The diagnosis of VWD is made by the combination of (1) signs or symptoms of clinical bleeding and (2) laboratory-based evidence of quantitative or qualitative deficiencies of VWF. VWD is commonly diagnosed in childhood or adolescence, especially for adolescent girls because VWD can lead to significant menorrhagia. However, it is not uncommon for individuals to go many years before diagnosis, thus there should be a high index of suspicion even in adults who present with symptoms of bleeding. MCB is the most common type of clinical bleeding, often manifesting as epistaxis, oral bleeding, purpura, petechiae, menorrhagia, and gastrointestinal bleeding. To standardize the reporting and consideration of varied bleeding symptoms, the International Society of Thrombosis and Haemostasis (ISTH) subcommittee on VWF has published generalized guidelines on bleeding symptoms to be reviewed when considering the diagnosis of VWD.[8] Further research has led to the development of validated questionnaires that can screen individuals for a diagnosis of VWD. These question-naires, often referred to as bleeding scores or bleeding assessment tools, have been shown to have relatively high sensitivities (85%–100%) and specificity (69%–87%). Most bleeding assessment tools reported to date demonstrate high negative predictive value.[9–11] They are often time-consuming and may have fundamental limi-tations in the pediatric population (in which most patients may have not undergone he-mostatic challenges), although condensed and pediatric-specific versions have been validated for clinical use.[12,13] To date, bleeding questionnaires have had limited suc-cess to accurately predict bleeding, although in a recent report it was shown that a bleeding score of greater than 10 predicted future clinical bleeding in a cohort of pa-tients with VWD.[14] Despite these potential limitations, bleeding questionnaires offer a standardized, comprehensive approach to the assessment of clinical bleeding symp-toms and are effective in assessing the need for further evaluation for VWD.

LABORATORY-BASED DIAGNOSTIC CRITERIA FOR VON WILLEBRAND DISEASE
Common Assays

As previously mentioned, the diagnosis of VWD requires the presence of clinical criteria, as well as laboratory-based evidence of VWF deficits. After a thorough history and physical, many clinicians will order both common and specialized laboratory tests to diagnose VWD.

Common laboratory testing in the evaluation for VWD includes a complete blood count, specifically to assess the platelet count and hematocrit, as well as the pro-thrombin time and the partial thromboplastin time. These tests are not likely to be pre-dictive in the diagnosis of VWD except in certain rare types of VWD, such as type 2N, 2B, and 3 (see later discussion). Another common assay widely used is the closure time in the Platelet Function Analyzer (PFA 100, Siemens, Tarrytown, NY), which tests the ability of platelets to adhere to a collagen-epinephrine–coated or collagen-adenosine diphosphate–coated aperture and generate a platelet clot. The PFA100 has been shown to have some efficacy in screening for VWD but it is unable to differ-entiate quantitative versus qualitative deficiencies of VWF.[15–18] Given the inability of these common screening tests to reliably and specifically identify deficiencies in VWF, if VWD is suspected, further VWF-specific testing is always recommended.

von Willebrand Factor–Specific Assays

von Willebrand factor to antigen
The VWF:antigen (Ag) level (VWF:Ag) measures the total amount of VWF protein pre-sent in plasma samples and has been traditionally performed via enzyme-linked immunosorbent assays (ELISA). However, more recently, many manufacturers have switched to latex immunoassay (LIA) testing to facilitate more rapid testing and ease of use. Normal values are typically between 50 and 200 IU/dL. Levels less than 50 IU/dL are considered to be low, although many national and international guidelines suggest that only levels less than 30 IU/dL should be considered diagnostic of VWD.

Platelet-dependent von Willebrand factor activity measurements The ISTH subcom-mittee on VWF recently published nomenclature guidelines on platelet-dependent VWF activity measurements.[19] Overall, these measurements compromise a wide range of assays (all used in the clinical setting) that include

1. VWF:ristocetin cofactor (RCo) assay (VWF:RCo), which uses the antibiotic ristoce-tin to activate VWF and spontaneously agglutinate platelets as a measure of VWF

function. This test is commonly used although it has been shown to have several limitations, including a known sensitivity to a specific VWF polymorphism (D1472H) that makes VWF nonreactive to ristocetin but does not alter its in vivo activity.[20] The presence of this polymorphism, which is highly prevalent in African Americans, commonly leads to a misdiagnosis of VWD despite having no clinical significance.

2. VWF to ristocetin-triggered GPIb–binding assays use ristocetin to activate VWF; however, instead of using platelets to detect VWF-A1-GPIb binding, a recombinant GPIb fragment is used. This assay was shown to have high correlation with traditional VWF/RCo assays and eliminates the concerns of platelet-dependent variation in the measurement of platelet-dependent VWF activity.

3. VWF to gain-of-function mutant GPIb binding assays are a further advancement to the use of recombinant GPIb fragments instead of platelets. It involves the use of a gain-of-function mutation in GPIb to eliminate the need for ristocetin to activate VWF because the gain-of-function mutation spontaneously binds to VWF. This assay has demonstrated excellent correlation with standard VWF/RCo assays.

4. VWF to monoclonal antibody binding-based VWF activity uses a monoclonal antibody the VWF A1 domain to mimic VWF-A1-GPIb-platelet binding. It has been shown to correlate well with VWF/RCo but, because it does not directly measure GPIb binding (as occurs in vivo), there remain concerns about the physiologic nature of this assay.

von Willebrand Factor Multimer Evaluation

Given the effects of multimer status on VWF function, the assessment of VWF multimer size and distribution is critical in certain types of VWD. Multimer analysis, which is technically similar to a western blot, is typically run on sodium dodecyl sulfate agarose gels with agarose concentrations that are varied for specific applications. Many smaller clinical laboratories do not have the technical expertise to conduct these assays; therefore, this testing is often a send-out laboratory evaluation. The typical pattern for VWF multimers is an even distribution of small to large bands that demonstrate a relative even distribution of multimeric sizes of VWF. Certain types of VWF may be represented by changes in multimeric patterns, these changes thus affect hemostatic function. Importantly, multimer evaluation is still qualitative but efforts to standardize the quantification of the assay are ongoing.

von Willebrand Factor Collagen Binding

Another important function to test is the ability of VWF to bind specifically to collagen. Several ELISA-based assays have been developed that assess the ability of VWF to bind to different types of human collagen, such as collagen type 1, 3, 4, and 6.[21] It has also been shown that large multimers are the most active in promoting VWF collagen-binding capacity; therefore, these assays are used as a proxy for VWF multimeric status.[22] Although the optimal use of these assays in the workup of VWD is yet to be determined, they are also used when traditional VWF testing (VWF/Ag, VWF/RCo) are negative despite a strong suspicion for VWD because families with mutations in *VWF* that correspond to collagen-binding defects (commonly in the A1 and A3 domains) have been recently described.[23]

von Willebrand Factor Propeptide

A few specialized laboratories offer VWF propeptide (VWFpp) assay. As previously mentioned, the VWFpp is synthesized and released on an equimolar ratio to the mature VWF, so it can serve as a useful marker for VWF clearance because the increased clearance of VWF that leads to lower levels of plasma VWF, as seen in type 1C VWD, primarily affects the full molecule and not the propeptide. By calculating the VWFpp/VWF:Ag ratio, which should be close to 1:1:1 in most individuals, clinicians can identify those with increased clearance of VWF/Ag as compared with the VWFpp.[3,24]

Stabilizing Factor VIII

FVIII levels play an important diagnostic role in the evaluation of VWD. Because VWF is the carrier for FVIII, protecting it from proteolysis, abnormally low levels of VWF can predispose individuals with VWD to have lower plasma levels of FVIII. In severe forms of VWD, such as type 3 in which there are little to no VWF present, the level of FVIII can be depressed to levels equivalent to moderate or severe hemophilia A.

Factor VIII–Binding Capacity

Although severe deficiency of VWF levels can decrease FVIII levels and mimic hemophilia A, VWD type 2N is the result of mutations in the FVIII-binding domains (D′D3) in VWF and results in normal quantitative and platelet-dependent VWF activity levels but with a severely decreased ability to bind and chaperone FVIII in the plasma.[25] The VWF/FVIIIB assay measures the ability of a patient's VWF to bind to FVIII in an ELISA-based assay and can be useful in distinguishing VWD type 2N and mild hemophilia.

Low-Dose Ristocetin-Induced Platelet Aggregation

The low-dose ristocetin-induced platelet aggregation (LD-RIPA) is an assay that is technically similar to the original VWF/RCo, whereby ristocetin is used to spontaneously agglutinate platelets in the presence of VWF in a platelet aggregometer.[26] In the LD-RIPA, the smaller dose of ristocetin as compared with the VWF/RCo is primarily used to test for VWF hyperreactivity, which is seen in type 2B platelet-type VWD (or pseudo-VWD). If patient plasma combined with control platelets demonstrates the increased aggregation, then type 2B VWD is diagnosed. If patient platelets with control plasma demonstrate the increased aggregation, then the more likely diagnosis is platelet-type VWD (or pseudo-VWD).[27]

Laboratory-Based Diagnostic Criteria: Focus on Pediatrics

Although VWD symptoms and diagnostic criteria are not age-specific, there do remain specific factors in the pediatric population that bear further mentioning. First, the lack of significant hemostatic challenges can often render the bleeding questionnaire falsely low in young children. Clinicians who choose to use bleeding questionnaires in the pediatric population are strongly encouraged to use a validated pediatric bleeding questionnaire. Similarly, children are often deemed to be at risk for VWD due to a strong family history of VWD, which often leads to testing at a young age, perhaps before the onset of symptoms. In the situation in which a child is found to have low VWF levels, a strong family history, but no MCB symptoms, published ISTH guidelines suggest that these individuals are labeled as having possible VWD.[8]

In terms of laboratory studies, it is critical to point out that VWF is an acute phase reactant and can be increased in times of exercise, stress, or inflammation.[28,29] Comparably, young children who are frightened in clinical settings or have high anxiety or discomfort for laboratory venous sampling may have higher levels of VWF. Therefore, if there remains a strong suspicion for VWD despite normal levels, repeat testing should be considered once or twice to ensure knowledge of a patient's baseline levels of VWF/Ag and VWF activity.

In terms of clinical symptoms that are highlighted in the pediatric population, epistaxis and menorrhagia are often presenting symptoms, and these often cause the most morbidity. As such, pediatric providers are strongly encouraged to provide anticipatory guidance on what to expect at the onset of menses for individuals with VWD. Finally, relatively routine procedures that are commonly done in pediatric populations, such as dental extraction, tonsillectomy, and adenoidectomy, are often the most extreme hemostatic challenges for patients in this age range. The propensity of VWD to affect areas of mucosal tissue contributes to the increased morbidity that can be seen with these otherwise common procedures. Clinicians should plan appropriate medical treatment plans, in conjunction with pediatric hematologists, to ensure effective medical interventions (**Fig. 1**).

VON WILLEBRAND DISEASE CLASSIFICATION

Laboratory findings help classify the different types of VWD and, although most of them are treated similarly, there are unique clinical and diagnostic criteria for certain types that make classification important in clinical management.

Quantitative Deficiencies of von Willebrand Disease

Type 1 von Willebrand disease
Type 1 VWD is the most common form of VWD, comprising 60% to 70% of VWD with levels that are less than 40 IU/dL (often <30 IU/dL). It is characterized by symmetric decreases in VWF/Ag and platelet-dependent VWF activity[30] with a ratio of VWF/RCo to VWF/Ag that is often greater than 0.6. It is usually inherited in an autosomal dominant manner and the mechanism of disease is mostly due to a dominant negative effect. There is normal multimer distribution but often with decreased intensity of all bands due to the overall decreased amount of VWF protein. The pathophysiology of

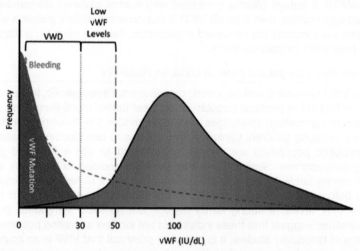

Fig. 1. Distribution of VWF levels in the general population. The distribution of VWF in the population is a continuum but is influenced by the ABO blood type. Individuals with VWF levels less than 30 IU/dL are more likely to have VWF mutations, as demonstrated in gray shading, and as VWF levels go down the risk of bleeding increases. (*Adapted from* Sadler JE. Low von Willebrand factor: sometimes a risk factor and sometimes a disease. Hematology Am Soc Hematol Educ Program 2009:107; with permission.)

type 1 VWD is commonly highlighted by packaging, secretion, or trafficking defects of the VWF protein. Contrary to some other types of VWD, further specialized testing is rarely required in type 1 VWD.

Type 1C von Willebrand disease

Type 1-clearance (type 1C) VWD exhibits unique laboratory and clinical characteristics. Type 1C VWD is the result of increased VWF clearance that leads to low VWF levels and a shortened half-life of the protein.[3] One treatment option available for VWD, 1-desamino-8-D-arginine vasopressin (DDAVP), increases endogenous release of VWF. However, due to the shortened half-life of VWF in type 1C, the effect can be transient and may not be an effective therapeutic option. The diagnosis of type 1C VWD often requires evaluation of VWF clearance by determining the ratio of the VWFpp/VWF/Ag, as previously mentioned.[31]

Type 3 von Willebrand disease

Type 3 VWD is characterized by severe deficiency of VWF that leads to significantly low VWF/Ag, platelet-dependent VWF activity, and low FVIII levels.[32] Patients present with the classic MCB pattern of VWD but also with deep muscle and joint bleeds that are characteristic of hemophilia. Most patients with VWD Type 3 exhibit recessive or compound heterozygous mutations in *VWF*.

Low von Willebrand factor levels

Patients with MCB and VWF levels between 30 and 50 IU/dL are usually characterized as belonging to the group of patients with low VWF levels. It is known that VWF levels less than 50 IU/dL likely represent a risk factor for MCB, with very low levels (<30 IU/dL) presenting the highest risk for bleeding complications.[33] Interestingly, most individuals in the general population with VWF levels between 30 and 50 IU/dL do not bleed, suggesting that other factors contribute to bleeding. Patients in the low-VWF level cohort, in contrast to those with VWD, usually do not have mutations in the *VWF* gene, leading to the hypothesis that alternative mechanisms are modifying VWF levels in these patients. The best characterized modifier of VWF levels is the ABO blood type. Individuals with blood type O have 25% lower levels than those with blood type A, B, or AB.[34] Interestingly, 14% of individuals with blood type O have VWF levels lower than 50 IU/dL. Other mechanisms that have been demonstrated to affect VWF levels involve increased clearance due to changes in glycosylation or carbohydrate processing.[35] Although the treatment of patients in this group is often similar to those with VWD, the classification of these patients is critical not only on a large scale for comparative studies or clinical trials but also on an individual level for clinical situations, such as enrollment in military service or athletics, in which individuals may be barred from participating based on historical diagnoses.

Qualitative Deficiencies of von Willebrand Factor

The qualitative deficiencies of VWF comprise type 2 VWD although the specific mechanistic deficiency highly depends on the location of the mutation.

Type 2A von Willebrand disease

Type 2A is the most common subtype of type 2 VWD and represents a functional deficit of VWF due to the loss of high molecular weight multimers due to either increased susceptibility to ADAMTS13 cleavage or abnormal multimer formation before endothelial cell release. Typical laboratory findings are notable for a platelet-dependent VWF activity level less than 30 IU/dL with a slightly low or normal VWF/Ag level; the ratio of VWF/RCo to VWF/Ag is usually less than 0.6. The multimeric pattern demonstrates the loss of high molecular weight multimers with preservation of the smaller multimers.

Type 2B and platelet-type (or pseudo) von Willebrand disease

Type 2B VWD is characterized by a gain-of-function mutation in *VWF* that increases the binding of the A1 domain to platelet GPIbα.[26] Although this may seem to be beneficial for promoting hemostasis, in vivo VWF-platelet aggregates are cleared from the circulation, which leads to overall decrease in the plasma VWF and significant loss of the high molecular weight multimers. In addition to VWF-specific abnormalities, thrombocytopenia (due to platelet clearance) can add an additional risk factor for bleeding, although thrombocytopenia is not universally present.[36]

For those individuals with type 2B VWD who do not seem to respond well to VWF concentrates, it is critically important to further investigate the possibility of the rare condition platelet-type (or pseudo) VWD.[27] In this particular subtype, the mutation does not reside in the VWF A1 domain but rather in the platelet GPIbα (*GP1BA*). As previously mentioned, the use of the LD-RIPA assay is crucial in this differentiation. When conducting an LD-RIPA assay, if increased aggregation is seen with patient plasma (a source of VWF), then the diagnosis is likely to be type 2B VWD. Conversely, if the increased aggregation is seen with patient platelets (likely due to a gain-of-function mutation in *GP1BA*), then the diagnosis is platelet-type or pseudo-VWD. DNA sequencing of *VWF* and *GP1BA* will confirm the diagnosis. Although they will present very similarly to those with traditional type 2B VWD, the bleeding phenotype in these patients is ameliorated by the transfusion of platelets as opposed to VWF-specific therapy.

Type 2M von Willebrand disease

Type 2M VWD is a result of loss-of-function mutations in the platelet-binding region of VWF, most commonly in the A1 domain. These mutations create decreased platelet-dependent VWF activity with a low VWF/RCo to VWF/Ag ratio but, in comparison with type 2A VWD, the multimer pattern in this type is normal because the defect is isolated to the A1 domain platelet-binding capacity. Due to the variability that can be seen in measurements of platelet-dependent VWF activity, this type can be often confused with type 1 VWD because the differentiating value is only a lower level of VWF activity. Thus, a poorly handled sample or the relatively high coefficient of variation seen in VWF activity can lead to falsely low VWF activity levels in a type 1 VWD patient, mimicking type 2 disease.

Type 2N von Willebrand disease

Type 2N VWD is a unique qualitative deficit of VWF whereby the FVIII-binding capacity of VWF is significantly decreased.[25] Patients exhibit normal platelet-dependent VWF function and normal VWF/Ag and VWF activity levels but severely decreased FVIII levels in plasma due to increased proteolysis, which could lead to the misdiagnosis of mild hemophilia A. Symptomatic individuals with type 2N VWD are usually heterozygous for mutations in the D'D3 region of VWF, which is the FVIII-binding region and heterozygotes for a type 1 VWD mutation.[37] Because there is a significant clinical overlap with mild hemophilia A, individuals with mild hemophilia A without significant family history, those with affected female family members, or those who have unusual shortened FVIII half-lives after factor replacement, should be tested for type 2N VWD via the VWF/FVIIIB.

von Willebrand Disease Classification: Effect of Age on von Willebrand Factor Levels

Although the classification of VWD does not significantly change as individuals transition from childhood to adulthood, an aspect that can affect the diagnosis of VWD is the natural history of VWF levels increasing with age; the average increase is approximately 10 IU/dL per decade of life.[34] The underlying mechanism that drives the increased VWF levels in older adults is unclear but is thought to be associated with other changes with aging, such as increased inflammation and changes in epigenetic patterning. As such, individuals who were diagnosed as type 1 VWD as children may in time become low-VWF level individuals later in life, with normalization to the lower population levels in their elderly years (**Table 1**).

GENETIC TESTING IN VON WILLEBRAND DISEASE

VWD mostly follows Mendelian inheritance patterns, with most VWD cases (type 1 and most of type 2) being autosomal dominant. This autosomal dominant pattern often causes dominant-negative effects in which the presence of mutated VWF significantly affects quantity or function of the wild-type VWF due to alterations in packaging or multimeric structure.[38] Type 3 VWD is often inherited in an autosomal recessive pattern and is usually represented by compound heterozygosity of 2 type 1 VWD mutations.

The use of next-generation sequencing has significantly improved the ability to sequence large regions of the genome at decreased cost. Several large studies are ongoing in which these modern genomic techniques are being used to identify new *VWF* variants and associate them with cellular, animal, and human clinical phenotypes. Therefore, a great deal of information is being generated. However, at this point, genetic testing is indicated only in a few key situations, especially in those situations in which genetic counseling or therapeutic management may change based on the results of findings. For example, individuals with type 3 VWD and with large deletions may be at higher risk for developing inhibitors after exposure to exogenous VWF.[39] In certain cases of VWD, such as in type 2B VWD, mutations may be clustered and specific sequencing of a few domains may prove to be more cost-efficient and time-efficient than sequential specialized VWD testing.

TREATMENT OF VON WILLEBRAND DISEASE

The basic treatment of VWD is focused on (1) increasing the amount of functional VWF available for hemostasis and (2) providing adjunctive therapies to promote or stabilize hemostasis (**Table 2**).

Increase in von Willebrand Factor

DDAVP (desmopressin acetate) is a synthetic version of vasopressin that can be administered either intravenous or intranasal. DDAVP stimulates endothelial cells to release VWF from Weibel-Palade bodies, increasing the plasma concentration of VWF. Responses to DDAVP are typically 2-fold to 4-fold the basal level of plasma VWF and DDAVP can be used to safely manage situations in which short-term increases in VWF are necessary for mild to moderate hemostatic needs; that is, simple dental extractions, nosebleeds, and menorrhagia.[39] Due to its function primarily as a signal to release VWF, repeated doses of DDAVP may cause tachyphylaxis. Side effects of DDAVP involve hyponatremia due to water retention (strict precautions should be followed on fluid intake and patients should be guided on the signs or symptoms of hyponatremia, particularly in children), as well as facial flushing and headaches. It is

Table 1
von Willebrand disease classification

	VWF/Ag	Platelet-Dependent VWF Activity	Ratio of Platelet-Dependent VWF Activity to VWF/Ag	FVIII	Multimer Pattern	Collagen Binding Ratio (Ratio of VWF Collagen Binding to VWF/Ag)	Notes
Type 1	Mild decrease	Mild decrease	>0.6	Normal to mild decrease	Normal, decreased band intensity due to decreased protein	>0.5	Typically VWF/Ag and VWF activity <30–40
Type 1C	Mild decrease	Mild decrease	>0.6	Normal to mild decrease	Normal, decreased band intensity due to decreased protein	>0.5	Increased VWF clearance or increased VWFpp/VWF/Ag ratio
Type 3	Severe decrease	Severe decrease	>0.6	Severe decrease	Absent	>0.5	Severe bleeding
Low VWF Levels	Mild decrease	Mild decrease	>0.6	Normal to mild decrease	Normal	>0.5	Typically VWF/Ag and VWF activity between 30–50
Type 2A	Mild decrease	Moderate decrease	<0.6	Normal to mild decrease	Absence of high molecular weight multimers	<0.5	Increased proteolysis by ADAMTS13 or decrease secretion
Type 2B	Mild decrease	Moderate decrease	<0.6	Normal to mild decrease	Absence of high molecular weight multimers	<0.5	Thrombocytopenia often noted Consider platelet-type VWD if not responsive to VWF concentrates
Type 2M	Mild decrease	Moderate decrease	<0.6	Normal to mild decrease	Normal	<0.5	No GP1b binding or mutations in the collagen-binding domain of VWF mimic type 2M
Type 2N	Mild decrease	Mild decrease	>0.6	Mild to moderate decrease	Normal	>0.5	Decreased FVIII binding

Table 2
von Willebrand disease treatment

Brand Name	Vonvendi	Wilate	Humate-P	Alphanate
Manufacturer	Shire	Octapharma	CSL Behring	Grifols
Initial approval date	2015	2009	1986	1978
Source	Recombinant expressed in CHO cells	Plasma-derived	Plasma-derived	Plasma-derived
Sterilization	—	Solvent treatment Terminal dry heat treatment	Cryoprecipitation, additional combination therapy, heat treatment, lyophilization	Solvent treatment Terminal dry heat treatment
Forms and strengths	Lyophilized powder for reconstitution	Lyophilized powder for reconstitution	Lyophilized powder for reconstitution	Lyophilized powder for reconstitution
Vial size (dose in VWF/RCo)	650 or 1300	500 and 1000	600, 1200, 2400	250, 500, 1000, 1500 (based on FVIII) Vials are colabeled with VWF/RCo amounts
Storage	2–8°C or room temperature for 12 mo	2–8°C for 36 mo or 6 mo at room temperature	25°C for 36 mo	2 and 8°C or <30°C for up to 2 mo
VWF/Rco/FVIII	No FVIII	1:1	2.4:1	Varied

usually recommended that individuals who are candidates for using DDAVP as a therapeutic option undergo a DDAVP challenge or testing to ensure that (1) there is an adequate response to DDAVP in terms of VWF increase (10% of patients do not respond) and (2) to ensure that the effect does not rapidly dissipate as seen in type 1C VWD.[40] Finally, clinicians and patients should be aware that the concentration used for intranasal use in VWD is higher than that used for the treatment of enuresis.

The administration of VWF concentrates is recommended for patients who do not respond to DDAVP or for patients who need sustained normal levels of VWF in situations such as trauma or surgeries. Although cryoprecipitate contains VWF, commercially available concentrates enriched for VWF are preferred owing to their portability, decreased risk of viral transmission, and more consistent dosing. Almost all VWF concentrates are plasma-derived and have varying amounts of VWF as compared with FVIII in their product. Many of these products may be dual-approved for the treatment of VWD and hemophilia A.[41] When using a product that contains both FVIII and VWF, dosing in VWD should be based on the standardized VWF/RCo available in the product and not the FVIII. Because different products have different VWF/FVIII ratios, it is imperative that clinicians using these products be familiar with the general ratios of each product to avoid confusion and subtherapeutic or supratherapeutic levels in varying clinical situations. A recombinant VWF product has been recently approved by the US Food and Drug Administration for use in VWD.[42] This product does not contain any FVIII, thus clinicians are advised to consider whether their patients may need a dose of FVIII in addition to VWF initially if their FVIII levels are low at baseline.[42] Over time, most individuals who receive recombinant VWD that does not contain FVIII will stabilize out to normal levels of FVIII because the increased amount of VWF will then chaperone the patient's endogenous FVIII (which should be produced at a normal amount). Most individuals require at least 50 IU/dL for normal hemostasis and higher levels close to 100 IU/dL for invasive surgical procedures.

The use of intravenous concentrates and DDAVP has dramatically improved the ability to rapidly correct VWF deficiencies and achieve hemostasis; however, caution must be exercised when using such medications to not drive VWF levels, as well as FVIII levels, to supratherapeutic levels that may potentiate thrombosis. This is particularly relevant for older adults.[43] Thus, when using these medications, consideration should be given to the dose and frequency, and, if necessary, follow-up laboratory evaluations, to ensure that VWF/FVIII levels are in the appropriate range.

Prophylaxis

Regular prophylactic schedules and extensive collaborative research has demonstrated that individuals with significant bleeding phenotypes, especially those with type 3 or severe type 2 VWD, can benefit from regular infusions of VWF concentrates.[44,45] The optimal dose and schedule of prophylaxis has not been clearly defined; however, large multicenter clinical trials are underway to assess this question.[46]

Adjunctive Therapies

Although the correction of either quantitative or qualitative deficiency of VWF focuses on increasing the amount of functional VWF, there are several other therapies that are beneficial in the treatment of VWD. Chief among these are the antifibrinolytic agents aminocaproic acid and tranexamic acid. Both of these agents are analogues of the amino acid lysine and inhibit the activation of plasminogen to plasmin at the site of active clot formation. Common uses for antifibrinolytic agents are mild to moderate bleeding situations, such as epistaxis, mild oral bleeding, or menorrhagia.[40] They are often used as an adjunctive therapy in addition to DDAVP or VWF concentrates at times of surgery or childbirth.

Treatment of von Willebrand Disease: Focus on Pediatrics

In the pediatric context, there are a few important considerations to treatment of VWD. First, with young children it is often difficult to ascertain and appropriately coordinate the timing of intranasal DDAVP delivery and inhalation. For this reason, many centers delay the use of intranasal DDAVP until the child demonstrates the developmental ability to coordinate and follow such coordinated tasks. Second, there have been reports of hyponatremia seizures in children younger than 2 years of age taking Amicar; therefore, its use should be limited in this population unless serial sodium measurements are performed. Finally, tranexamic acid is currently only available in tablet form and the use of this medication in younger children may be limited by their inability to orally take this form.

SUMMARY

The diagnosis and treatment of VWD has improved significantly over the last decades. New diagnostic tests, as well as novel treatments, give clinicians and patients more options. Despite advancements in the biologic function of VWF and the pathophysiology of VWD, there remain many unanswered questions worthy of further research. From a clinical perspective, further understanding into the variation of VWF levels and individuals with low VWF levels will further understanding in the contribution of VWF to hemostasis.

REFERENCES

1. Willebrand von E. Hereditar pseudohemofili. Finska Lakarsallskapets 1926;67: 7–112.
2. Ng C, Motto DG, Di Paola J. Diagnostic approach to von Willebrand disease. Blood 2015;125(13):2029–37.
3. Haberichter SL, Haberichter SL, Castaman G, et al. Identification of type 1 von Willebrand disease patients with reduced von Willebrand factor survival by assay of the VWF propeptide in the European study: molecular and clinical markers for the diagnosis and management of type 1 VWD (MCMDM-1VWD). Blood 2008; 111(10):4979–85.
4. Zhou Y-F, Eng ET, Zhu J, et al. Sequence and structure relationships within von Willebrand factor. Blood 2012;120(2):449–58.
5. Fowler WE, Fretto LJ, Hamilton KK, et al. Substructure of human von Willebrand factor. J Clin Invest 1985;76(4):1491–500.
6. Fujikawa K, Suzuki H, McMullen B, et al. Purification of human von Willebrand factor-cleaving protease and its identification as a new member of the metalloproteinase family. Blood 2001;98(6):1662–6.
7. Dong J-F, Moake JL, Bernardo A, et al. ADAMTS-13 rapidly cleaves newly secreted ultralarge von Willebrand factor multimers on the endothelial surface under flowing conditions. Blood 2002;100(12):4033–9.
8. Sadler JE, Rodeghiero F. Provisional criteria for the diagnosis of VWD type 1: on behalf of the ISTH SSC Subcommittee on von Willebrand factor. J Thromb Haemost 2005;3(4):775–7.
9. Tosetto A, Rodeghiero F, Castaman G, et al. A quantitative analysis of bleeding symptoms in type 1 von Willebrand disease: results from a multicenter European study (MCMDM-1 VWD). J Thromb Haemost 2006;4(4):766–73.
10. Tosetto A, Castaman G, Plug I, et al. Prospective evaluation of the clinical utility of quantitative bleeding severity assessment in patients referred for hemostatic evaluation. J Thromb Haemost 2011;9(6):1143–8.
11. O'Brien SH. Bleeding scores: are they really useful? Hematol Am Soc Hematol Educ Program 2012;2012:152–6.
12. Bowman M, Mundell G, Grabell J, et al. Generation and validation of the condensed MCMDM-1VWD bleeding questionnaire for von Willebrand disease. J Thromb Haemost 2008;6(12):2062–6.
13. Bowman M, Riddel J, Rand ML, et al. Evaluation of the diagnostic utility for von Willebrand disease of a pediatric bleeding questionnaire. J Thromb Haemost 2009;7(8):1418–21.
14. Federici AB, Bucciarelli P, Castaman G, et al. The bleeding score predicts clinical outcomes and replacement therapy in adults with von Willebrand disease. Blood 2014;123(26):4037–44.
15. Dean JA, Blanchette VS, Carcao MD, et al. von Willebrand disease in a pediatric-based population–comparison of type 1 diagnostic criteria and use of the PFA-100 and a von Willebrand factor/collagen-binding assay. Thromb Haemost 2000;84(3):401–9.

16. Posan E, McBane RD, Grill DE, et al. Comparison of PFA-100 testing and bleeding time for detecting platelet hypofunction and von Willebrand disease in clinical practice. Thromb Haemost 2003;90(3):483–90.

17. Castaman G, Tosetto A, Goodeve A, et al. The impact of bleeding history, von Willebrand factor and PFA-100® on the diagnosis of type 1 von Willebrand disease: results from the European study MCMDM-1VWD. Br J Haematol 2010;151(3): 245–51.

18. Cattaneo M, Federici AB, Lecchi A, et al. Evaluation of the PFA-100 system in the diagnosis and therapeutic monitoring of patients with von Willebrand disease. Thromb Haemost 1999;82(1):35–9.

19. Bodó I, Eikenboom J, Montgomery R, et al. Platelet-dependent von Willebrand factor activity. Nomenclature and methodology: communication from the SSC of the ISTH. J Thromb Haemost 2015;13(7):1345–50.

20. Flood VH, Friedman KD, Gill JC, et al. No increase in bleeding identified in type 1 VWD subjects with D1472H sequence variation. Blood 2013;121(18):3742–4.

21. Flood VH, Gill JC, Christopherson PA, et al. Comparison of type I, type III and type VI collagen binding assays in diagnosis of von Willebrand disease. J Thromb Haemost 2012;10(7):1425–32.

22. Flood VH, Flood VH, Gill JC, et al. Collagen binding provides a sensitive screen for variant von Willebrand disease. Clin Chem 2013;59(4):684–91.

23. Flood VH, Lederman CA, Wren JS, et al. Absent collagen binding in a VWF A3 domain mutant: utility of the VWF: CB in diagnosis of VWD. J Thromb Haemost 2010;8(6):1431–3.

24. Haberichter SL, Balistreri M, Christopherson P, et al. Assay of the von Willebrand factor (VWF) propeptide to identify patients with type 1 von Willebrand disease with decreased VWF survival. Blood 2006;108(10):3344–51.

25. Mazurier C, Dieval J, Jorieux S, et al. A new von Willebrand factor (vWF) defect in a patient with factor VIII (FVIII) deficiency but with normal levels and multimeric patterns of both plasma and platelet vWF. Characterization of abnormal vWF/FVIII interaction. Blood 1990;75(1):20–6.

26. Ruggeri ZM, Pareti FI, Mannucci PM, et al. Heightened interaction between platelets and factor VIII/von Willebrand factor in a new subtype of von Willebrand's disease. N Engl J Med 1980;302(19):1047–51.

27. Miller JL, Kupinski JM, Castella A, et al. von Willebrand factor binds to platelets and induces aggregation in platelet-type but not type IIB von Willebrand disease. J Clin Invest 1983;72(5):1532–42.

28. Branchford BR, Ruegg K, Villalobos-Menuey E, et al. FVIII/VWF ratio is not a reliable predictor of VWD in children. Pediatr Blood Cancer 2014;61(5):936–9.

29. Stibbe J. Effect of exercise on F VIII-complex: proportional increase of ristocetin cofactor (Von Willebrand factor) and F VIII-AGN, but disproportional increase of F VIII-AHF. Thromb Res 1977;10(1):163–8.

30. Castaman G, Federici AB, Rodeghiero F, et al. Von Willebrand's disease in the year 2003: towards the complete identification of gene defects for correct diagnosis and treatment. Haematologica 2003;88(1):94–108.

31. Haberichter SL. von Willebrand factor propeptide: biology and clinical utility. Blood 2015;126(15):1753–61.

32. Eikenboom JC. Congenital von Willebrand disease type 3: clinical manifestations, pathophysiology and molecular biology. Best Pract Res Clin Haematol 2001; 14(2):365–79.

33. Sadler JE. Low von Willebrand factor: sometimes a risk factor and sometimes a disease. Hematology Am Soc Hematol Educ Program 2009;106–12.

34. Gill JC, Endres-Brooks J, Bauer PJ, et al. The effect of ABO blood group on the diagnosis of von Willebrand disease. Blood 1987;69(6):1691–5.
35. Casari C, Lenting PJ, Wohner N, et al. Clearance of von Willebrand factor. J Thromb Haemost 2013;11(Suppl 1):202–11.
36. Federici AB, Mannucci PM, Castaman G, et al. Clinical and molecular predictors of thrombocytopenia and risk of bleeding in patients with von Willebrand disease type 2B: a cohort study of 67 patients. Blood 2009;113(3):526–34.
37. Mazurier C, Goudemand J, Hilbert L, et al. Type 2N von Willebrand disease: clinical manifestations, pathophysiology, laboratory diagnosis and molecular biology. Best Pract Res Clin Haematol 2001;14(2):337–47.
38. Sadler JE, Budde U, Eikenboom JCJ, et al. Update on the pathophysiology and classification of von Willebrand disease: a report of the Subcommittee on von Willebrand Factor. J Thromb Haemost 2006;4(10):2103–14.
39. Mannucci PM. Desmopressin (DDAVP) in the treatment of bleeding disorders: the first 20 years. Blood 1997;90(7):2515–21.
40. Nichols WL, Hultin MB, James AH, et al. von Willebrand disease (VWD): evidence-based diagnosis and management guidelines, the National Heart, Lung, and Blood Institute (NHLBI) Expert Panel report (USA). Haemophilia 2008;14(2):171–232.
41. Budde U, Metzner HJ, Müller H-G. Comparative analysis and classification of von Willebrand factor/factor VIII concentrates: impact on treatment of patients with von Willebrand disease. Semin Thromb Hemost 2006;32(6):626–35.
42. Ragni M, Obermann-Slupetzky O, Fritsch S, et al. Hemostatic efficacy, safety, and pharmacokinetics of a recombinant von Willebrand factor in severe von Willebrand disease. Blood 2015;126(17):2038–46.
43. Mannucci PM. Venous thromboembolism in von Willebrand disease. Thromb Haemost 2002;88(3):378–9.
44. Berntorp E. Prophylaxis and treatment of bleeding complications in von Willebrand disease type 3. Semin Thromb Hemost 2006;32(6):621–5.
45. Berntorp E. Prophylaxis in von Willebrand disease. Haemophilia 2008;14(Suppl 5):47–53.
46. Abshire T, Cox-Gill J, Kempton CL, et al. Prophylaxis escalation in severe von Willebrand disease: a prospective study from the von Willebrand disease prophylaxis network. J Thromb Haemost 2015;13(9):1585–9.

Abnormal Uterine Bleeding in Young Women with Blood Disorders

Kathryn E. Dickerson, MD[a], Neethu M. Menon, MD[b],
Ayesha Zia, MD[a],*

KEYWORDS

- Adolescents • Blood disorders • Heavy periods • Abnormal uterine bleeding

KEY POINTS

- Abnormal uterine bleeding is common in adolescents with blood disorders but remains underrecognized.
- Most data on management approaches is extrapolated from adult guidelines.
- A multidisciplinary approach is needed to address gynecologic morbidity associated with blood disorders in young women for optimal outcomes.

INTRODUCTION

Abnormal uterine bleeding (AUB) is common in adolescents.[1] Immaturity of the hypothalamic pituitary ovarian axis is the most common cause of AUB in this age group.[2] Certain aspects of underlying inherited or acquired blood disorders, as discussed herein, exacerbate the "expected" hormonal imbalance at this age, thereby increasing the morbidity of the underlying problem.[3,4] Even though blood disorders may induce AUB, uterine structural and/or endocrine abnormalities tend to be overlooked in the presence of a blood disorder.[5] A multifactorial etiology demands a collaborative approach between hematologists and gynecologists or adolescent medicine physicians.[6,7] In this article, we discuss the management of AUB in adolescents within 4 clinical contexts: AUB while on anticoagulant therapy, and with inherited bleeding disorders (BDs), bleeding management with cytopenias (specifically, thrombocytopenia), and in sickle cell disease (SCD). Throughout, areas of controversy and opportunities for further research are highlighted.

Disclosure Statement: The authors have no commercial or financial conflict of interests to disclose.

Funding: Funded by: NIH: Grant number(s): 1K23HL132054-01.

[a] Division of Hematology/Oncology, The University of Texas Southwestern, 5323 Harry Hines Boulevard, Dallas, TX 75390, USA; [b] Pediatric Hematology Oncology, Division of Hematology/Oncology, The University of Texas Southwestern, 5323 Harry Hines Boulevard, Dallas, TX 75390, USA

* Corresponding author.

E-mail address: Ayesha.zia@utsouthwestern.edu

There has been a long-standing confusion concerning terminologies and definitions surrounding female reproductive tract bleeding.[5] Menorrhagia, a loosely defined term, is used for heavy menstrual bleeding (HMB). Dysfunctional uterine bleeding is associated with adolescents and often implies anovulatory bleeding. We will use the International Federation of Gynecology and Obstetrics terminologies and classification system throughout this article, and strongly recommend them for use in every day practice.[5] These have been published after years of robust international cooperation and consensus forming in 2011.[5] AUB or HMB are the preferred overarching terms, and the workup of HMB or AUB proceeds within the realm of PALM-COEIN classification, irrespective of age. PALM indicates structural causes—polyp, adenomyosis, leiomyoma, and malignancy—and COEIN indicates nonstructural causes—coagulopathy, ovulatory dysfunction, endometrial, iatrogenic, and not yet classified.[5] HMB is defined as periods lasting more than 7 days, soaking through a pad or tampon in less than 2 hours or soaking through bed clothes, passing clots, and ferritin below normal limits or anemia.[8] AUB refers to any departure from normal uterine bleeding, either in volume or duration of flow, regularity or frequency, and in theory, encompasses HMB.

Abnormal Uterine Bleeding During Treatment of Venous Thromboembolism

The number of adolescents in need of antithrombotic therapy has gradually increased over the past decades.[9] Anticoagulation is associated with AUB in 20% to 70% of patients.[10] One retrospective study of 90 women aged 15 to 49 years found that frequency of HMB increased from 17.8% before anticoagulation to 29.5% thereafter.[11]

Another consideration is that heavy periods, often the reason for hormone-induced venous thromboembolism (VTE) in the first place, are associated with stopping hormonal therapy and may be intensified by anticoagulants. Estrogens are known to increase the risk for VTE 2-fold to 4-fold in a dose-dependent way.[12,13] The risk is also increased with third-generation progestins when compared with the first- or second-generation progestins.[13] Patients with hormone-induced VTE are instructed to discontinue hormones, generally at the time of diagnosis. There is controversy regarding whether discontinuation should be immediate upon diagnosis of the VTE or deferred to the time point of discontinuation of anticoagulant therapy. The former recommendation is found in a World Health Organization publication from 2010, stating that estrogen-containing oral contraceptives (OCs) should not be used, even on established oral anticoagulation.[14] In contrast, the Scientific and Standardization Committee of the International Society on Thrombosis and Haemostasis in a guidance document suggested that hormonal therapy can be continued in selected patients, but that anticoagulants should be continued for the duration of hormonal therapy.[15] This recommendation is based on the premise that the anticoagulant effect trumps the thrombogenic potential of estrogens.

Key implications in this clinical context, therefore, include (a) the risk of recurrence with hormones while on anticoagulation, and (b) medication options for AUB control and pregnancy prevention while on anticoagulants.

Risk of recurrent venous thromboembolism with hormonal therapy while on anticoagulant therapy

The risk of continuing hormonal therapy in women younger than 60 years of age (mean age, 41.3 years) with VTE was investigated in those treated with either low-molecular-weight heparin followed by vitamin K antagonists or with a direct oral anticoagulant, Rivaroxaban, in one landmark study: 1888 women were analyzed, evenly distributed between the 2 anticoagulant regimens.[16] Of those, 475 women were taking concomitant hormonal treatment, either remaining on it despite the VTE diagnosis (n = 402) or initiated during the study period (n = 73). The key finding of this study was the similar incidence rate during the time periods at risk, among those on hormonal therapy (3.7% per year) and those off/without hormonal therapy (4.7% per year), even after adjustment for age, prior hormonal therapy, assigned anticoagulant treatment, and cancer at baseline. In addition, there was no difference in the crude incidence densities between women taking estrogen versus progestin (3.7% per year and 3.8% per year, respectively), suggesting that the patient may continue with the type of hormones of her choice while on anticoagulation. Only 7 VTE events occurred on hormonal therapy (4 on estrogen-containing and 3 on progestin-only therapy).[16] Despite these findings, there is reluctance among physicians to prescribe estrogen-containing OCs to women on anticoagulation. Moreover, there are no data to guide such management decisions in adolescents with AUB on anticoagulation. A recent systematic review highlighted that anticoagulant dose reduction or temporal cessation for controlling AUB while on anticoagulation was associated with a greater risk of recurrent VTE, although this was based on findings from only 1 study in this systematic review.[10]

Treatment options for abnormal uterine bleeding while on anticoagulant therapy

Treatment of AUB/HMB in adolescents taking anticoagulants, like in older women, depends on comorbidities, hormonal imbalance, either owing to immaturity of the hypothalamic pituitary ovarian axis or polycystic ovarian syndrome, the need for contraception, and, rarely, the presence of structural uterine changes. Other general principles, specific to adolescents, are discussed in **Box 1**. In women of childbearing potential who receive vitamin K antagonists (eg, warfarin), adequate contraception is required because these drugs cross the placenta, potentially leading to bleeding in the fetus and/or severe embryopathy.[17] The direct oral anticoagulants, currently in phase III trials in pediatrics, have as yet unknown adverse effects on fetal

---

Box 1
General principles for AUB management on anticoagulation

- Assess pregnancy status before initiating anticoagulation, especially, if there are plans to transition to VKAs or DOACs (either in the setting of a clinical trial or in anticipation of meeting FDA-approved age criteria for DOAC use during therapy duration).

- Assess and document menstrual bleeding pattern (frequency, duration, flow, and volume) before initiating anticoagulation.

- Consider hormonal suppression or regulation at the time of VTE diagnosis, if there is a history of AUB or HMB before VTE, irrespective of whether VTE was hormone induced or not.

- Assess anticoagulation (LMWH anti-Xa or INR) and hematology parameters (hemoglobin and ferritin) at the time AUB or HMB is reported.

- Determine if current anticoagulant needs to be changed in view of AUB or HMB (eg, fluctuating INRs with warfarin, or a different DOAC).

- Initiate treatment for AUB based on personal preference and needs.

- Consider a multidisciplinary, collaborative management approach, with inclusion of gynecology or adolescent medicine for improved patient outcomes.

Abbreviations: AUB, abnormal uterine bleeding; DOAC, direct oral anticoagulant; HMB, heavy menstrual bleeding; FDA, US Food and Drug Administration; INR, international normalized ratio; LMWH, low-molecular-weight heparin; VKA, vitamin K antagonist; VTE, venous thromboembolism.

development.[18] Even without the teratogenic effects, anticoagulants in therapeutic doses increase the duration and severity of menstrual bleeding, which often requires medical management. In adolescents with AUB on anticoagulants, options such as nonsteroidal antiinflammatory drugs and estrogen-containing OCs, as discussed elsewhere in this article, are either contraindicated or not used. A recent systematic review shows that insertion of a progestin-releasing intrauterine device (IUD) seems to decrease the duration and severity of menses in most women on anticoagulation. The investigators of this review also acquired the clinical judgment of 2 panels of key opinion leaders (10 international AUB and 10 thrombosis experts) and compared expert opinion to current practice patterns by surveying approximately 300 international physicians (hematology, gynecology, internal medicine cardiology, pulmonology, etc). The expert recommendations were divergent and different in several important points from actual clinical practice, which was quite heterogenous. Only the following aspects of combined expert opinion analyses met the predefined threshold of 70% or greater agreement: (1) hormonal contraception was not judged to be a risk factor for recurrent VTE during active/ongoing anticoagulation, (2) progestin-only pills and progestin-releasing IUDs were suggested to be best options for patients wishing to initiate contraception on anticoagulants, (3) tranexamic acid was suggested to be useful for treatment of anticoagulant associated AUB, and (4) anticoagulant dose reduction and inferior vena cava filter placement were not recommended management options for AUB, especially not in the first month after a VTE.

Invasive approaches such as endometrial ablation are an alternative to hysterectomy in older women with refractory or life-threatening HMB on anticoagulation.[19] However, as opposed to the "general" principles of AUB management in older women that conceivably can be applied to young women with AUB on anticoagulants, invasive management approaches require careful consideration given the lack of recent or any data, respectively.

To summarize, key management points include the following.

- Women of reproductive age may suffer from HMB when treated with anticoagulants. Adequate information regarding this risk should be given to the patient when initiating anticoagulation.
- Women taking oral anticoagulants for VTE may use estrogen or progestin hormonal therapy to control menstrual bleeding without an increased risk for recurrent VTE.[16]
- For women with HMB on anticoagulant therapy, tranexamic acid is an alternative to hormonal therapy to reduce the bleeding. The latter does not provide a contraceptive effect.
- The thrombogenic effect of estrogens does not disappear precipitously upon the discontinuation of estrogen-containing OCs. The World Health Organization Collaborative Study had noted that the effect disappeared 3 months after stopping OCs.[13] It, therefore, seems reasonable to recommend discontinuing OCs or oral estrogen substitution at least 1 month before planned discontinuation of anticoagulation rather than at the same time.
- A collaborative, multidisciplinary approach between thrombosis and AUB experts is paramount for effective health care delivery.

During anticoagulation, adequate measures to control AUB and prevent pregnancy, and reproductive toxicity to a fetus, are indicated for all women with reproductive potential, including adolescents. Research on this subject is desperately needed to guide clinical practice in young women.

ABNORMAL UTERINE BLEEDING IN INHERITED BLEEDING DISORDERS

Menstruation disrupts blood vessels, the restoration of which requires an intact hemostatic system and successful interaction of platelets, clotting factors, and fibrinolytic proteins.[20] Although less likely to present with spontaneous bleeding, inherited BDs can become particularly severe after hemostatic challenges such as surgery, trauma, menses, or childbirth. Mounting evidence suggests that 10% to 62% adolescents with HMB may have an underlying BD (**Table 1**).[7] The average age of women identified with an underlying BD, however, is 35 years. In other words, the diagnosis of a BD is a relatively late one. Wide ranges of reported prevalence, difficulty in discerning normal menstrual bleeding from HMB and the semiempiric use of hormonal therapy makes BDs in adolescents challenging to identify.[21] There have been awareness efforts by the American College of Obstetricians and Gynecologists (ACOG) in 2001, and in 2006, by the American Academy of Pediatrics in collaboration with ACOG advising that hematologic disorders (particularly, von Willebrand disease [VWD]) be considered in HMB, especially at menarche.[22,23] VWD is reviewed in Christopher J. Ng and Jorge Di Paola's article, "Von Willebrand Disease: Diagnostic Strategies and Treatment Options," in this issue. However, despite awareness efforts, BDs remain underdiagnosed in women.[7]

Historically, clinical questions that discriminate individuals with BDs from those without have been bleeding after hemostatic challenges such as tonsillectomy or dental extraction and the presence of a BD in the family; however, such exposures are often absent in the pediatrics. Generic bleeding assessment tools (BATs) that quantify bleeding symptoms in adults improve diagnostic accuracy and predict bleeding phenotype for a variety of BDs.[24–26] The International Society on Thrombosis and Haemostasis BAT was specifically designed to incorporate pediatric-specific bleeding symptoms, including the frequency and severity of bleeding.[27] Even though the International Society on Thrombosis and Haemostasis BAT can discriminate between no BD and a possible BD with acceptable accuracy, it has not been tested in adolescents.[28] The pictorial blood assessment chart (PBAC) is a semiquantitative method and allows women to track the number of pads or tampons during a menstrual period, and the degree of soiling.[29] A score is generated based on that information, and PBAC scores of 100 or greater correlate with 80 mL or more of menstrual blood loss, the classic definition of HMB. The sensitivity and specificity of the PBAC is 86% and 89%, respectively, in adult women with HMB.[30,31] PBAC was evaluated in adolescents.[32] The mean PBAC score for the entire cohort was 195, but notably different when 3 groups were analyzed separately: 362, 136, and 44 for subjects in heavy, normal, or light periods group, respectively. Twenty percent of subjects in the heavy group were diagnosed with a BD, although there were no patients with a BD in the other 2 groups. Although analysis of diagnostic usefulness was not performed, this is the first study in adolescents investigating PBAC.[32] More recently, another HMB specific BAT called the Phillip screening tool was evaluated to screen for BDs in women aged 18 to 50 years with a PBAC score of greater than 100 and a normal pelvic ultrasound examination.[33] This tool has a sensitivity of 89% for a BD. The sensitivity was lower (62%) for the 25 adolescents included in the study. The overall sensitivity improved to 93% by adding iron deficiency, and to 95%, when the PBAC score was increased to greater than 185.[34] The usefulness of this tool is yet to be studied in an exclusive adolescent population.

The initial laboratory evaluation of patients with a suspected BD should start with a complete blood count, review of peripheral blood smear for platelet morphology, prothrombin time, partial thromboplastin time, and optionally either fibrinogen or thrombin time.[35] The ACOG and American Academy of Pediatrics recommend testing for VWD

Table 1

Overview of published prevalence studies of bleeding disorders in adolescents with HMB

Lead Authors, Year (Study Period)	Study Design/ Study Setting	Study Population	n	Age (y)	BD Frequency (%)	VWD (n)	PFD (n)	Clotting Factor Deficiency (n)	Fibrinolytic Disorders (n)	D Definition of BD	L Limitations
Gursel & Albayrak[76], 2014	Cross-sectional/ university students selected by survey	Adolescents with PBAC scores >100	76	17–25	14.5	5	4	2 (FXI and FVII deficiencies)	NT	• VWF: Ag and/or VWF: RCo <45 for O and <50 for non-O blood types • Decreased platelet aggregation to ADP and/or collagen	• Platelet aggregation performed without release
Diaz & Srivaths[41], 2014 (2009–2011)	Retrospective/ young women's BD clinic	Adolescents referred for HMB	131	10–14	21	−7 −32 with low VWF	11	2	1* (PAI-1 deficiency)	• VWF: Ag and/or VWF: RCo <30 • Two abnormalities in platelet aggregation and/or secretion	• Clotting factors and fibrinolytic protein testing when deemed necessary
Rodriguez & Simmons[77], 2013	Retrospective/ primary care, hematology clinics; inpatient or outpatient	Adolescents referred for HMB	160	10–19	16	12	10	Not described	NA	• Not provided	
Seravalli & Bruni[78], 2013 (2007–2011)	Retrospective/ pediatric and adolescent gynecology clinic	Adolescents referred for HMB	113	11–20	48	15	20	14	NA	• Not provided	• Platelet aggregation performed without release

Study	Setting	Population	N	Age						Definitions	Comments
Vo & O'Brien[79], 2012 (2009–2011)	Retrospective/young women's BD clinic	Adolescents referred for HMB	105	8–18	62	9	−36 PSPD −8 other PFDs	NT	NT	• VWF: Ag and/or VWF: RCo <40 • PSPD: ≤3.68 granules per platelet • Other PFD: not clearly defined	• Platelet aggregation was not performed uniformly • Diagnosis of PFD based mainly on platelet EM
Mikhail & Kouides[40], 2007 (2001–2004)	Retrospective/hemophilia treatment center or hematology outpatient clinic	Adolescents referred for HMB	61	11–19	41	36	7	NT	NT	• VWF: RCo <40% and/or VWF: Ag <50% • PFD: dec in agg to ≥1 agonists <2 SD of local lab range and/or abnormal PFA	• Platelet aggregation was not performed uniformly • Platelet aggregation performed without release
Jayasinghe & Grover[80], 2005 (2001–2003)	Retrospective/inpatient outpatient gynecology clinic	Adolescents referred for HMB	106	9–19	10.4	5	8	NT	NT	• VWF: RCo < and/or VWF: Ag below local laboratory reference range. • PFD: Abnormalities to ADP, collagen, ristocetin, or epinephrine	
Philipp & Saidi[81], 2005 (1999–2004)	Prospective/outpatient primary care clinic	Adolescents referred for HMB	25	≤ 19	56	4	44	8	NT	• Clear definitions of BD not provided	

(continued on next page)

Table 1 *(continued)*

Lead Authors, Year (Study Period)	Study Design/ Study Setting	Study Population	n	Age (y)	BD Frequency (%)	VWD (n)	PFD (n)	Clotting Factor Deficiency (n)	Fibrinolytic Disorders (n)	Definition of BD	Limitations
Bevan & Scott[67], 2001 (1990–1998)	Retrospective/ ED, urgent care, inpatient	Adolescents referred for HMB	71	10–19	11	2	6	NT	NT	• VWF: RCo or VWF: Ag <45% • Platelet agg <50% with ADP, collagen, TRAP, ristocetin and AA	• 9 cases had ITP • Only 14 girls in this series had hemostatic evaluation performed
Oral & Ocer[82], 2001 (1988–1995)	Retrospective/ inpatient	Adolescents hospitalized for HMB	25	11–17	8	2	NT	NT	NT	• Clear definitions of BD not provided	• An additional 4 cases were diagnosed with ITP
Smith & Hertzberg[83], 1998 (1979–1995)	Retrospective/ inpatient	Adolescents hospitalized for HMB	37	10–20	13	5	NT	NT	NT	• Clear definitions of BD not provided	
Claessens & Cowell,[3] 1981 (1971–1981)	Retrospective/ inpatient	Adolescents hospitalized for HMB	59		19	3	2	NT	NT	• Clear definitions of BD not provided	

Abbreviations: AA, arachidonic acid; ADP, adenosine diphosphate; Ag, antigen; agg, aggregated; BD, bleeding disorder; ED, emergency department; EM, electron microscopy; FVII, factor VII; FXI, factor XI; HMB, heavy menstrual bleeding; ITP, immune thrombocytopenia; NT, not tested; PAI-1, plasminogen activator-1 activity; PBAC, pictorial blood assessment chart; PFD, platelet functional disorders; PSPD, platelet storage pool disorder; RCo, ristocetin cofactor activity; SD, standard deviation; TRAP, thrombin receptor activation peptide; VWF, von Willebrand factor.

in adolescents with HMB, especially at menarche.[23,36] Ideally, testing should be repeated at least twice for those with a high suspicion of a BD, and subnormal results should be confirmed.[35] Testing on OCs containing 30 to 35 μg of estrogen does not affect the laboratory diagnosis of VWD.[37,38] However, testing should not be performed during an OC taper or after high dose estrogen pulses because von Willebrand factor (VWF) levels are elevated with OCs containing 50 μg or more of estrogen.[39] If these tests are normal, further testing should include screening for qualitative platelet disorders with a platelet aggregation and secretion study.[40,41] The authors propose a management algorithm, including laboratory testing (**Fig. 1**), developed in the context of multidisciplinary management of young women with HMB.[6]

Recommended gynecologic testing for HMB includes screening for pregnancy, *Chlamydia trachomatis*, and *Neisseria gonorrhea* in this age group.[42] A history of irregular bleeding before the onset of heavy bleeding should prompt hormone testing to screen for polycystic ovarian syndrome and hypothyroidism.[2,43] The role of pelvic examination is debated but an external genital examination is generally undertaken to detect anatomic abnormalities.[1,44] A pelvic ultrasound examination is generally performed in cases that are refractory to therapy.[45,46]

A multidisciplinary approach to management, with involvement from a hematologist, an adolescent medicine specialist, and/or a gynecologist results in optimal treatment outcomes.[47,48] OCs, the prototype for other combined hormonal contraceptives, offer both contraceptive and noncontraceptive benefits in adolescents with HMB, and include reduction of menstrual flow.[49,50] The 2008 National Heart, Lung, and Blood Institute VWD treatment guidelines recommend OCs as the first choice for HMB in an adolescent who does not desire pregnancy but may desire future child bearing.[51] The effectiveness of OCs in adolescents with platelet function defects remains to be studied. Extended cycling of OCs to reduce withdrawal bleeding that would otherwise occur every 28 days with conventional OCs is promising.[52] Studies in adult women have demonstrated that menstruating less frequently than monthly is highly acceptable.[52] Use of progesterone-only hormonal therapy, such as progesterone-only pills, medroxyprogesterone acetate (MPA), and the progestin implant, also may reduce menstrual flow and are another alternative to OCs in adolescents with HMB but seem less preferable owing to weight gain.[49] Increasingly used in adolescents, the levonorgestrel intrauterine system steadily releases 20 μg of levonorgestrel per 24 hours for 5 years into the endometrial cavity.[53] IUDs are safe in nulliparous adolescents, but require the expertise of an experienced gynecologist.[54] The levonorgestrel intrauterine system was shown to be an effective option in adolescents in a number of BDs with minimal complications, a high compliance rate, and improvements in HMB and anemia.[50,55]

Antifibrinolytics decrease the fibrinolytic activity observed in the endometrial tissue of women with HMB.[56] Two antifibrinolytics, epsilon aminocaproic acid (Amicar) and tranexamaic acid have well-established safety profiles,[57] and both decrease menstrual flow and improved quality of life among females with HMB and abnormal laboratory hemostasis.[58]

Data on the use of nonsteroidal antiinflammatory drugs for the management of HMB in adolescents are nonexistent. Expert guidelines suggest they should not be used as first-line therapy for HMB, because they affect platelet function and may further increase menstrual blood loss in patients with undiagnosed BDs.[35] Because menstrual pain is common in adolescents with BDs, the use of nonsteroidal antiinflammatory drugs in those with severe menstrual cramps with hemostatic therapy deserves further study. In contrast with BDs, such as severe hemophilia reviewed in Stacy E. Croteau's article, "Evolving Complexity in Hemophilia Management," in this issue, in which prophylaxis is the accepted standard of care, factor replacement such as von

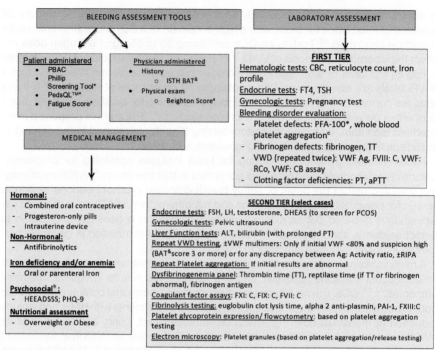

Fig. 1. Testing and management algorithm for young women with heavy menstrual bleeding (HMB). The current management protocol is being tested prospectively in the setting of a research study. Asterisks (*) denote research assessments. Ag, antigen; ALT, alanine transaminase; aPTT, activated partial thromboplastin time; BAT, bleeding assessment tool; CB, collagen binding assay; CBC, complete blood count; DHEAS, dehydroepiandrosterone; FSH, follicle stimulating hormone; FT4, free T4; FIX, factor IX; FVII, factor VII; FVIII, factor VIII; FXI, factor XI; ISTH, International Society of Thrombosis and Haemostasis; LH, luteinizing hormone; PAI-1, plasminogen activator inhibitor-1; PBAC, pictorial blood assessment tool; PCOS, polycystic ovarian syndrome; PFA, platelet function analyzer; PT, prothrombin time; RCo, ristocetin cofactor activity; RIPA, ristocetin induced platelet aggregation; TSH, thyroid-stimulating hormone; TT, thrombin time; VWD, von Willebrand disease; VWF, von Willebrand factor. [a] The Beighton score is a 9-point evaluation to assess joint hypermobility, with attribution of 1 point in the presence of any of the following: (A) Passive apposition of the thumb to the flexor aspect of the forearm (1 point for each hand), (B) passive dorsiflexion of the V finger beyond 90° (1 point for each hand), (C) hyperextension of the elbow beyond 10° (1 point for each arm), (D) hyperextension of the knees beyond 10° (1 point for each leg), (E) forward flexion of the trunk with the knees extended and the palms resting flat on the floor.[75] [b] A psychosocial assessment using the HEEADSSS (Home environment, Education, Eating, peer-related Activities, Drugs, Sexuality, Suicide/depression, and Safety from injury and violence) format is recommended for adolescents during preventive health screening to identify depression and other high-risk behavior, which may need to be addressed given that these may be underlying causes of HMB. Similarly, a Patient Health Questionnaire (PHQ) screen is performed to screen, diagnose, and measure the severity of depression. [c] Whole bleed aggregation is suggested as part of this algorithm because of the availability at our institution. Light transmission aggregometry remains the gold standard method for measurement of platelet function at this time.

Willebrand factor replacement for VWD, is less frequently used in women with HMB and is another area in need of investigation.

The need for surgery in adolescents with HMB is based on the clinical stability of the patient. Examination under general anesthesia, evacuation of blood clots from the uterine cavity, and curettage should be considered for serious or refractory menstrual bleeding. Endometrial ablation is not considered in adolescents owing to concerns for future fertility preservation.[59] Endometrial balloon tamponade using a Foley catheter may provide a temporary measure to control bleeding in a hemodynamically unstable patient.[60] Readers are encouraged to refer to other reviews for management protocols for acute HMB on an inpatient and outpatient basis.[6,35]

ABNORMAL UTERINE BLEEDING IN CYTOPENIAS/THROMBOCYTOPENIA

There are many conditions in childhood that feature thrombocytopenia, of which those with moderate to severe thrombocytopenia may likely experience AUB. Thrombocytopenia can arise from a production problem, such as that associated with inherited bone marrow failure syndromes, idiopathic aplastic anemia (which is reviewed in Süreyya Savaşan's article, "Acquired Aplastic Anemia: What Have We Learned and What Is in the Horizon?," in this issue), and chemotherapy-induced thrombocytopenia, or because of platelet destruction such as with immune thrombocytopenia (ITP). The treatment of AUB in patients with thrombocytopenia should always include the treatment of the underlying disorder (**Box 2**), but there are some unique differences in the approach to those with impaired production versus increased destruction.

Impaired Platelet Production

The most logical therapy for platelet production disorders may seem to be platelet transfusion, but given the risk of alloimmunization and transfusion-related complications,

---

Box 2
General principles for AUB management in the setting of thrombocytopenia

- Assess pregnancy status before initiating therapy, especially, if there is clinical concern that thrombocytopenia is possibly secondary to SLE or that the use of possible antibiologics such as rituximab may be needed.

- Assess and document menstrual bleeding pattern (frequency, duration, flow, and volume) before presumed onset of thrombocytopenia. Determine if AUB or HMB predates thrombocytopenia.

- Consider hormonal suppression or regulation at the time of thrombocytopenia diagnosis, especially if there is a history of AUB or HMB before thrombocytopenia.

- Assess the severity of thrombocytopenia and hematology parameters (hemoglobin and ferritin) at the time AUB or HMB is reported.

- Determine the underlying cause of thrombocytopenia and if current severity of thrombocytopenia would be improved by/responsive to platelet transfusion.

- Treat underlying cause of thrombocytopenia as indicated by standard of care for each underlying entity.

- Initiate treatment for AUB based on personal preference and needs.

- Consider a multidisciplinary, collaborative management approach, with inclusion of gynecology or adolescent medicine for improved patient outcomes.

Abbreviations: AUB, abnormal uterine bleeding; HMB, heavy menstrual bleeding; SLE, systemic lupus erythematosus.

it may be desirable to pursue adjunctive therapies, especially in disorders that may require future hematopoietic stem cell transplant or in which one might choose to reserve platelet transfusion for life-threatening bleeding. Other therapeutic modalities include hormonal and hemostatic agents. There is little to no evidence in inherited bone marrow failure syndromes and idiopathic aplastic anemia for the use of antifibrinolytics such as aminocaproic acid and tranexamaic acid.[61] The induction of amenorrhea with hormone-based therapies or luteinizing hormone-releasing hormone agonist or MPA may be useful. In conditions in which it is not expected for the production to improve or when the thrombocytopenia is moderate, one could consider the use of an IUD for induction of amenorrhea.[62] Desmopressin acetate can also increase the release of von Willebrand factor, making what few platelets are in circulation more effective, but given the limited literature in these disorders, this measure should be considered when other methods are not effective.[63]

Chemotherapy-induced thrombocytopenia often leads to a transient window of risk of AUB. Platelet transfusion is recommended prophylactically when platelet count is less than 10,000/mm^3.[64] The incidence of moderate to severe HMB is 40% in patients receiving ablative chemotherapy for hematopoietic stem cell transplantation.[62] The induction of amenorrhea is commonly pursued in oncology and hematopoietic stem cell transplant patients because the severity and duration of thrombocytopenia is expected to be quite long and the impact of chemotherapy on the ovaries may additionally lead to AUB owing to hypothalamic pituitary ovarian axis disruption. Scarce evidence exists for aminocaproic acid and tranexamaic acid in patients undergoing chemotherapy in conjunction with platelet transfusion for the treatment of abnormal bleeding, but this is not specific to menstrual bleeding.[61] Luteinizing hormone-releasing hormone agonist and MPA are commonly used in advance of conditioning chemotherapy with or without radiation,[62,65] with the recommendation that a luteinizing hormone-releasing hormone agonist is more effective than MPA for menstrual suppression and reduction of HMB.[62,66] Owing to the risk of VTE in patients with cancer, providers may choose to avoid estrogen-based hormonal therapy. Additionally, whether a foreign body such as an IUD serves as a nidus of infection in patients with prolonged immunosuppression is controversial and no studies have been done to determine the exact risk.

Increased Platelet Destruction

In ITP, platelet transfusion should be reserved for life-threatening bleeding when all the mainstays of ITP therapy have been exhausted. In persistent or chronic ITP, it is important to consider the use of hormonal suppression of menses or slowing of menstrual flow with the use of antifibrinolytic agents.[61] For those with a history of HMB before the diagnosis of ITP, it is important to exclude VWD and qualitative platelet dysfunction with a thorough hemostatic evaluation.[67]

ABNORMAL UTERINE BLEEDING IN SICKLE CELL DISEASE

The gynecologic issues in adolescents with SCD include a later onset of menarche, AUB, and vasoocclusive pain associated with menstrual cycles.[68] Menstrual patterns are reported to be normal.[69] An important feature, exclusive to women, is the association of SCD-related pain with menstrual cycles.[69] Readers should refer to Emily Riehm Meier's article, "Treatment Options for Sickle Cell Disease," in this issue, which is focused on current therapies for women with SCD. Although hormonal fluctuations seem to underlie the painful SCD episodes associated with menses,[69] there is a paucity of data investigating HMB in this group of adolescents. Conceivably, etiologic factors underlying HMB in non-SCD patients should also be present in SCD patients. It is possible that mild BDs are mitigated by the SCD related hypercoagulability, but a more pronounced bleeding phenotype is present in those who experience HMB and manifests with the monthly challenge of menstruation.

Adolescents with SCD and HMB are also at higher risk of iron deficiency anemia that may be masked in the presence of the underlying chronic anemia. This finding is especially true for the patients on hydroxycarbamide whose higher mean corpuscular volume[70] masks the microcytosis characteristic of iron deficiency. Low ferritin levels, the hallmark of iron deficiency anemia,[71] are not present in SCD owing to the underlying inflammatory state, making diagnosis difficult.

AUB in adolescents with SCD, like other blood disorders, requires a systematic approach that begins with a thorough menstrual history. A careful consideration of other blood disorders, such as underlying VWD, systemic medical illnesses like hypothyroidism, polycystic ovarian syndrome, or structural uterine abnormalities, is paramount. Iron deficiency should be screened with ferritin level; however, caution should be exercised with interpretation. A better marker of iron deficiency in SCD may be a percent transferrin saturation of less than 25%.[72] There is reluctance to use estrogen-containing OCs for hormonal suppression in an already hypercoagulable state; however, the World Health Organization guidelines on contraceptives in SCD, also endorsed by ACOG, state that the benefits of combined injectable contraceptives, low-dose OCs, and IUDs outweigh the risks associated with the increased morbidity and mortality associated with pregnancy.[73] Additionally, progesterone-only pills can be used without restriction.[14] It should be noted that data are based on the high unplanned pregnancy risk rather than the safety profile of these pills.[74] Longitudinal, prospective studies on etiology of AUB, uses and complications of contraception, risk of unplanned pregnancy, and the prevalence of other reproductive issues are urgently needed for adolescents with SCD.

SUMMARY

Several issues for adolescents with AUB remain to be studied. A correct appreciation of the importance of AUB and its management are skills that all pediatricians should strive to achieve. It is quite clear that failure to do so could result in suffering and risk of serious bleeding. Despite advances in the clinical investigation and management of adult women with AUB and blood disorders, several areas need to be studied in adolescents as covered herein. These gaps urgently require future research and should be filled in the next years by multicenter collaborative studies.

REFERENCES

1. Gray SH, Emans SJ. Abnormal vaginal bleeding in adolescents. Pediatrics in Review 2007;28(5):175–82.
2. Benjamins LJ. Practice guideline: evaluation and management of abnormal vaginal bleeding in adolescents. J Pediatr Health Care 2009;23(3):189–93.
3. Claessens EA, Cowell CA. Acute adolescent menorrhagia. Am J Obstet Gynecol 1981;139(3):277–80.
4. Khosla AH, Devi L, Goel P, et al. Puberty menorrhagia requiring inpatient admission. JNMA J Nepal Med Assoc 2010;49(178):112–6.
5. Munro MG, Critchley HO, Broder MS, et al, FIGO Working Group on Menstrual Disorders. FIGO classification system (PALM-COEIN) for causes of abnormal uterine bleeding in nongravid women of reproductive age. Int J Gynaecol Obstet 2011;113(1):3–13.

6. Zia A, Lau M, Journeycake J, et al. Developing a multidisciplinary Young Women's Blood Disorders Program: a single-centre approach with guidance for other centres. Haemophilia 2016;22:199–207.

7. Zia A, Rajpurkar M. Challenges of diagnosing and managing the adolescent with heavy menstrual bleeding. Thromb Res 2016;143:91–100.

8. Warner PE, Critchley HO, Lumsden MA, et al. measured blood loss, clinical features, and outcome in women with heavy periods: a survey with follow-up data. Am J Obstet Gynecol 2004;190(5):1216–23.

9. Raffini L, Huang YS, Witmer C, et al. Dramatic increase in venous thromboembolism in children's hospitals in the United States from 2001 to 2007. Pediatrics 2009;124(4):1001–8.

10. Klok FA, Schreiber K, Stach K, et al. Oral contraception and menstrual bleeding during treatment of venous thromboembolism: expert opinion versus current practice: combined results of a systematic review, expert panel opinion and an international survey. Thromb Res 2017;153:101–7.

11. Sjalander A, Friberg B, Svensson P, et al. Menorrhagia and minor bleeding symptoms in women on oral anticoagulation. J Thromb Thrombolysis 2007;24(1): 39–41.

12. Lidegaard O, Lokkegaard E, Svendsen AL, et al. Hormonal contraception and risk of venous thromboembolism: national follow-up study. BMJ 2009; 339:b2890.

13. Venous thromboembolic disease and combined oral contraceptives: results of international multicentre case-control study. World Health Organization Collaborative Study of Cardiovascular Disease and Steroid Hormone Contraception. Lancet 1995;346(8990):1575–82.

14. Centers for Disease Control and Prevention. U S. Medical Eligibility Criteria for Contraceptive Use, 2010. MMWR Recomm Rep 2010;59(RR-4):1–86.

15. Baglin T, Bauer K, Douketis J, et al. Duration of anticoagulant therapy after a first episode of an unprovoked pulmonary embolus or deep vein thrombosis: guidance from the SSC of the ISTH. J Thromb Haemost 2012;10(4):698–702.

16. Martinelli I, Lensing AW, Middeldorp S, et al. Recurrent venous thromboembolism and abnormal uterine bleeding with anticoagulant and hormone therapy use. Blood 2016;127(11):1417–25.

17. Bates SM, Greer IA, Hirsh J, et al. Use of antithrombotic agents during pregnancy: the seventh ACCP conference on antithrombotic and thrombolytic therapy. Chest 2004;126(3 Suppl):627S–44S.

18. Ginsberg JS, Hirsh J, Turner DC, et al. Risks to the fetus of anticoagulant therapy during pregnancy. Thromb Haemost 1989;61(2):197–203.

19. Farley TM, Rosenberg MJ, Rowe PJ, et al. Intrauterine devices and pelvic inflammatory disease: an international perspective. Lancet 1992;339(8796):785–8.

20. Kulkarni R. Improving care and treatment options for women and girls with bleeding disorders. Eur J Haematol 2015;95(Suppl 81):2–10.

21. Sramek A, Eikenboom JC, Briet E, et al. Usefulness of patient interview in bleeding disorders. Arch Intern Med 1995;155(13):1409–15.

22. ACOG Committee on Adolescent Health Care. ACOG Committee Opinion No. 349, November 2006: menstruation in girls and adolescents: using the menstrual cycle as a vital sign. Obstetrics Gynecol 2006;108(5):1323–8.

23. ACOG Committee on Gynecologic Practice. Committee Opinion: number 263, December 20001. von Willebrand's disease in gynecologic practice. Obstetrics Gynecol 2001;98(6):1185–6.

24. Marcus PD, Nire KG, Grooms L, et al. The power of a standardized bleeding score in diagnosing paediatric type 1 von Willebrand's disease and platelet function defects. Haemophilia 2011;17(2):223-7.

25. Rodeghiero F, Castaman G, Tosetto A, et al. The discriminant power of bleeding history for the diagnosis of type 1 von Willebrand disease: an international, multicenter study. J Thromb Haemost 2005;3(12):2619-26.

26. Biss TT, Blanchette VS, Clark DS, et al. Quantitation of bleeding symptoms in children with von Willebrand disease: use of a standardized pediatric bleeding questionnaire. J Thromb Haemost 2010;8(5):950-6.

27. Bidlingmaier C, Grote V, Budde U, et al. Prospective evaluation of a pediatric bleeding questionnaire and the ISTH bleeding assessment tool in children and parents in routine clinical practice. J Thromb Haemost 2012;10(7):1335-41.

28. Elbatarny M, Mollah S, Grabell J, et al. Normal range of bleeding scores for the ISTH-BAT: adult and pediatric data from the merging project. Haemophilia 2014; 20(6):831-5.

29. Higham JM, O'Brien PM, Shaw RW. Assessment of menstrual blood loss using a pictorial chart. Br J Obstet Gynaecol 1990;97(8):734-9.

30. Zakherah MS, Sayed GH, El-Nashar SA, et al. Pictorial blood loss assessment chart in the evaluation of heavy menstrual bleeding: diagnostic accuracy compared to alkaline hematin. Gynecol Obstet Invest 2011;71(4):281-4.

31. Janssen CA, Scholten PC, Heintz AP. A simple visual assessment technique to discriminate between menorrhagia and normal menstrual blood loss. Obstetrics Gynecol 1995;85(6):977-82.

32. Sanchez J, Andrabi S, Bercaw JL, et al. Quantifying the PBAC in a pediatric and adolescent gynecology population. Pediatr Hematol Oncol 2012;29(5):479-84.

33. Philipp CS, Faiz A, Dowling NF, et al. Development of a screening tool for identifying women with menorrhagia for hemostatic evaluation. Am J obstetrics Gynecol 2008;198(2):163.e1-8.

34. Philipp CS, Faiz A, Heit JA, et al. Evaluation of a screening tool for bleeding disorders in a US multisite cohort of women with menorrhagia. Am J obstetrics Gynecol 2011;204(3):209.e1-7.

35. James AH, Kouides PA, Abdul-Kadir R, et al. Von Willebrand disease and other bleeding disorders in women: consensus on diagnosis and management from an international expert panel. Am J Obstet Gynecol 2009;201(1):12.e1-18.

36. American College of Obstetricians and Gynecologists Committee on Adolescent Health Care, American College of Obstetricians and Gynecologists Committee Gynecologic Practice. ACOG Committee opinion No. 451: Von Willebrand disease in women. Obstetrics Gynecol 2009;114(6):1439-43.

37. Kadir RA, Economides DL, Sabin CA, et al. Variations in coagulation factors in women: effects of age, ethnicity, menstrual cycle and combined oral contraceptive. Thromb Haemost 1999;82(5):1456-61.

38. Zia A, Callaghan MU, Callaghan JH, et al. Hypercoagulability in adolescent girls on oral contraceptives- global coagulation profile and estrogen receptor polymorphisms. Am J Hematol 2015;90(8):725-31.

39. Alperin JB. Estrogens and surgery in women with von Willebrand's disease. Am J Med 1982;73(3):367-71.

40. Mikhail S, Varadarajan R, Kouides P. The prevalence of disorders of haemostasis in adolescents with menorrhagia referred to a haemophilia treatment centre. Haemophilia 2007;13(5):627-32.

41. Diaz R, Dietrich JE, Mahoney D Jr, et al. Hemostatic abnormalities in young females with heavy menstrual bleeding. J Pediatr Adolesc Gynecol 2014;27(6): 324–9.

42. Committee on Practice Bulletins—Gynecology. Practice bulletin no. 128: diagnosis of abnormal uterine bleeding in reproductive-aged women. Obstetrics Gynecol 2012;120(1):197–206.

43. Azziz R, Carmina E, Dewailly D, et al. The Androgen Excess and PCOS Society criteria for the polycystic ovary syndrome: the complete task force report. Fertil Steril 2009;91(2):456–88.

44. Westhoff CL, Jones HE, Guiahi M. Do new guidelines and technology make the routine pelvic examination obsolete? J Women's Health (Larchmt) 2011;20(1): 5–10.

45. Snook ML, Nayak S, Lara-Torre E, et al. Adolescent gynecology: special considerations for special patients. Clin Obstet Gynecol 2012;55(3):651–61.

46. Tayal VS, Crean CA, Norton HJ, et al. Prospective comparative trial of endovaginal sonographic bimanual examination versus traditional digital bimanual examination in nonpregnant women with lower abdominal pain with regard to body mass index classification. J Ultrasound Med 2008;27(8):1171–7.

47. Lee CA, Chi C, Shiltagh N, et al. Review of a multidisciplinary clinic for women with inherited bleeding disorders. Haemophilia 2009;15(1):359–60.

48. Winikoff R, Amesse C, James A, et al. The role of haemophilia treatment centres in providing services to women with bleeding disorders. Haemophilia 2004; 10(Suppl 4):196–204.

49. Ott MA, Sucato GS. Committee on A. Contraception for adolescents. Pediatrics 2014;134(4):e1257–81.

50. Chi C, Pollard D, Tuddenham EG, et al. Menorrhagia in adolescents with inherited bleeding disorders. J Pediatr Adolesc Gynecol 2010;23(4):215–22.

51. Nichols WL, Hultin MB, James AH, et al. von Willebrand disease (VWD): evidence-based diagnosis and management guidelines, the National Heart, Lung, and Blood Institute (NHLBI) Expert Panel report (USA). Haemophilia 2008;14(2):171–232.

52. Miller L, Notter KM. Menstrual reduction with extended use of combination oral contraceptive pills: randomized controlled trial. Obstetrics Gynecol 2001;98(5 Pt 1):771–8.

53. Sivin I, Stern J, Coutinho E, et al. Prolonged intrauterine contraception: a seven-year randomized study of the levonorgestrel 20 mcg/day (LNg 20) and the Copper T380 Ag IUDS. Contraception 1991;44(5):473–80.

54. Finer LB, Jerman J, Kavanaugh ML. Changes in use of long-acting contraceptive methods in the United States, 2007-2009. Fertil sterility 2012;98(4):893–7.

55. Adeyemi-Fowode OA, Santos XM, Dietrich JE, et al. Levonorgestrel-releasing intrauterine device use in female adolescents with heavy menstrual bleeding and bleeding disorders: single institution review. J Pediatr Adolesc Gynecol 2017; 30(4):479–83.

56. Dockeray CJ, Sheppard BL, Daly L, et al. The fibrinolytic enzyme system in normal menstruation and excessive uterine bleeding and the effect of tranexamic acid. Eur J Obstet Gynecol Reprod Biol 1987;24(4):309–18.

57. Lethaby A, Farquhar C, Cooke I. Antifibrinolytics for heavy menstrual bleeding. Cochrane Database Syst Rev 2000;(4):CD000249.

58. Srivaths LV, Dietrich JE, Yee DL, et al. Oral tranexamic acid versus combined oral contraceptives for adolescent heavy menstrual bleeding: a pilot study. J Pediatr Adolesc Gynecol 2015;28(4):254–7.

59. Rubin G, Wortman M, Kouides PA. Endometrial ablation for von Willebrand disease-related menorrhagia–experience with seven cases. Haemophilia 2004; 10(5):477–82.
60. Hamani Y, Ben-Shachar I, Kalish Y, et al. Intrauterine balloon tamponade as a treatment for immune thrombocytopenic purpura-induced severe uterine bleeding. Fertil sterility 2010;94(7):2769.e13-5.
61. Estcourt LJ, Desborough M, Brunskill SJ, et al. Antifibrinolytics (lysine analogues) for the prevention of bleeding in people with haematological disorders. Cochrane Database Syst Rev 2016;(3):CD009733.
62. Kirkham YA, Ornstein MP, Aggarwal A, et al. Menstrual suppression in special circumstances. J Obstet Gynaecol Can 2014;36(10):915–24.
63. Kobrinsky NL, Tulloch H. Treatment of refractory thrombocytopenic bleeding with 1-desamino-8-D-arginine vasopressin (desmopressin). J Pediatr 1988;112(6): 993–6.
64. Barkhan P. Blood and neoplastic diseases. Thrombocytopenia. Br Med J 1974; 2(5914):324–5.
65. Ghalie R, Porter C, Radwanska E, et al. Prevention of hypermenorrhea with leuprolide in premenopausal women undergoing bone marrow transplantation. Am J Hematol 1993;42(4):350–3.
66. Quaas AM, Ginsburg ES. Prevention and treatment of uterine bleeding in hematologic malignancy. Eur J obstetrics, Gynecol Reprod Biol 2007;134(1):3–8.
67. Bevan JA, Maloney KW, Hillery CA, et al. Bleeding disorders: a common cause of menorrhagia in adolescents. The J Pediatr 2001;138(6):856–61.
68. Stimpson SJ, Rebele EC, DeBaun MR. Common gynecological challenges in adolescents with sickle cell disease. Expert Rev Hematol 2016;9(2):187–96.
69. Smith-Whitley K. Reproductive issues in sickle cell disease. Hematology Am Soc Hematol Educ Program 2014;2014(1):418–24.
70. Kattamis A, Lagona E, Orfanou I, et al. Clinical response and adverse events in young patients with sickle cell disease treated with hydroxyurea. Pediatr Hematol Oncol 2004;21(4):335–42.
71. Powers JM, Buchanan GR. Potential for improved screening, diagnosis, and treatment for iron deficiency and iron deficiency anemia in young children. The J Pediatr 2017;188:8–10.
72. Killip S, Bennett JM, Chambers MD. Iron deficiency anemia. Am Fam Physician 2007;75(5):671–8.
73. ACOG Committee on Practice Bulletins-Gynecology. ACOG practice bulletin. No. 73: use of hormonal contraception in women with coexisting medical conditions. Obstetrics Gynecol 2006;107(6):1453–72.
74. O'Brien SH, Klima J, Reed S, et al. Hormonal contraception use and pregnancy in adolescents with sickle cell disease: analysis of Michigan Medicaid claims. Contraception 2011;83(2):134–7.
75. van der Giessen LJ, Liekens D, Rutgers KJ, et al. Validation of beighton score and prevalence of connective tissue signs in 773 Dutch children. J Rheumatol 2001;28:2726–30.
76. Gursel T, Biri A, Kaya Z, et al. The frequency of menorrhagia and bleeding disorders in university students. Pediatr Hematol Oncol 2014;31:467–74.
77. Rodriguez V, Alme C, Killian JM, et al. Bleeding disorders in adolescents with menorrhagia: an institutional experience. Haemophilia 2013;19:e101–2.
78. Seravalli V, Linari S, Peruzzi E, et al. Prevalence of hemostatic disorders in adolescents with abnormal uterine bleeding. J Pediatr Adolesc Gynecol 2013;26: 285–9.

79. Vo KT, Grooms L, Klima J, et al. Menstrual bleeding patterns and prevalence of bleeding disorders in a multidisciplinary adolescent haematology clinic. Haemophilia 2013;19:71–5.

80. Jayasinghe Y, Moore P, Donath S, et al. Bleeding disorders in teenagers presenting withmenorrhagia. Aust N Z J Obstet Gynaecol 2005;45:439–43.

81. Philipp CS, Faiz A, Dowling N, et al. Age and the prevalence of bleeding disorders in women with menorrhagia. Obstet Gynecol 2005;105:61–6.

82. Oral E, Cagdas A, Gezer A, et al. Hematological abnormalities in adolescent menorrhagia. Arch Gynecol Obstet 2002;266:72–4.

83. Smith YR, Quint EH, Hertzberg RB. Menorrhagia in adolescents requiring hospitalization. J Pediatr Adolesc Gynecol 1998;11:13–5.

Congenital Disorders of Platelet Function and Number

Ruchika Sharma, MD[a], Juliana Perez Botero, MD[b],
Shawn M. Jobe, MD, PhD[c],*

KEYWORDS

- Congenital platelet disorder • Thrombocytopenia • Platelet function
- Thrombasthenia

KEY POINTS

- New research and diagnostic tools continue to expand understanding of the genetic and molecular causes of disorders of platelet number and function.
- Congenital disorders of both platelet number and function have been associated with multiple hematologic and clinical manifestations, including auditory, musculoskeletal, cardiac, immunologic, and oncologic complications and disease.
- Delineation of the molecular cause of the platelet disorder can aid the practitioner in the early detection and prevention of disorder-associated manifestations and guide appropriate treatment and anticipatory care for the patient and family.

CLINICAL MANIFESTATIONS OF PLATELET-RELATED BLEEDING

Bleeding associated with platelet disorders primarily involves the skin and mucous membranes. The distribution and other characteristics of petechiae and bruising can be helpful in distinguishing bleeding related to platelet disorders from other causes, such as vasculitic disease or nonaccidental injury. For example, the lesions associated with Henoch-Schönlein purpura, a vasculitic disease, are raised and primarily involve dependent surfaces and the lower extremities. Unusual or regular patterns of skin lesions (eg, handprint, linear) may suggest the possibility of nonaccidental injury.

Disclosure Statement: No relevant disclosures.
[a] BloodCenter of Wisconsin, Medical College of Wisconsin, 8733 Watertown Plank Road, Milwaukee, WI 53226, USA; [b] BloodCenter of Wisconsin, 8733 Watertown Plank Road, Milwaukee, WI 53226, USA; [c] Blood Center of Wisconsin, Blood Research Institute, Medical College of Wisconsin, 8733 Watertown Plank Road, Milwaukee, WI 53226, USA
* Corresponding author.
E-mail address: Shawn.jobe@bcw.edu

Pediatr Clin N Am 65 (2018) 561–578
https://doi.org/10.1016/j.pcl.2018.02.009
0031-3955/18/© 2018 Elsevier Inc. All rights reserved.

Mucosal surfaces that can be involved in platelet-related bleeding include the nasal membranes; oral cavity; gastrointestinal hemorrhage; hematuria; and, in young women, menorrhagia. (See discussion of heavy menstrual bleeding in Kathryn E. Dickerson and colleagues' article, "Abnormal Uterine Bleeding in Young Women with Blood Disorders,"in this issue.) Platelet dysfunction should also be considered in the presence of increased bleeding following dental extraction, tonsillectomy, or other surgical procedures.

Differential Diagnosis of Platelet-Related Bleeding

A careful medical history, physical examination, and evaluation of the platelet count and smear can rapidly narrow the diagnostic possibilities in the setting of platelet-related bleeding. History should be obtained regarding medication usage, particularly aspirin or nonsteroidal antiinflammatory drugs. Detailed evaluation of the family and past medical history may provide clues about whether the bleeding disorder is acquired or congenital. Careful evaluation of the peripheral blood smear and blood count, as well as assessment of hepatosplenomegaly and lymphadenopathy, may reveal the need for further evaluation for the presence of myeloproliferative disease, malignancy, or aplastic anemia.

Differentiation of immune thrombocytopenic purpura (ITP) from a congenital platelet disorder can sometimes be problematic. The persistence of neonatal thrombocytopenia or a low platelet count despite the use of several standard therapies (eg, intravenous immunoglobulin, steroids) for ITP should prompt consideration of a congenital cause for the thrombocytopenia. Patients with ITP typically have minimal bleeding until their platelet count decreases to below 10,000 to 20,000/μL. Bleeding observed at platelet counts greater than 30,000/μL suggests the presence of an underlying platelet dysfunction.

Many congenital platelet disorders are associated with other diseases, unique physical characteristics, or findings on the peripheral blood smear. These additional characteristics can assist in narrowing the differential diagnosis. For example, thrombocytopenia in the presence of auditory or renal dysfunction suggests an MYH-9–related thrombocytopenia, and the presence of skeletal abnormalities may lead to the diagnosis of thrombocytopenia with absent radii or amegakaryocytic thrombocytopenia with radioulnar synostosis.

Diagnostic Evaluation of Platelet-Related Bleeding

Initial laboratory evaluation of individuals with platelet-related bleeding should include a complete blood count with differential and von Willebrand factor (vWF) studies (including activity and antigen) to rule out this primary cause of mucocutaneous bleeding. (See Christopher J. Ng and Jorge Di Paola's article, "Von Willebrand disease: Diagnostic Strategies and Treatment Options, in this issue.") Utilization of a platelet function analyzer can identify individuals with severe defect in platelet number or function; however, this test has poor sensitivity and specificity for less severe defects of platelet function.[1] Standard evaluation of platelet dysfunction should include evaluation of platelet aggregation to multiple platelet agonists. Aggregation studies are often performed in concert with luminometry studies that evaluate for the presence and functional release of platelet-dense granules. Finally, electron microscopy, genetic testing, and other specialized studies (see later discussion) can be used to identify a definitive syndrome or molecular cause for a dysfunction in platelet count or number.

Estimation of platelet size can assist in narrowing the differential diagnosis in patients with a suspected inherited thrombocytopenia. Light microscopy can further identify abnormalities in platelet granularity or inclusions in white blood cells that are characteristic of certain disorders. Although there is great variability between instruments reporting mean platelet volume and clear cutoffs of normal platelet size in the general population have not been established,[2] a mean platelet volume greater than 12.4 fL and mean platelet diameter greater than 3.3 μm have a sensitivity of 97% in differentiating inherited macrothrombocytopenia from large platelets seen in ITP[3] (see later discussion of select platelet disorders of number and function). These are categorized by average platelet size in disorders classically associated with thrombocytopenia and mild platelet dysfunction (**Table 1**) and by the nature of the defect in those disorders with primary effects on platelet function independent of platelet count (**Table 2**).

CONGENITAL DISORDERS WITH THROMBOCYTOPENIA AND SMALL PLATELET SIZE
Wiskott-Aldrich Syndrome and X-linked Thrombocytopenia

Wiskott-Aldrich syndrome (WAS) and X-linked thrombocytopenia are X-linked disorders caused by mutations in *WAS*, which is located on the X chromosome. The WAS protein (WASp) is required to maintain the integrity of the actin cytoskeleton in multiple cell types. The clinical phenotype is heterogeneous with variable severity of eczema, immunodeficiency (humoral and cellular), and microthrombocytopenia.[4] Autoimmune complications, such as autoimmune cytopenias, and increased risk of B-cell lymphoma have been reported.[5] Thrombocytopenia occurs due to ineffective thrombopoiesis and increased platelet clearance.[6] Mutations in *WAS* can also lead to isolated microthrombocytopenia without syndromic associations[7] Mutations affecting the WASp-interacting protein can also result in a phenotype resembling WAS that is inherited in an autosomal recessive fashion.[8]

The platelet phenotype consists of small platelets with normal granularity. No additional functional or ultrastructural abnormalities have been reported. Treatment is based on supportive care for infection, including prevention of infection using antibiotics and immunoglobulin therapy. Splenectomy has been shown to improve platelet counts[9]; however, it significantly increases infectious risk in these already immunocompromised patients. Allogeneic stem cell transplantation with reduced intensity conditioning is curative and retroviral-based gene therapy is under investigation.[10]

CONGENITAL DISORDERS WITH THROMBOCYTOPENIA AND NORMAL PLATELET SIZE
ANKRD26-related Thrombocytopenia

Ankyrin repeat domain 26 (ANKRD26)-RT is an autosomal dominant disorder caused by mutations in *ANKRD26*. Most of the pathogenic mutations described are in the 5′ untranslated region of the gene.[11] This mutation results in increased expression of *ANKRD26* due to ineffective downregulation of transcription from the *ANKRD26* gene loci. The subsequent accumulation of *ANKRD26* protein in megakaryocytes leads to defects in proplatelet formation and an increased risk of myeloid transformation though its impact on TPO-MPL and MAPK-ERK signaling pathways.[12]

Patients present with moderate thrombocytopenia. Erythrocytosis has been described in some patients. Importantly, individuals with ANKRD26-RT have a 20-fold to 30-fold increased risk of developing myeloid malignancies (acute myeloid leukemia [AML], myelodysplastic syndrome [MDS], chronic myeloid leukemia [CMML], and chronic myelomonocytic leukemia [CML]) relative to that of the general population.[13] Although there is complete penetrance in the thrombocytopenic phenotype, the risk of transformation is variable even within families. Increased

Table 1
Average platelet size in disorders classically associated with thrombocytopenia and mild platelet dysfunction

	Genes	Inheritance	Clinical Associations	Platelet Phenotype
Small platelet size				
Wiskott-Aldrich or X-linked thrombocytopenia	WAS, WIPF-1	X linked recessive	Eczema, immunodeficiency (cellular and humoral), autoimmune disease, bleeding, increased risk of B-cell lymphoma	Small platelets with normal granularity
Normal platelet size				
ANKRD26-related thrombocytopenia	ANKRD26	Autosomal dominant	Risk of myeloid malignancy	Variable platelet aggregation abnormalities, decreased alpha granules, complex canalicular network
Congenital amegakaryocytic thrombocytopenia (CAMT)	MPL	Autosomal recessive	Bleeding, bone marrow failure	No known abnormalities
CYCS-related thrombocytopenia[79]	CYCS	Autosomal dominant	None	No known abnormalities
ETV6-related thrombocytopenia	ETV6	Autosomal dominant	Risk of myeloid and lymphoid malignancy, microcytosis, mild or moderate bleeding	Elongated alpha granules
Familial platelet disorder with predisposition to acute myelogenous leukemia (FPD-AML)	RUNX1	Autosomal dominant	Risk of myeloid malignancy, moderate bleeding	Dense granule deficiency
Platelet type von Willebrand disease (vWD)	GPIBA	Autosomal dominant	Bleeding	Platelet aggregates
Radioulnar synostosis with amegakaryocytic thrombocytopenia (RUSAT)[80,81]	HOXA11, MECOM	Autosomal dominant	Bleeding, MSK abnormalities, hearing loss	No known abnormalities
Thrombocytopenia absent radii (TAR)	RBM8A	Autosomal recessive	MSK abnormalities, cardiac and renal malformations, milk-protein allergy	No known abnormalities

Large platelet size

22q deletion syndromes	22q11.2 deletion	Autosomal dominant	MSK abnormalities, deafness	BSS phenotype if glycoprotein (GP)-IBA deleted
ACTN1-related thrombocytopenia[82]	ACTN1	Autosomal dominant	None	Platelet anisocytosis
Arthrogryposis-renal dysfunction-cholestasis	VPS33B, VIPAS39	Autosomal recessive	MSK abnormalities, renal tubular acidosis, cholestasis, early mortality	Absent alpha granules, impaired aggregation with adenosine diphosphate (ADP)
Bernard-Soulier syndrome (BSS)	GP1BA, GP1BB, GP9	Autosomal dominant or autosomal recessive	Bleeding	Absent aggregation with ristocetin, decreased GPIb-alpha and GPIX
DIAPH1-related thrombocytopenia[83]	DIAPH1	Autosomal dominant	Deafness, mild bleeding	Elongated platelets with vacuoles and abnormal distribution of alpha granules
FLNA-related thrombocytopenia[84]	FLNA	X-linked recessive	Mild or moderate bleeding	Variably decreased alpha granules
Integrin (ITG)-A2B or ITG3B-related thrombocytopenia	ITGA2B, ITG3B	Autosomal dominant	Mild bleeding	Mild decrease in GPIIb or IIa
Gray platelet syndrome	NBEAL2, GF11B	Autosomal recessive	Bleeding, risk of bone marrow fibrosis, splenomegaly	Platelet anisocytosis alpha granule deficiency
MYH-9-related disorders	MYH9	Autosomal dominant	Deafness, renal failure, cataracts, transaminitis	Protein aggregates (Döhle body-like inclusions) in white cells
Paris-Trousseau thrombocytopenia	FLI1, 11q23 deletion	Autosomal recessive	Bleeding, MSK abnormalities,	Giant or fused alpha granules
Sitosterolemia[85]	ABCG5, ABCG9	Autosomal recessive	Abnormal serum lipids, hemolysis, splenomegaly	Reduced aggregation with ristocetin
PRKACG-related macrothrombocytopenia	PRKACG	Autosomal recessive	Spontaneous bleeding	Impaired platelet activation
TUBB1-related thrombocytopenia[86]	TUBB1	Autosomal dominant	None	Absent circumferential microtubules
X-linked thrombocytopenia with or without dyserythropoietic anemia	GATA1	X linked recessive	Bleeding, beta thalassemia, neutropenia, congenital erythropoietic porphyria	Alpha granule deficiency, increased endoplasmic reticulum
York platelet syndrome[87]	STIM1	Autosomal dominant	Proximal myopathy, functional asplenia, moderate bleeding	Giant electron-opaque organelles and target organelles, absent alpha granules

Abbreviations: ACTN1, actinin alpha 1; CYCS, cytochrome C; DIAPH, diaphanous-related formin; FLNA, filamin A; MSK, musculoskeletal; TUBB1, tubulin beta 1 class VI.

Table 2
Platelet disorders resulting in thrombocytopenia

	Genes	Inheritance	Clinical Associations	Platelet Abnormality
Disorders of platelet adhesion				
Bernard-Soulier syndrome	GP1BA, GP1BB, GP9	Autosomal recessive	None	No response to ristocetin on platelet aggregation studies
Disorders of platelet aggregation				
Glanzmann thrombasthenia	ITGA2B, ITGB3, FERMT3	Autosomal recessive	FERMT3 may be associated with leukocyte adhesion deficiency–III	Absent or greatly diminished response to all physiologic agonists
Platelet granule defects				
Hermansky-Pudlak syndrome	HPS 1–10	Autosomal recessive	Depending on type: oculocutaneous albinism, pulmonary fibrosis, nystagmus, cataracts, granulomatous colitis, immune defects	Absent second-wave on light-based aggregation and luminometry with no or markedly diminished response Electron micrographs with absence or extreme paucity of dense granules
Chediak-Higashi syndrome	LYST	Autosomal recessive	Neutropenia, immunodeficiencies, nonmalignant lymphohistiocytic infiltration	Granulocytes with very large cytoplasmic granules
Gray platelet syndrome	NBEAL2, GF11B	Autosomal recessive	Bleeding, risk of bone marrow fibrosis, splenomegaly	Gray platelets
Quebec platelet syndrome	PLAU	Autosomal dominant	Delayed onset of bleeding	Abnormal aggregation with epinephrine

Platelet receptor defects

P2Y12 receptor deficiency	P2YR12	Autosomal recessive	None	Rapidly reversible and reduced platelet aggregation to ADP
Thromboxane A2 receptor deficiency	TBXA2R	Autosomal recessive	None	Defective platelet aggregation with arachidonic acid and thromboxane A2
Defects in signaling pathways				
Thromboxane-A synthase (Ghosal syndrome)	TBXAS1	Autosomal recessive	None	Defective platelet aggregation with arachidonic acid
Cytosolic phospholipase A2	PLA2G4A	Autosomal recessive	None	Decreased platelet aggregation with ADP, collagen
Defects in platelet procoagulant activity				
Scott syndrome	ANO6 (TMEM16F)	Autosomal dominant	None	Platelet aggregation normal. flow cytometry of activated platelets with absent binding of annexin V
Stormorken syndrome[88]	STIM1	—	Miosis, myopathy, ectodermal dysplasia	Increased platelet procoagulant activity, defects in platelet adhesiveness

References are provided for disorders not described in the text.

megakaryocytes with small hypolobated nuclei, as well as normal micromegakaryo-cytes, are seen in the bone marrow.[11] Variable but inconsistent aggregation abnormalities have been described.

Management involves surveillance of counts for early identification of changes that suggest myeloid transformation. If stem cell transplantation is required, donor selection should ensure a related donor does not harbor the same mutation.

Congenital amegakaryocytic thrombocytopenia

Congenital amegakaryocytic thrombocytopenia is an autosomal recessive disorder caused by mutations in the thrombopoietin receptor gene MPL, which is essential for thrombopoiesis and maintenance of hematopoietic stem cells.[14] Patients present with severe thrombocytopenia at birth with clinically significant bleeding (skin, mucosae, gastrointestinal tract) without other syndromic associations. Megakaryocytes are absent in the bone marrow. Evolution to bone marrow failure occurs later in childhood (median 3.7 years).[15] Treatment is supportive with platelet transfusions. Allogeneic bone marrow transplantation is the only curative strategy.

ETV6-related thrombocytopenia

Mutations in ETV6 (also known as TEL) lead to autosomal dominant nonsyndromic thrombocytopenia. ETV6 is a transcriptional repressor that participates in hematopoietic regulation and germline mutations lead to impaired megakaryocyte maturation.[16] Somatic mutations in ETV6 and translocations involving the gene are well-described in MDS, CML, CMML, and acute lymphoblastic leukemia (ALL).

Patients present with mild to moderate thrombocytopenia and an elevated mean corpuscular volume of 92.5 to 101.5 fL.[17] The bleeding tendency is mild to moderate. Patients have an increased risk of both myeloid and lymphoid disorders with variable penetrance, depending on the type of mutation. Of known patients with ETV6-RT, 30% have developed a hematologic malignancy.[18] In vitro, the ability of platelets to spread on fibrinogen is reduced, suggesting impaired signaling of glycoprotein (GP) IIb-IIIa. At the platelet ultrastructural level, elongated alpha granules have been described.[16]

Management involves surveillance of counts for early identification of changes that suggest myeloid transformation. If stem cell transplantation is required, donor selection should ensure a related donor does not harbor the same mutation.

Familial platelet disorder with predisposition to acute myelogenous leukemia

Familial platelet disorder (FPD)-AML is an autosomal dominant disorder caused by germline mutations in RUNX1, leading to nonsyndromic thrombocytopenia with normal platelet size and increased risk of MDS and AML. RUNX1 encodes the alpha subunit of core binding factor, a key transcriptional regulator of genes participating in hematopoiesis, T-cell development, and thrombopoiesis.[19]

Patients present with mild to moderate thrombocytopenia; however, some can have platelet counts in the lower range of normal. The bleeding phenotype is more pronounced compared with other thrombocytopenias of normal platelet size. Approximately 35% of patients develop transformation to MDS or AML.[20] The risk of transformation largely depends on the type of mutation and acquisition of somatic mutations that promote myeloid clonal evolution.[21] Reduced or absent adenosine triphosphate (ATP) release and decreased delta granules on platelet transmission electron microscopy compatible with a dense granule storage pool disorder have been consistently observed, explaining the increased bleeding tendency in this disorder.[22]

Management involves surveillance of counts for early identification of changes that suggest myeloid transformation. If stem cell transplantation is required, donor selection should ensure a related donor does not harbor the same mutation.

Thrombocytopenia with absent radii

Thrombocytopenia with absent radii is an autosomal recessive disorder caused by mutations in the RBM8A gene, usually a large deletion (200-kb and involving at least 10 other genes) in 1 allele combined with a noncoding single-nucleotide polymorphism on the other.[23] Patients present at birth with a severe but sometimes transient thrombocytopenia, absent radii with various upper and lower limb abnormalities, renal and cardiac defects, and a high incidence of milk-protein allergy.[24] Treatment includes supportive platelet transfusions, orthopedic interventions to maximize limb function, and a therapeutic trial of avoidance of cow's milk.[25]

CONGENITAL DISORDERS WITH THROMBOCYTOPENIA AND LARGE PLATELET SIZE
Arthrogryposis-renal Dysfunction-cholestasis

Arthrogryposis-renal dysfunction-cholestasis is a gray platelet-like syndrome with an autosomal recessive inheritance caused by mutations in VPS33B or VIPAS39. These genes code for proteins that are involved in vesicle-mediated protein sorting and trafficking in the Golgi network. The defect leads to absence of alpha granules due to impaired maturation of their precursors and also causes decreased dense granule secretion.

Patients present with joint defects, renal tubular dysfunction, and cholestasis. They usually die within the first year of life. At the ultrastructural level, platelets lack alpha granules or contain only vestigial structures. Dense granule secretion is impaired and leads to decreased platelet aggregation with adenosine diphosphate (ADP) and decreased ATP release.[26]

Integrin A2B and integrin B3–related thrombocytopenia

Loss of functions mutations in integrin (ITG)-A2B and ITGB3 cause Glanzmann thrombasthenia (GT), an autosomal recessive disorder of platelet function. However, heterozygous mutations in these genes can lead to nonsyndromic autosomal dominant macrothrombocytopenia through gain of function mutations that lead to constitutive activation of the affected ITG without induction of platelet activation. This activation leads to incorrect platelet sizing and causes thrombocytopenia by increased platelet turnover. Patients present with mild bleeding. At the structural level, platelets have decreased expression of GPIIb-IIIa.[27,28]

Myosin heavy chain 9–related disorders

Mutations in the nonmuscle myosin heavy chain 9 (MYH9) lead to autosomal dominant syndromic thrombocytopenia. Previously described as May-Hegglin anomaly, Sebastian syndrome, Fechtner syndrome, and Epstein syndrome, according to the platelet phenotype and syndromic associations, they are now collectively known as MYH9RD.[29] Dysfunctional MYH9 affects cytoskeletal structure and function leading to defective megakaryocyte maturation and abnormal cytoplasmic transport.[30]

Patients present with macrothrombocytopenia with giant platelets and varying degrees of sensorineural hearing loss, renal dysfunction, cataracts, and transaminitis. Bleeding is usually not a prominent clinical concern. Recent data suggest a strong genotype-phenotype correlation between the type of mutation and protein domain affected and the development of end-organ damage.[31] At the platelet structural level, pathognomonic basophilic leukocyte inclusions (Döhle-like bodies) can be observed on light microscopy. Immunofluorescence analysis is the gold standard with 100% sensitivity and 95% specificity.[32]

Prophylactic management of hemostasis before a high-risk surgical procedure is based on platelet transfusions and adjunct hemostatic agents. Eltrombopag has been successfully used in a small group of patients to elevate platelet counts.[33] Molecular confirmation is important to provide effective genetic counseling because it allows for more precise prognostication of extrahematologic complications. Surveillance for extrahematologic complications such as hearing loss with audiogram, periodic urine studies to evaluate for proteinuria, and liver function tests are recommended.[34]

Paris-Trousseau thrombocytopenia

Paris-Trousseau thrombocytopenia was initially described in patients with macrothrombocytopenia with giant alpha granules, in the context of 11q deletion syndrome, which causes craniofacial abnormalities, cardiac malformations, and intellectual disability.[35] Subsequently, all patients affected with thrombocytopenia in this context were found to have heterozygous deletions of *FLI1*, a protooncogene encoding a member of the ETS family of transcription factors that has a role in embryogenesis, vascular development, and megakaryopoiesis.[36] Homozygous missense mutations in *FLI1* outside of a deletion syndrome have also been reported.[37]

Patients present with chronic thrombocytopenia; however, cases of resolution of thrombocytopenia during the early years of life have been reported. At the structural level, abnormal platelets with giant alpha granules can be seen by light microscopy and confirmed by electron microscopy to be fused granules.[38]

Gamma catalytic protein kinase gene–related thrombocytopenia

Homozygous mutations in the cyclic adenosine monophosphate (cAMP)-dependent gamma catalytic protein kinase gene (*PRKACG*) lead to autosomal recessive macrothrombocytopenia through defects in proplatelet formation and platelet activation. Patients present with spontaneous bleeding (mucocutaneous and muscular). Flow cytometric studies show inability of platelets to undergo activation. This impaired platelet function can explain the severity of the bleeding phenotype.[39]

X-linked thrombocytopenia with or without dyserythropoietic anemia

X-linked thrombocytopenia with or without dyserythropoietic anemia is caused by germline mutations in *GATA1* and has X-linked recessive inheritance. *GATA1* encodes a zinc finger DNA-binding transcription factor that participates in hematopoietic cell development.[40] Patients present with thrombocytopenia with or without anemia and can also have mild beta thalassemia, neutropenia, or congenital erythropoietic porphyria. Clinically significant bleeding can be present. Platelet aggregation shows variable defects with reduced aggregation to collagen. Decreased to absent alpha granules and cytoplasmic cluster of smooth endoplasmic reticulum are seen.[41] Management is supportive and, for severe cases, allogeneic stem cell transplantation may be required.

DISORDERS OF PLATELET ADHESION
Glycoprotein Ib-IX Receptor Defects (Bernard-Soulier, Mediterranean Macrothrombocytopenia, and Velocardiofacial [DiGeorge] Syndrome)

The GPIb-IX complex is the primary platelet receptor for vWF and is composed of the products of 3 separate genes (*GP1BA, GP1BB, and GP9*). Mutations in the genes that encode for the components of this receptor have been implicated in several thrombocytopenic syndromes, including Bernard-Soulier syndrome (BSS), Mediterranean macrothrombocytopenia, and the thrombocytopenia observed in velocardiofacial (22q11 microdeletion) syndrome.

BSS is an autosomal recessive disorder characterized by the presence of giant platelets and thrombocytopenia, ranging from 20,000/μL to near normal.[42] Homozygous or compound heterozygous mutations of each of GPIbα, GPIbβ, and GPIX have been demonstrated in BSS.[43] Platelet aggregation studies exhibit a lack of response to ristocetin and platelet glycoprotein expression studies demonstrate absence or markedly decreased expression of the receptor on the platelet surface. Patients with BSS typically exhibit mucocutaneous bleeding manifestations. Life-threatening bleeding may occur and necessitate platelet transfusions.[44] There may be a risk for alloimmunization; however, this risk is usually not as profound as in GT (see later discussion).[45] Desmopressin and rVIIa have been used with success in BSS patients.[20]

Autosomal dominant Mediterranean macrothrombocytopenia and velocardiofacial syndromes are disorders in which only a single allele of a component of the GPIb-IX-V complex is mutated.[46–48] Unlike BSS, these syndromes are characterized by large but not giant platelets and a mild bleeding diathesis. Interestingly, only 60% of patients heterozygous for the absence of the GPIb-IX-V complex exhibit macrothrombocytopenia. Accordingly, the manifestations of the heterozygote carriers of mutations known to cause BSS are quite variable.

Platelet-type von Willebrand disease (gain of function mutation of glycoprotein Ib-IX)
Platelet-type von Willebrand disease (vWD), also known as pseudo-vWD, is an autosomal dominant disorder characterized by gain of function mutations in GP1bα, leading to spontaneous binding of vWF to platelets and increased clearance of vWF-platelet complexes.[44,49] Patients present with mild to moderate mucocutaneous bleeding, mild macrothrombocytopenia, and decreased vWF activity due to a decrease in high molecular weight multimers of vWF.

It is critical to differentiate platelet type vWD from type 2B vWD because the treatment of these 2 entities is different. Platelet replacement is the treatment of choice for platelet-type vWD, whereas desmopressin or vWF concentrates are used to treat the latter. This distinction may be made by using mixing studies with platelet aggregometry or, alternatively, by genetic testing of *GPIBA* and vWF.

DISORDERS OF PLATELET AGGREGATION: GLANZMANN THROMBASTHENIA

GT is an autosomal recessive disorder occurring as a result of mutations in genes coding for the platelet fibrinogen receptor, integrin $\alpha_{IIb}\beta_3$. In most patients, the causative mutation results in an absence of expression of the receptor on the platelet surface.[50] However, functional defects in the integrin proteins that have minimal effect on surface expression can also result in GT[51] and such mutations have been reported in the intracellular and extracellular domains of these proteins. A GT-phenotype is also present in patients with leukocyte adhesion deficiency–III (LAD-III), a disorder associated with elevated leukocyte counts, immunodeficiency and bleeding in infancy. In LAD-III, the absence of kindlin-3 prevents normal inside-out activation of β1, β2, and β3 ITGs.[52,53]

Patients with GT typically present with moderate to severe mucocutaneous bleeding. Platelet aggregation studies show absent or greatly diminished response to all agonists except ristocetin. Flow cytometry most often shows significantly low or absent surface levels of $\alpha_{IIb}\beta_3$. However, in the case of functional defects, flow cytometry may be normal or only slightly reduced. Genetic studies may show mutations within the genes *ITGA2B* (that encodes for α_{IIb}), *ITGB3* (that encodes for β_3), or *FERMT3* (that codes for kindlin-3).[54]

Platelet transfusion is the treatment of choice for severe bleeding episodes in GT. However, alloimmunization to ITG integrin $\alpha_{IIb}\beta_3$ frequently complicates platelet transfusion, especially in the context of absent integrin surface expression. This may necessitate the use of rVIIa to limit potential alloimmunization and when platelet refractoriness is observed.[55,56] A few patients with extremely severe bleeding due to alloimmunization have undergone bone marrow transplantation with full engraftment and resolution of the platelet defect.[57]

Platelet Granule Defects

Hermansky-Pudlak syndrome

Hermansky-Pudlak syndrome (HPS) is an autosomal recessive disease that is characterized by an absence of platelet-dense granules and oculocutaneous albinism.[58] The hypopigmentation derives from impaired melanosome formation and trafficking. There are 10 different subtypes caused by mutations in 10 different genes, out of which HPS1 is the most common and most cases occur in patients of Puerto Rican descent.

The bleeding diathesis in HPS is frequently mild. Light-transmission–based platelet aggregation studies demonstrate an absent second wave of aggregation, and luminometry studies demonstrate absent or minimal response to all agonists due to the absence of dense granules. Accordingly, electron micrographs show absence or an extreme paucity of dense granules.

Other characteristic features are subtype-specific and may include pulmonary fibrosis occurring typically in the fourth decade of life in HPS-1 and HPS-4, ophthalmologic complications, such as nystagmus and cataracts, and granulomatous colitis in HPS-1.[59] In patients with HPS-2, an innate immune defect and neutropenia have been seen.[60]

Chediak-Higashi syndrome

Chediak-Higashi syndrome (CHS) is a rare autosomal recessive disorder characterized by a paucity of dense granules, leading to a mild bleeding diathesis and oculocutaneous albinism. Patients have immune defects with neutropenia, impaired chemotaxis and bactericidal activity, and abnormal natural killer cell function. These patients may develop a nonmalignant lymphohistiocytic infiltration of multiple organs.[61,62] The underlying defect in CHS is a mutation in the gene *LYST*. The peripheral blood smear shows granulocytes with very large cytoplasmic granules, which is a hallmark of this disorder.

Gray platelet syndrome

Gray platelet syndrome (GPS) is an autosomal recessive bleeding disorder with large platelets that lack α-granules. Clinically, GPS is usually characterized by mild to moderate bleeding. GPS is also associated with myelofibrosis and splenomegaly as a consequence of myelofibrosis.[26,63]

GPS is characterized by a typical gray appearance of platelets by light microscopy due to a paucity of basophilic α -granules. Mutations in the neurobeachin-like 2 (*NBEAL2*) gene have been identified as the genetic cause of GPS.[64–66] *NBEAL2* encodes a protein containing a BEACH domain that is predicted to be involved in vesicular trafficking and may be critical for the development of platelet α-granules. An autosomal dominant form of GPS due to a mutation in the gene *GF1B* has recently been described.[67]

OTHER DISORDERS OF PLATELET FUNCTION
Quebec Platelet Disorder

Quebec platelet disorder (QPD) is an autosomal dominant bleeding disorder associated with a unique gain-of-function defect in fibrinolysis associated with ectopic expression of urokinase plasminogen activator (uPA) within the developing platelet α-granule.[68,69] The causative genetic defect is a tandem duplication of the *PLAU* gene, which encodes the uPA protein.[70] Bleeding in QPD occurs secondary to release and localization of ectopically expressed uPA in the newly forming hemostatic plug and subsequently accelerated clot lysis.

This disorder is classically characterized by delayed-onset bleeding following hemostatic challenges and the salutary effects of pharmacologic inhibitors of fibrinolysis.[71] Platelet aggregation studies show very abnormal aggregation with epinephrine. Genetic testing for the *PLAU* duplication is diagnostic.

Receptor defects
Adenosine diphosphate receptor defects Platelets possess multiple ADP receptors; among these the P2Y12 receptor, which is responsible for aggregate growth and stabilization of the hemostatic plug.[72] Patients with defects a decreased and rapidly reversible platelet aggregation to ADP have been described with mutations in the *P2RY12* gene affecting ADP binding and even receptor trafficking.[73]

Thromboxane receptor defects An inherited defect of platelet aggregation to thromboxane (TX)-A2 was first reported in Japanese families with a mild bleeding disorder. This defect is characterized by loss of aggregation response to both arachidonic acid and TXA2 receptor agonist.[74] Other mutations of *TBXA2R* have been reported to physiologically mimic the effect of aspirin that blocks arachidonic acid metabolism by irreversibly inhibiting cyclooxygenase.[75]

Defects in intracellular signaling pathways
This group of disorders is associated with selective or suboptimal functional responses to specific agonists. These include defects in GTP-binding proteins, phospholipase C activation, calcium mobilization, lineage-specific $G\alpha_q$ subunit deficiency with impaired $\alpha_{IIb}\beta_3$ activation, and defective phospholipase C expression and activation.[76]

Defects in platelet procoagulant activity
Scott syndrome is a rare inherited bleeding disorder caused by defective scrambling of phospholipids on blood cells. The defect is characterized by normal platelet aggregation and platelet counts with markedly decreased platelet procoagulant activity.[77] Scott syndrome is the result of loss of function mutations in *TMEM16F*, which encodes a transmembrane protein involved in Ca^{2+}-dependent phospholipid scrambling.[78]

SUMMARY

Almost with complete certainty, this list will be viewed as incomplete, and perhaps even grossly lacking, by the next generation of practicing pediatric hematologists. New genetic defects accounting for low platelet counts and platelet-related bleeding continue to be identified. However, diagnostic curiosity, a careful history, guided physical examination, and the careful utilization of newly-developed diagnostic tools (eg, genetic panels, -omic studies) will continue to guide the pediatrician and consultant in the diagnosis and anticipatory or medical management of patients with too few or dysfunctional platelets.

REFERENCES

1. Quiroga T, Goycoolea M, Munoz B, et al. Template bleeding time and PFA-100 have low sensitivity to screen patients with hereditary mucocutaneous hemorrhages: comparative study in 148 patients. J Thromb Haemost 2004;2(6):892–8.

2. Latger-Cannard V, Hoarau M, Salignac S, et al. Mean platelet volume: comparison of three analysers towards standardization of platelet morphological phenotype. Int J Lab Hematol 2012;34(3):300–10.

3. Noris P, Klersy C, Zecca M, et al. Platelet size distinguishes between inherited macrothrombocytopenias and immune thrombocytopenia. J Thromb Haemost 2009;7(12):2131–6.

4. Sullivan KE, Mullen CA, Blaese RM, et al. A multiinstitutional survey of the Wiskott-Aldrich syndrome. J Pediatr 1994;125(6 Pt 1):876–85.

5. Shcherbina A, Candotti F, Rosen FS, et al. High incidence of lymphomas in a subgroup of Wiskott-Aldrich syndrome patients. Br J Haematol 2003;121(3):529–30.

6. Ochs HD, Slichter SJ, Harker LA, et al. The Wiskott-Aldrich syndrome: studies of lymphocytes, granulocytes, and platelets. Blood 1980;55(2):243–52.

7. Villa A, Notarangelo L, Macchi P, et al. X-linked thrombocytopenia and Wiskott-Aldrich syndrome are allelic diseases with mutations in the WASP gene. Nat Genet 1995;9(4):414–7.

8. Lanzi G, Moratto D, Vairo D, et al. A novel primary human immunodeficiency due to deficiency in the WASP-interacting protein WIP. J Exp Med 2012;209(1):29–34.

9. Mullen CA, Anderson KD, Blaese RM. Splenectomy and/or bone marrow transplantation in the management of the Wiskott-Aldrich syndrome: long-term follow-up of 62 cases. Blood 1993;82(10):2961–6.

10. Hacein-Bey Abina S, Gaspar HB, Blondeau J, et al. Outcomes following gene therapy in patients with severe Wiskott-Aldrich syndrome. JAMA 2015;313(15):1550–63.

11. Noris P, Perrotta S, Seri M, et al. Mutations in ANKRD26 are responsible for a frequent form of inherited thrombocytopenia: analysis of 78 patients from 21 families. Blood 2011;117(24):6673–80.

12. Bluteau D, Balduini A, Balayn N, et al. Thrombocytopenia-associated mutations in the ANKRD26 regulatory region induce MAPK hyperactivation. J Clin Invest 2014;124(2):580–91.

13. Noris P, Favier R, Alessi MC, et al. ANKRD26-related thrombocytopenia and myeloid malignancies. Blood 2013;122(11):1987–9.

14. Savoia A, Dufour C, Locatelli F, et al. Congenital amegakaryocytic thrombocytopenia: clinical and biological consequences of five novel mutations. Haematologica 2007;92(9):1186–93.

15. King S, Germeshausen M, Strauss G, et al. Congenital amegakaryocytic thrombocytopenia: a retrospective clinical analysis of 20 patients. Br J Haematol 2005;131(5):636–44.

16. Melazzini F, Palombo F, Balduini A, et al. Clinical and pathogenic features of ETV6-related thrombocytopenia with predisposition to acute lymphoblastic leukemia. Haematologica 2016;101(11):1333–42.

17. Noetzli L, Lo RW, Lee-Sherick AB, et al. Germline mutations in ETV6 are associated with thrombocytopenia, red cell macrocytosis and predisposition to lymphoblastic leukemia. Nat Genet 2015;47(5):535–8.

18. Feurstein S, Godley LA. Germline ETV6 mutations and predisposition to hematological malignancies. Int J Hematol 2017;106(2):189–95.

19. Song WJ, Sullivan MG, Legare RD, et al. Haploinsufficiency of CBFA2 causes familial thrombocytopenia with propensity to develop acute myelogenous leukaemia. Nat Genet 1999;23(2):166–75.

20. Owen CJ, Toze CL, Koochin A, et al. Five new pedigrees with inherited RUNX1 mutations causing familial platelet disorder with propensity to myeloid malignancy. Blood 2008;112(12):4639–45.

21. Langabeer SE, Owen CJ, McCarron SL, et al. A novel RUNX1 mutation in a kindred with familial platelet disorder with propensity to acute myeloid leukaemia: male predominance of affected individuals. Eur J Haematol 2010;85(6):552–3.
22. Perez Botero J, Chen D, Cousin MA, et al. Clinical characteristics and platelet phenotype in a family with RUNX1 mutated thrombocytopenia. Leuk Lymphoma 2017;58(8):1963–7.
23. Albers CA, Paul DS, Schulze H, et al. Compound inheritance of a low-frequency regulatory SNP and a rare null mutation in exon-junction complex subunit RBM8A causes TAR syndrome. Nat Genet 2012;44(4):435–9. S431-432.
24. Greenhalgh KL, Howell RT, Bottani A, et al. Thrombocytopenia-absent radius syndrome: a clinical genetic study. J Med Genet 2002;39(12):876–81.
25. Toriello HV. Thrombocytopenia absent radius syndrome. 2009 Dec 8 [Updated 2016 Dec 8]. In: Adam MP, Ardinger HH, Pagon RA, et al, editors. GeneReviews® [Internet]. Seattle (WA): University of Washington, Seattle; 1993-2018. Available at: https://www.ncbi.nlm.nih.gov/books/NBK23758/.
26. Nurden AT, Nurden P. Should any genetic defect affecting alpha-granules in platelets be classified as gray platelet syndrome? Am J Hematol 2016;91(7): 714–8.
27. Kunishima S, Kashiwagi H, Otsu M, et al. Heterozygous ITGA2B R995W mutation inducing constitutive activation of the alphaIIbbeta3 receptor affects proplatelet formation and causes congenital macrothrombocytopenia. Blood 2011;117(20): 5479–84.
28. Kobayashi Y, Matsui H, Kanai A, et al. Identification of the integrin beta3 L718P mutation in a pedigree with autosomal dominant thrombocytopenia with anisocytosis. Br J Haematol 2013;160(4):521–9.
29. Kunishima S, Kojima T, Tanaka T, et al. Mapping of a gene for May-Hegglin anomaly to chromosome 22q. Hum Genet 1999;105(5):379–83.
30. Pecci A, Canobbio I, Balduini A, et al. Pathogenetic mechanisms of hematological abnormalities of patients with MYH9 mutations. Hum Mol Genet 2005;14(21): 3169–78.
31. Pecci A, Klersy C, Gresele P, et al. MYH9-related disease: a novel prognostic model to predict the clinical evolution of the disease based on genotype-phenotype correlations. Hum Mutat 2014;35(2):236–47.
32. Savoia A, De Rocco D, Panza E, et al. Heavy chain myosin 9-related disease (MYH9 -RD): neutrophil inclusions of myosin-9 as a pathognomonic sign of the disorder. Thromb Haemost 2010;103(4):826–32.
33. Pecci A, Gresele P, Klersy C, et al. Eltrombopag for the treatment of the inherited thrombocytopenia deriving from MYH9 mutations. Blood 2010;116(26):5832–7.
34. Savoia A, Pecci A. MYH9-related disorders. 2008 Nov 20 [Updated 2015 Jul 16]. In: Adam MP, Ardinger HH, Pagon RA, et al, editors. GeneReviews® [Internet]. Seattle (WA): University of Washington, Seattle; 1993-2018. Available from: https://www.ncbi.nlm.nih.gov/books/NBK2689/.
35. Favier R, Douay L, Esteva B, et al. A novel genetic thrombocytopenia (Paris-Trousseau) associated with platelet inclusions, dysmegakaryopoiesis and chromosome deletion AT 11q23. C R Acad Sci III 1993;316(7):698–701.
36. Hart A, Melet F, Grossfeld P, et al. Fli-1 is required for murine vascular and megakaryocytic development and is hemizygously deleted in patients with thrombocytopenia. Immunity 2000;13(2):167–77.
37. Stevenson WS, Rabbolini DJ, Beutler L, et al. Paris-Trousseau thrombocytopenia is phenocopied by the autosomal recessive inheritance of a DNA-binding domain mutation in FLI1. Blood 2015;126(17):2027–30.

38. Favier R, Jondeau K, Boutard P, et al. Paris-Trousseau syndrome: clinical, hematological, molecular data of ten new cases. Thromb Haemost 2003;90(5):893–7.
39. Manchev VT, Hilpert M, Berrou E, et al. A new form of macrothrombocytopenia induced by a germ-line mutation in the PRKACG gene. Blood 2014;124(16): 2554–63.
40. Calligaris R, Bottardi S, Cogoi S, et al. Alternative translation initiation site usage results in two functionally distinct forms of the GATA-1 transcription factor. Proc Natl Acad Sci U S A 1995;92(25):11598–602.
41. Freson K, Matthijs G, Thys C, et al. Different substitutions at residue D218 of the X-linked transcription factor GATA1 lead to altered clinical severity of macrothrombocytopenia and anemia and are associated with variable skewed X inactivation. Hum Mol Genet 2002;11(2):147–52.
42. Nurden AT, Nurden P. Inherited defects of platelet function. Rev Clin Exp Hematol 2001;5(4):314–34 [quiz following 431].
43. Savoia A, Kunishima S, De Rocco D, et al. Spectrum of the mutations in Bernard-Soulier syndrome. Hum Mutat 2014;35(9):1033–45.
44. Othman M, Notley C, Lavender FL, et al. Identification and functional characterization of a novel 27-bp deletion in the macroglycopeptide-coding region of the GPIBA gene resulting in platelet-type von Willebrand disease. Blood 2005; 105(11):4330–6.
45. Lopez JA, Andrews RK, Afshar-Kharghan V, et al. Bernard-Soulier syndrome. Blood 1998;91(12):4397–418.
46. Savoia A, Balduini CL, Savino M, et al. Autosomal dominant macrothrombocytopenia in Italy is most frequently a type of heterozygous Bernard-Soulier syndrome. Blood 2001;97(5):1330–5.
47. Kato T, Kosaka K, Kimura M, et al. Thrombocytopenia in patients with 22q11.2 deletion syndrome and its association with glycoprotein Ib-beta. Genet Med 2003;5(2):113–9.
48. Lambert MP, Arulselvan A, Schott A, et al. The 22q11.2 deletion syndrome: cancer predisposition, platelet abnormalities and cytopenias. Am J Med Genet A 2017. [Epub ahead of print].
49. Miller JL, Castella A. Platelet-type von Willebrand's disease: characterization of a new bleeding disorder. Blood 1982;60(3):790–4.
50. Nurden AT, Pillois X, Wilcox DA. Glanzmann thrombasthenia: state of the art and future directions. Semin Thromb Hemost 2013;39(6):642–55.
51. Ruiz C, Liu CY, Sun QH, et al. A point mutation in the cysteine-rich domain of glycoprotein (GP) IIIa results in the expression of a GPIIb-IIIa (alphaIIbbeta3) integrin receptor locked in a high-affinity state and a Glanzmann thrombasthenia-like phenotype. Blood 2001;98(8):2432–41.
52. Kuijpers TW, van de Vijver E, Weterman MA, et al. LAD-1/variant syndrome is caused by mutations in FERMT3. Blood 2009;113(19):4740–6.
53. Svensson L, Howarth K, McDowall A, et al. Leukocyte adhesion deficiency-III is caused by mutations in KINDLIN3 affecting integrin activation. Nat Med 2009; 15(3):306–12.
54. Buitrago L, Rendon A, Liang Y, et al. alphaIIbbeta3 variants defined by next-generation sequencing: predicting variants likely to cause Glanzmann thrombasthenia. Proc Natl Acad Sci U S A 2015;112(15):E1898–907.
55. Di Minno G, Zotz RB, d'Oiron R, et al. The international, prospective Glanzmann Thrombasthenia registry: treatment modalities and outcomes of non-surgical bleeding episodes in patients with Glanzmann thrombasthenia. Haematologica 2015;100(8):1031–7.

56. Poon MC, d'Oiron R, Zotz RB, et al. The international, prospective Glanzmann Thrombasthenia registry: treatment and outcomes in surgical intervention. Haematologica 2015;100(8):1038–44.

57. Bellucci S, Damaj G, Boval B, et al. Bone marrow transplantation in severe Glanzmann's thrombasthenia with antiplatelet alloimmunization. Bone Marrow Transplant 2000;25(3):327–30.

58. Seward SL Jr, Gahl WA. Hermansky-Pudlak syndrome: health care throughout life. Pediatrics 2013;132(1):153–60.

59. Brantly M, Avila NA, Shotelersuk V, et al. Pulmonary function and high-resolution CT findings in patients with an inherited form of pulmonary fibrosis, Hermansky-Pudlak syndrome, due to mutations in HPS-1. Chest 2000;117(1):129–36.

60. Fontana S, Parolini S, Vermi W, et al. Innate immunity defects in Hermansky-Pudlak type 2 syndrome. Blood 2006;107(12):4857–64.

61. Introne W, Boissy RE, Gahl WA. Clinical, molecular, and cell biological aspects of Chediak-Higashi syndrome. Mol Genet Metab 1999;68(2):283–303.

62. Kaplan J, De Domenico I, Ward DM. Chediak-Higashi syndrome. Curr Opin Hematol 2008;15(1):22–9.

63. Chen CH, Lo RW, Urban D, et al. alpha-granule biogenesis: from disease to discovery. Platelets 2017;28(2):147–54.

64. Kahr WH, Hinckley J, Li L, et al. Mutations in NBEAL2, encoding a BEACH protein, cause gray platelet syndrome. Nat Genet 2011;43(8):738–40.

65. Albers CA, Cvejic A, Favier R, et al. Exome sequencing identifies NBEAL2 as the causative gene for gray platelet syndrome. Nat Genet 2011;43(8):735–7.

66. Gunay-Aygun M, Falik-Zaccai TC, Vilboux T, et al. NBEAL2 is mutated in gray platelet syndrome and is required for biogenesis of platelet alpha-granules. Nat Genet 2011;43(8):732–4.

67. Monteferrario D, Bolar NA, Marneth AE, et al. A dominant-negative GFI1B mutation in the gray platelet syndrome. N Engl J Med 2014;370(3):245–53.

68. Blavignac J, Bunimov N, Rivard GE, et al. Quebec platelet disorder: update on pathogenesis, diagnosis, and treatment. Semin Thromb Hemost 2011;37(6): 713–20.

69. Hayward CP, Rivard GE, Kane WH, et al. An autosomal dominant, qualitative platelet disorder associated with multimerin deficiency, abnormalities in platelet factor V, thrombospondin, von Willebrand factor, and fibrinogen and an epinephrine aggregation defect. Blood 1996;87(12):4967–78.

70. Paterson AD, Rommens JM, Bharaj B, et al. Persons with Quebec platelet disorder have a tandem duplication of PLAU, the urokinase plasminogen activator gene. Blood 2010;115(6):1264–6.

71. McKay H, Derome F, Haq MA, et al. Bleeding risks associated with inheritance of the Quebec platelet disorder. Blood 2004;104(1):159–65.

72. Hechler B, Gachet C. Purinergic receptors in thrombosis and inflammation. Arterioscler Thromb Vasc Biol 2015;35(11):2307–15.

73. Lecchi A, Femia EA, Paoletta S, et al. Inherited dysfunctional platelet P2Y12 receptor mutations associated with bleeding disorders. Hamostaseologie 2016; 36(4):279–83.

74. Hirata T, Ushikubi F, Kakizuka A, et al. Two thromboxane A2 receptor isoforms in human platelets. Opposite coupling to adenylyl cyclase with different sensitivity to Arg60 to Leu mutation. J Clin Invest 1996;97(4):949–56.

75. Mumford AD, Dawood BB, Daly ME, et al. A novel thromboxane A2 receptor D304N variant that abrogates ligand binding in a patient with a bleeding diathesis. Blood 2010;115(2):363–9.

76. Rao AK. Inherited defects in platelet signaling mechanisms. J Thromb Haemost 2003;1(4):671–81.

77. Sims PJ, Wiedmer T, Esmon CT, et al. Assembly of the platelet prothrombinase complex is linked to vesiculation of the platelet plasma membrane. Studies in Scott syndrome: an isolated defect in platelet procoagulant activity. J Biol Chem 1989;264(29):17049–57.

78. Suzuki J, Umeda M, Sims PJ, et al. Calcium-dependent phospholipid scrambling by TMEM16F. Nature 2010;468(7325):834–8.

79. Morison IM, Cramer Borde EM, Cheesman EJ, et al. A mutation of human cyto-chrome c enhances the intrinsic apoptotic pathway but causes only thrombocy-topenia. Nat Genet 2008;40(4):387–9.

80. Niihori T, Ouchi-Uchiyama M, Sasahara Y, et al. Mutations in MECOM, encoding oncoprotein EVI1, cause radioulnar synostosis with amegakaryocytic thrombocy-topenia. Am J Hum Genet 2015;97(6):848–54.

81. Thompson AA, Nguyen LT. Amegakaryocytic thrombocytopenia and radio-ulnar synostosis are associated with HOXA11 mutation. Nat Genet 2000;26(4):397–8.

82. Kunishima S, Okuno Y, Yoshida K, et al. ACTN1 mutations cause congenital mac-rothrombocytopenia. Am J Hum Genet 2013;92(3):431–8.

83. Stritt S, Nurden P, Turro E, et al. A gain-of-function variant in DIAPH1 causes dominant macrothrombocytopenia and hearing loss. Blood 2016;127(23): 2903–14.

84. Nurden P, Debili N, Coupry I, et al. Thrombocytopenia resulting from mutations in filamin A can be expressed as an isolated syndrome. Blood 2011;118(22): 5928–37.

85. Rees DC, Iolascon A, Carella M, et al. Stomatocytic haemolysis and macrothrom-bocytopenia (Mediterranean stomatocytosis/macrothrombocytopenia) is the haematological presentation of phytosterolaemia. Br J Haematol 2005;130(2): 297–309.

86. Kunishima S, Kobayashi R, Itoh TJ, et al. Mutation of the beta1-tubulin gene asso-ciated with congenital macrothrombocytopenia affecting microtubule assembly. Blood 2009;113(2):458–61.

87. Markello T, Chen D, Kwan JY, et al. York platelet syndrome is a CRAC channelop-athy due to gain-of-function mutations in STIM1. Mol Genet Metab 2015;114(3): 474–82.

88. Misceo D, Holmgren A, Louch WE, et al. A dominant STIM1 mutation causes Stor-morken syndrome. Hum Mutat 2014;35(5):556–64.

Red Blood Cell Enzyme Disorders

Rachael F. Grace, MD, MMSc[a],*, Bertil Glader, MD, PhD[b]

KEYWORDS

- Glucose-6-phosphate dehydrogenase deficiency • Pyruvate kinase deficiency
- Other red cell enzyme disorders • Anemia • Splenectomy • Cholecystectomy

KEY POINTS

- Red blood cell enzyme disorders are important to recognize and diagnose for proper supportive care, monitoring, and treatment.
- Glucose-6-phosphate dehydrogenase (G6PD) deficiency is an X-linked disorder most commonly characterized by episodic hemolysis in the setting of oxidative triggers, such as fava beans, infections, and certain medications.
- Enzymopathies, such as pyruvate kinase deficiency, should be suspected in patients of all ages with a chronic hemolytic anemia in the absence of immune-mediated hemolysis, a hemoglobinopathy, or evidence of a red cell membrane disorder.
- Splenectomy partially ameliorates the anemia in most patients with pyruvate kinase deficiency and other red blood cell enzyme disorders.
- Glycolytic red cell disorders cause congenital hemolytic anemia with wide clinical heterogeneity and frequent complications, including neonatal jaundice, gallstones, and both transfusion-related and transfusion-independent iron loading.

INTRODUCTION

Mature red blood cells (RBC) are anucleate and devoid of ribosomes and mitochondria. Despite these limitations, RBCs survive 100 to 120 days in the circulation and effectively deliver oxygen to peripheral tissues. Glucose is the main metabolic substrate of RBCs, and it is metabolized by 2 major pathways: the glycolytic or "energy-producing" pathway and the hexose monophosphate (HMP) shunt or "protective" pathway (**Fig. 1**). The major products of glycolysis are ATP (a source of energy for numerous RBC membrane and metabolic reactions), nicotinamide adenine

Disclosure Statement: The authors are scientific advisors and receive research funding from Agios Pharmaceuticals.
[a] Department of Pediatric Hematology/Oncology, Dana-Farber/Boston Children's Cancer and Blood Disorders Center, Harvard Medical School, 450 Brookline Avenue, Dana 3-106, Boston, MA 02215, USA; [b] Department of Pediatric Hematology/Oncology, Lucile Packard Children's Hospital, Stanford University School of Medicine, 1000 Welch Road # 300, Palo Alto, CA 94304, USA
* Corresponding author.
E-mail address: Rachael.Grace@childrens.harvard.edu

dinucleotide (a necessary cofactor for methemoglobin reduction by cytochrome b5 reductase), and 2,3-diphosphoglycerate (2,3-DPG; an important intermediate that modulates hemoglobin-oxygen affinity).

The consequence of red cell enzymopathies is hemolysis, and although these diagnoses are clinically diverse, the general laboratory findings, symptoms, and complications are similar. In these disorders, RBCs have a shortened life span, and clinical features vary from absent or mild anemia with episodic hemolysis to severe, chronic anemia requiring transfusions. Patients have a compensatory erythropoiesis, often with reticulocytosis, and, because of ongoing hemolysis, typically have scleral icterus or jaundice from elevation of the unconjugated bilirubin.

A hemolytic disorder should be suspected in the setting of a low hemoglobin, normal to elevated mean cell volume, elevated reticulocyte count, elevated indirect bilirubin level, and/or elevated lactate dehydrogenase (LDH). Testing for a RBC enzyme disorder should be pursued in patients with chronic hemolysis who have a negative direct Coombs test, no evidence of red cell consumption or a membranopathy, and a normal hemoglobin electrophoresis (**Fig. 2**). Suspicion for these

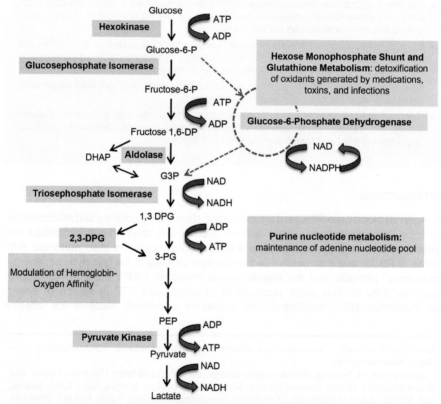

Fig. 1. Summary of overall glycolysis, hexose monophosphate shunt, glutathione metabolism, and red blood cell nucleotide metabolism. Blue boxes contain enzymes in glycolytic pathway that correlate with the more common glycolytic enzymopathies. 1,3-DPG, 1,3-diphosphoglycerate; 2,3-DPG, 2,3-diphosphoglycerate; 3-PG, 3-phosphoglycerate; DHAP, dihydroxyacetone phosphate; Fructose 1,6-DP, fructose 1,6-diphosphate; Fructose-6-P, fructose-6-phophate; G3P, glyceraldehyde-3-phosphate; Glucose-6-P, glucose-6-phosphate; PEP, phosphoenolpyruvate. *Dotted arrows* show the hexose monosphosphate shunt and glutathione metabolism pathway.

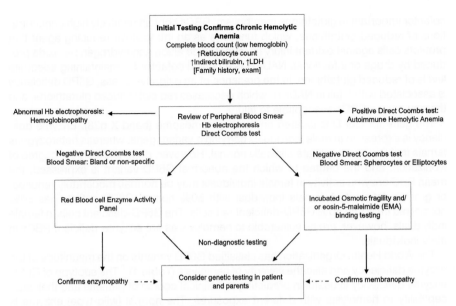

Fig. 2. Evaluation of chronic hemolytic anemia.

disorders should be raised in the setting of neonatal jaundice and/or nonimmune hemolysis. Symptoms and findings of glycolytic enzyme deficiencies include chronic hemolytic anemia, gallstones, and transfusion-related and transfusion-independent iron overload. Splenectomy can partially ameliorate the anemia and/or transfusion burden in some of these disorders. Diagnosis is important with regard to monitoring, supportive care, and the role of splenectomy.

GLUCOSE-6-PHOSPHATE DEHYDROGENASE DEFICIENCY

Deficiency of glucose-6-phosphate dehydrogenase (G6PD) is the most common metabolic disorder of RBCs and has been estimated to affect more than 400 million people worldwide.[1-3] Although global in its distribution, G6PD deficiency is encountered with greatest frequency in the tropical and subtropical zones of the Eastern Hemisphere. The incidence of the deficiency state is approximately 12% in African American men and as many as 20% of female African American individuals are heterozygous and 1% are homozygous for G6PD mutants.[4] Because of its high incidence among populations in which malaria was once endemic, G6PD deficiency is thought to have conferred a selective advantage against infection by falciparum malaria.[5]

It is important to recognize that in almost all individuals with G6PD deficiency, there is no anemia in the steady state, and reticulocyte counts are normal.[6] However, episodic exacerbations of hemolysis accompanied by anemia occur in association with the administration of certain drugs, with some infections, and with ingestion of fava beans. In a small minority of cases, G6PD deficiency can be associated with a chronic hemolytic process.

Pathophysiology

The HMP shunt pathway metabolizes 5% to 10% of glucose used by red cells, and this is critical for protecting red cells against oxidant injury. The HMP pathway is the only RBC source of reduced nicotinamide adenine dinucleotide phosphate (NADPH), a cofactor important in glutathione metabolism. RBCs contain relatively high concentrations of reduced glutathione, which functions as an intracellular reducing agent that protects cells against oxidant injury (ie, superoxide anion and hydrogen peroxide produced by drugs or infections). NADPH is a critical cofactor for maintaining adequate levels of reduced glutathione. In the presence of an oxidative stress, G6PD deficiency is associated with a fall in NADPH, which decreases red cell reduced glutathione, and thereby makes RBCs susceptible to injury.

The gene for G6PD is located on the X chromosome (band X q28). Enzyme deficiency is expressed in male individuals carrying a variant gene, whereas heterozygous female individuals usually are clinically normal. However, dependent on the degree of lyonization, and the degree to which the abnormal G6PD variant is expressed, the mean RBC enzyme activity in female individuals may be normal, moderately reduced, or grossly deficient. A female individual with 50% normal G6PD activity has 50% normal red cells and 50% G6PD-deficient red cells. The G6PD-deficient cells in female individuals, however, are as vulnerable to hemolysis as are enzyme-deficient RBCs in male individuals.

The World Health Organization has classified G6PD variants on the magnitude of the enzyme deficiency and also the severity of hemolysis (**Table 1**).[7] The subtype of G6PD enzyme deficiency is useful in predicting the clinical course of patients and their susceptibility to hemolysis with different exposures. The normal (wild-type) enzyme is referred to as G6PD B. The common G6PD deficiency subtypes with their degree of severity and classification are shown in **Table 2**.[2]

As red cells age, the activity of G6PD normally declines. Nevertheless, healthy RBCs contain sufficient G6PD activity to generate NADPH and avoid hemolysis in the setting of oxidant stress. However, in G6PD variants associated with hemolysis, the enzymes are unstable and have a much shorter half-life. The activity of G6PD A-declines rapidly with a half-life of only 13 days. The instability of G6PD Mediterranean is even more pronounced, with a half-life measured in hours.[11] The clinical correlate of this age-related enzyme instability is that hemolysis in patients with G6PD A-generally is mild and limited to older deficient erythrocytes. In contrast, the enzymatic defect in Class II variants, such as G6PD Mediterranean, G6PD Canton, and G6PD Gaohe, are due to much greater enzyme instability, and RBCs of all ages are grossly deficient.[10] Consequently, a large fraction of the RBC population of individuals with these G6PD variants is susceptible to oxidant-induced injury, and this can lead to severe hemolytic anemia.

The result of oxidative damage to red cells is the production of rigid, nondeformable erythrocytes that are susceptible to destruction by the reticuloendothelial system.[12] Both extravascular and intravascular hemolysis occur in acute hemolytic episodes in G6PD-deficient individuals. Thus, patients develop a low hemoglobin, increased

Table 1
The World Health Organization classification of glucose-6-phosphate dehydrogenase variants

Variant Type	Residual Enzyme Activity	Clinical Findings
Class I	Severe deficiency <10% normal	Chronic hemolytic anemia, occasional decreased white blood cell function
Class II	Severe deficiency <10% normal	Episodic severe hemolysis with oxidative triggers
Class III	Moderate deficiency 10%–60% normal	Episodic moderate hemolysis with oxidative triggers
Class IV	Normal activity >60%	None

Table 2
The common glucose-6-phosphate dehydrogenase (G6PD) deficiency subtypes and their degree of severity

G6PD Enzyme Subtypes	Common Demographic Features	Severity	Classification
G6PD B	Most common	Wild-type enzyme	Normal
G6PD A+	20%–30% of African Black individuals[8]	Normal, no hemolysis	Class IV
G6PD A–	10%–15% of African American and African Black individuals[9]	Mild to moderate hemolysis	Class III
G6PD Kaiping	Asian individuals[10]	Mild to moderate hemolysis	Class III
G6PD Mahidol	Southeast Asian individuals	Mild to moderate hemolysis	Class III
G6PD Mediterranean	Common in Mediterranean regions, Middle East, and India[1]	Severe hemolysis	Class II
G6PD Canton	Asian individuals	Severe hemolysis	Class II
G6PD Gaohe	Asian individuals	Severe hemolysis	Class II

indirect bilirubin, elevated LDH, free plasma hemoglobin, low haptoglobin, and hemoglobinuria.

Diagnosis

In many parts of the world with a high incidence of G6PD deficiency, there are neonatal screening programs. In the United States, however, there is no generalized neonatal screening program for G6PD deficiency. Because of its prevalence and worldwide distribution, and also considering the diversity of the population in the United States, G6PD deficiency should be given serious consideration in the differential diagnosis of any nonimmune hemolytic anemia (see **Fig. 2**). Most commonly, anemia is first recognized during or after an infectious illness, after exposure to one of several suspect drugs or chemicals (**Table 3**), or following exposure to fava beans. G6PD deficiency also should be considered in neonates with excessive and unexplained

Table 3
Drugs and chemicals associated with hemolysis in G6PD deficiency

Unsafe (Class 1, II, and III G6PD Variants)

Acetanilid	Thiazolesulfone
Diaminodiphenyl sulfone (Dapsone)	Phenazopyridine (Pyridium)
Furazolidone (Furoxone)	Phenylhydrazine
Glibenclamide	Primaquine
Henna (Lawsone)	Sulfacetamide
Isobutyl nitrate	Sulfanilamide
Methylene blue	Sulfapyridine
Nalidixic acid (Neg—Gram)	Thiazolesulfone
Naphthalene (Mothballs)	Trinitrotoluene (TNT)
Niridazole (Ambilhar)	Urate oxidase (Rasburicase)
Nitrofurantoin (Furadantin)	

Republished with permission of American Society of Hematology, *From* Beutler E. Glucose-6-phosphate dehydrogenase deficiency: a historical perspective. Blood 2008;111(1):16–24; permission conveyed through Copyright Clearance Center, Inc.

hyperbilirubinemia, even in the absence of anemia or hemolysis. Patients with G6PD deficiency in the midst of a hemolytic episode can have irregularly contracted erythrocytes and "bite" cells on the Wright-stained peripheral blood smear.

The diagnosis of G6PD deficiency is often made using a qualitative screening test, for example, using the fluorescence of NADPH after glucose-6-phosphate and NADP are added to a RBC hemolysate of test cells.[13] Also, G6PD is commonly evaluated in a spectrophotometric assay that provides a quantitative measure of enzyme activity. Regardless of the test used to detect G6PD deficiency, false-negative reactions can occur if the most severely enzyme-deficient RBCs have been removed by hemolysis. In many suspected cases of G6PD deficiency, it may be prudent to reevaluate the patient 3 months after the acute episode when the RBC mass is repopulated with cells of all ages.

Advances in molecular biology have further enhanced our understanding of G6PD deficiency, and now more than 160 different gene mutations or mutation combinations have been identified.[1,14–16] These DNA changes are almost all missense mutations, located throughout the coding region of the gene, leading to single amino acid substitutions in the enzyme. However, in Class I variants associated with chronic hemolysis, mutations are clustered around exon 10, an area that governs the formation of the active G6PD dimer. Molecular sequencing is not necessary in those with common clinical phenotypes with normal baseline blood counts and episodic hemolysis only with exposures to oxidative triggers. However, in those with chronic nonspherocytic hemolytic anemia, molecular analysis may be useful for verifying that the cause is due to a Class I G6PD deficiency versus a separate red cell mutation.

Clinical Features and Complications

In most affected individuals, G6PD deficiency is unrecognized; however, in some, it causes episodic or moderate to severe anemia. The common clinical entities encountered are neonatal hyperbilirubinemia and acute hemolytic anemia.

Neonatal hyperbilirubinemia

Hyperbilirubinemia resulting from G6PD deficiency are well documented in the newborn period. Hyperbilirubinemia related to G6PD deficiency is rarely present at birth and has a peak incidence of clinical onset between days 2 and 3. Although the cause of hyperbilirubinemia in G6PD-deficient infants occasionally reflects accelerated red cell breakdown, more often, there is no obvious RBC destruction. In most cases, there is more jaundice than anemia. Close monitoring of serum bilirubin levels in infants known to be G6PD deficient is warranted, as more than 30% of kernicterus cases in the United States are associated with G6PD deficiency.[17,18]

Acute hemolytic anemia

With most G6PD variants, hemolysis occurs only after exposure to oxidant stresses. In the steady state, there is no anemia and the hemolytic markers and RBC morphology are normal. Sudden destruction of enzyme-deficient RBCs is triggered by specific drugs, toxins, and/or infections. After exposure, jaundice, pallor, nausea, chills, and dark urine, with or without abdominal and back pain, are sudden in onset. An abrupt decrement in hemoglobin concentration occurs. The peripheral blood smear contains spherocytes and eccentrocytes or "blister" cells. In response to anemia, red cell production increases; an increase in reticulocytes is apparent within 5 days and is maximal by 7 to 10 days after onset of hemolysis. In G6PD A, with continued oxidant exposure, the acute hemolytic process ends spontaneously after approximately 1 week, and the hemoglobin concentration thereafter returns to normal levels. In contrast, in Class II variants, such as G6PD Mediterranean, there can be severe hemolysis affecting almost the entire RBC population. Hemolytic episodes can occur in both heterozygous female individuals as well as hemizygous male individuals.

Table 3 lists several drugs that are predictably injurious for all G6PD-deficient individuals. Other drugs and compounds, although sometimes producing a modest shortening of survival of G6PD-deficient red cells, can be given safely in usual therapeutic doses to individuals with Class II and III G6PD variants (**Table 4**). Certain drugs were historically labeled as unsafe in G6PD deficiency; however, for these medications, it is now clear that the hemolysis was due to oxidative stress from an infection for which the drugs were prescribed, rather than related to the actual drug.[19] Infection is probably the most common factor inciting hemolysis, particularly in children.[20] Exposure to fava beans is toxic and potentially fatal for some individuals. However, unlike other agents capable of inducing hemolysis, the fava bean is toxic for only some individuals with G6PD Class II variants; most frequently implicated are G6PD Mediterranean and Asian G6PD variants. African and African American individuals with G6PD deficiency are much less susceptible, although rare hemolytic episodes have been reported.[21] Favism has been observed in nursing infants of mothers who have eaten fava beans.[22] Symptoms of acute intravascular hemolysis occur within 5 to 24 hours of ingestion of fava beans. The drop in hemoglobin concentration is precipitous and often severe enough to require a red cell transfusion.

Congenital nonspherocytic hemolytic anemia

A very small fraction of G6PD-deficient individuals have chronic lifelong hemolysis in the absence of infection or drug exposure. The hemolytic anemia associated with Class I variants is indistinguishable from the congenital nonspherocytic hemolytic syndromes related to glycolytic enzyme deficiencies. The hemolytic process may be fully compensated, although mild to moderate anemia is the rule (hemoglobin 8–10 g/dL),

Table 4
Common medications and chemicals that are usually safe at usual doses in glucose-6-phosphate dehydrogenase deficiency

Safe Drugs in Usual Therapeutic Doses[a]	
Acetaminophen (Tylenol)	Phenylbutazone
Acetylsalicylic acid (aspirin)	Phenytoin
Antazoline (Antistine)	Probenecid (Benemid)
Antipyrine	Procainamide hydrochloride (Pronestyl)
Ascorbic Acid	Pyrimethamine (Daraprim)
Benzhexol (Artane)	Quinine
Chloramphenicol	Streptomycin
Chlorguanidine (Proguanil, Paludrine)	Sulfacytine
Chloroquine	Sulfadiazine
Colchicine	Sulfamethoxazole (Gantanol)
Cotrimoxazole (trimethoprim/sulfamethoxazole)	Sulfamethoxypyridazine (Kynex)
Diphenhydramine (Benadryl)	Sulfisoxazole (Gantrisin)
Isoniazid	Tiaprofenic acid
L-Dopa	Trimethoprim
p-Aminobenzoic acid	Tripelennamine (Pyribenzamine)
p-Aminosalicylic acid	Vitamin K
Trimethoprim	

[a] Safety for Class I glucose-6-phosphate dehydrogenase variants is not known.

Republished with permission of American Society of Hematology, *From* Beutler E. Glucose-6-phosphate dehydrogenase deficiency: a historical perspective. Blood 2008;111(1):16–24; permission conveyed through Copyright Clearance Center, Inc.

and, under basal conditions, the usual reticulocyte count is 10% to 15%. Splenectomy may be of benefit to some patients.[23]

Treatment

Therapy for neonatal hyperbilirubinemia resulting from G6PD deficiency includes phototherapy or exchange transfusion to prevent kernicterus. In some cases, RBC transfusion is indicated for symptomatic anemia. Avoidance of drugs or toxins and treatment of underlying infections that may be contributing to hemolysis are critical. In infants known to be G6PD deficient, prevention of severe hyperbilirubinemia by administration of 1 to 2 doses of an inhibitor of heme oxygenase appears highly effective but is not yet clinically available.[24,25]

Individuals having variants associated with acute, episodic hemolysis may have a significant fall in hemoglobin concentration, requiring a RBC transfusion, more common with Class II than Class III variants. All affected individuals should avoid exposure to medications and toxins known to trigger hemolysis. Pregnant and nursing women known to be heterozygous for the deficiency also should avoid ingestion of drugs with oxidant potential, because some gain access to the fetal circulation and to breast milk. If the indication for its use is critical, however, administration of an offending drug may be justifiable, despite modest shortening of red cell survival. Chronic nonspherocytic hemolytic anemia due to Class I G6PD variants may require more active intervention, similar to the other glycolytic enzyme defects, as outlined as follows.

OTHER DISORDERS OF THE HEXOSE MONOPHOSPHATE SHUNT AND GLUTATHIONE METABOLISM

In addition to G6PD, other enzymes of the HMP shunt pathway, the closely linked reactions of glutathione metabolism, and the glutathione synthetic pathway are important in protecting RBCs against oxidant injury. Rare abnormalities in these enzymes have been reported and have similar clinical findings to the glycolytic red cell enzyme disorders.[26]

GLYCOLYTIC ENZYME ABNORMALITIES: GENERAL CONSIDERATIONS

In contrast to G6PD deficiency, which affects millions of people, hemolytic anemias due to glycolytic enzymopathies are relatively rare, affecting thousands of individuals worldwide.[14,27,28] Abnormalities in virtually every glycolytic enzyme have been described, although more than 90% of cases associated with hemolysis are due to pyruvate kinase (PK) deficiency. Most glycolytic enzymopathies have an autosomal recessive pattern of inheritance. Heterozygotes almost always are hematologically normal, although their RBCs contain less than normal levels of enzyme activity. The vast majority of cases of hemolytic anemia due to glycolytic enzyme deficiencies are a consequence of compound heterozygosity for 2 different enzyme variants, thus accounting for the diverse biochemical and clinical heterogeneity of the red cell glycolytic enzymopathies.

Clinical manifestations of hemolysis due to glycolytic enzymopathies include chronic anemia, reticulocytosis, and indirect hyperbilirubinemia. In most cases, the hemolytic process is recognized and diagnosed in childhood. Most often, there is a history of neonatal jaundice, often requiring phototherapy or an exchange transfusion. The magnitude of chronic anemia varies; there may be accelerated hemolysis with infections or transient aplastic crises associated with parvovirus infection.

The possibility of a glycolytic defect is considered when a chronic hemolytic anemia cannot be explained by the more common causes (see **Fig. 2**). There are no specific RBC morphologic abnormalities in these disorders, although anisocytosis and poikilocytosis are common. A specific assay of RBC enzyme activity and/or RBC genetic testing is necessary to make the diagnosis. Identification of patients with glycolytic enzyme abnormalities can be complex, particularly in patients managed with regular transfusions, which confounds enzyme testing. Mutant erythrocytes also can be so unstable that they are rapidly removed from the circulation, whereas the remaining cells may be biochemically less abnormal. Consequently, "false-negative" assays can obscure the correct diagnosis.

Historically, specific enzyme assays have been considered the gold standard for the diagnosis of disorders of erythrocyte metabolism. The availability of clinical molecular testing has grown for disorders of glycolysis. There are advantages and disadvantages of molecular testing compared with direct enzyme assay, and these can be complementary techniques. In many patients, direct enzyme analysis is adequate for initial diagnosis, with molecular testing serving as a confirmatory test.

PYRUVATE KINASE DEFICIENCY

Of the enzymatic deficiencies involving glycolysis, PK deficiency is the most common and the most extensively studied. Although hundreds of cases have been reported, the prevalence is not known, but estimated to be 1 in 20,000 in the United States.[29] A particularly high frequency exists among the Pennsylvania Amish due to the founder effect.[30,31] The development of patient registries for PK deficiency has helped to better characterize the spectrum of symptoms and complications in patients with this anemia.[32]

Pathophysiology

PK catalyzes the conversion of phosphoenolpyruvate to pyruvate, which is one of the 2 glycolytic reactions resulting in net ATP production. PK deficiency results in impaired glucose utilization and a diminished capacity to generate ATP.[33] In addition, glycolytic intermediates proximal to the block accumulate in red cells, and, of particular interest, the levels of 2,3-DPG may increase up to threefold, and this important intermediate is known to enhance oxygen unloading from hemoglobin[34,35] As a result, patients with PK deficiency are hypothesized to have a greater exercise tolerance than would be expected from the degree of anemia.[35]

PK-deficient reticulocytes generate ATP through mitochondrial oxidative phosphorylation.[33,36] The advantage of oxidative phosphorylation for PK-deficient reticulocytes is that ATP can be generated without relying on glycolysis. When reticulocytes mature, mitochondria disappear, oxidative phosphorylation ceases, and ATP levels fall. In severely PK-deficient RBCs, the fall in ATP leads to membrane defects and RBC destruction in the spleen.[37,38] Given the unique metabolic abnormalities of PK-deficient reticulocytes, it is understandable why the spleen poses a problem where limited oxygen and glucose restrict effective oxidative phosphorylation.[36] Impaired ATP production leads to RBC destruction in the spleen or in the liver after escape from the spleen. Severely deficient reticulocytes are metabolically more stable in the absence of the spleen; therefore, a paradoxical, sustained and robust reticulocytosis follows splenectomy in this disorder.[39]

There are 2 different PK genes (PKM2 and PKLR). The PKLR gene is on chromosome 1(1q21), and the hemolytic anemia associated with PK deficiency is due to homozygous or compound heterozygous mutations in the PKLR gene. Heterozygous mutations in the PKLR gene are clinically silent with no hemolysis or anemia. More than 300 different mutations of the PKLR gene have been identified as causes of chronic hemolytic anemia. Most of these are missense mutations (approximately 70%).[14,40–42] Except for certain groups, such as the Amish and Romani population, most PK mutations are rare, occurring only once, and approximately 25% of patients diagnosed will have a newly described pathogenic variant. Current molecular biology studies are focused on determining the relationship of specific mutations with the clinical phenotype.[40,42]

Diagnosis

The hematologic features of PK deficiency are not distinct from many other hemolytic disorders and can vary between patients. The specific diagnosis rests on a low PK enzyme activity level and/or molecular analysis. Simple enzyme screening tests are available, but false-negative results are common. In cases in which PK deficiency is suspected, a direct quantitative assay of the enzyme is essential. Most deficient individuals have 5% to 25% of the normal mean enzyme activity. The diagnosis of PK deficiency also should be suspected when the PK enzyme activity is normal but relatively low in comparison with other age-dependent RBC enzymes. Thus, PK activity should always be measured along with another RBC age-dependent enzyme, such as hexokinase or G6PD. There is little or no relationship between the measured red cell PK activity in vitro and severity of hemolysis in vivo.[14,39]

In families with a child with PK deficiency, molecular diagnostic techniques are useful for prenatal diagnosis.[43] In addition, for patients who are transfused before the enzyme disorder is recognized, molecular testing is more straightforward. The increasing availability of clinical molecular testing for PK deficiency allows for molecular diagnosis in patients in whom enzyme analysis is challenging or confirmation testing is useful.

The peripheral blood smear reveals all the morphologic hallmarks of accelerated erythropoiesis: polychromatophilia, anisocytosis, poikilocytosis, and variable numbers of nucleated red cells. Irregularly contracted erythrocytes with surface spicules, ecchinocytes,[44] and acanthocytes[45] have been observed in the blood smears of some affected individuals. Before splenectomy, the reticulocyte count may be increased (5%–15%); after splenectomy, reticulocyte counts paradoxically increase and can be as high as 50% to 70%.[38] The robust reticulocytosis is due to the longer survival of reticulocytes following splenectomy.

Clinical Features and Complications

Anemia due to PK deficiency is mild to severe in degree with a hemoglobin concentration most commonly between 6 and 12 g/dL.[39] Approximately one-quarter of patients with PK deficiency will have complications in utero or at the time of birth, including intrauterine growth retardation, hydrops, preterm birth, and perinatal anemia. After birth, most newborns will develop severe jaundice and hemolysis requiring phototherapy and/or simple or exchange transfusions. Severe hepatic disease with evolution to liver failure has been reported in several neonates.[46]

Beyond the neonatal period, anemia of varying degree, jaundice, and splenomegaly characterize erythrocyte PK deficiency. Notably, some affected children have no jaundice at birth and only a mild or fully compensated, chronic hemolytic anemia. These patients are often diagnosed later in childhood or adulthood; thus, PK deficiency should be suspected in individuals of any age with a chronic hemolytic anemia without evidence of an immune-mediated process, red cell membrane disorder, or hemoglobinopathy.

The burden of transfusions in PK deficiency is quite variable and is dependent on both patient-specific and provider-specific factors. Young children are more often reliant on frequent transfusions to decrease symptoms and improve growth. For most children and adolescents, transfusion needs decrease after splenectomy. The anemia in PK deficiency may be better tolerated than similarly low hemoglobin levels in other anemias because of the increased RBC 2,3-DPG content, which is responsible for enhanced oxygen off-loading into the tissues.

Aplastic and hemolytic crises

Hemolytic crises present with worsening of baseline symptoms and findings including jaundice, splenomegaly, decreased hemoglobin, and increased reticulocytes. Hemolytic crises in PK deficiency are often triggered by infections. Pregnancy also is a common hemolytic trigger. In contrast, aplastic crises are characterized by decreased hemoglobin and reduced or absent reticulocytes and are caused by parvovirus B19 infection, which suppresses erythroid bone marrow progenitor cells. In PK deficiency, aplastic crises often necessitate blood transfusions.

Gallbladder disease

Gallstones are a frequent complication across the age continuum, with many children and adolescents requiring cholecystectomy.[39] The risk of gallstones is lifelong and continues even after splenectomy due to ongoing hemolysis. Given the lifelong risk of gallstones and their complications, some clinicians recommend cholecystectomy at the time of splenectomy, even in patients without evidence of gallstones.[47,48]

Iron overload

Iron overload is a predictable complication of chronic transfusion therapy, but iron loading also occurs in patients with PK deficiency in the absence of transfusions.[49] Transfusion-independent iron loading in PK deficiency is underrecognized, occurring at all ages and in patients with both mild and more severe anemia. Because iron loading is common in PK deficiency, patients should have iron monitoring at least annually with ferritin measurements and, when patients are able to have a nonsedated assessment, with MRI evaluation in those with ferritin greater than 500 ng/mL. Depending on the degree of iron burden, iron chelation may be prescribed in nontransfused patients through their lifetime.

Other complications

Bone changes associated with hyperplastic bone marrow, such as those seen in thalassemia, occasionally may result in frontal bossing.[50] Patients with PK deficiency are at risk for osteopenia; thus, close attention to vitamin D and calcium intake may be beneficial with consideration of monitoring with dual-energy X-ray absorptiometry scans for baseline assessment in late adolescence or early adulthood. Chronic leg ulcers and pulmonary hypertension occur as infrequent complications.[51,52]

Treatment

Current supportive care for PK deficiency and other RBC glycolytic defects is similar to that of other chronic hemolytic anemias.

Transfusions

RBC transfusions often are needed, particularly during the first years of life. The decision for transfusion therapy is dependent on the patient's tolerance of anemia rather than an arbitrary level of hemoglobin.

Splenectomy

Splenectomy is often beneficial in severely anemic patients because the spleen participates in the destruction of enzymatically abnormal cells. Splenectomy partially ameliorates the anemia in many patients and usually is beneficial in decreasing the transfusion need; however, in almost all patients, an incompletely compensated hemolytic process with reticulocytosis and indirect hyperbilirubinemia persists. Recent guidelines recommend splenectomy in those patients who are reliant on regular transfusions or are severely anemic.[48] Due to the well-known risk of postsplenectomy sepsis associated with encapsulated organism bacteremia in young children, surgery usually is delayed until 5 years of age. The risk of postsplenectomy thrombosis in this population is approximately 10%.[47]

Stem cell transplantation

Hematopoietic stem cell transplantation has been reported in only a few patients with PK deficiency with varying success. The clinical criteria for transplantation is not clear, and, despite the report of success with transplantation in several patients, in almost all cases of hemolytic anemia due to PK deficiency, the risk-benefit ratio for most hematologists currently remains weighted in favor of splenectomy over stem cell transplantation.[53]

Future therapies

New therapies for PK deficiency are under investigation. A pharmacologic activator of RBC PK, AG-348, is currently in clinical trials.[54] Early results from a phase II clinical trial in patients with PK deficiency demonstrate an increase in hemoglobin in a significant subset of patients with hemolysis.[55] PK deficiency is also considered a candidate disease for gene therapy, and, based on preclinical data, future trials in gene therapy may be feasible.[56]

OTHER GLYCOLYTIC DISORDERS
Glucose Phosphate Isomerase Deficiency

Glucose phosphate isomerase (GPI) deficiency is the second most common glycolytic enzymatic defect associated with hemolytic anemia.[57] GPI deficiency is an autosomal recessive disorder, caused by homozygous or compound heterozygous mutations. Definitive diagnosis requires a specific enzyme assay or molecular analysis. The clinical symptoms and complications are similar to PK deficiency, including neonatal complications, chronic anemia, aplastic and hemolytic crises, gallstones, and iron overload. However, neuromuscular impairment (ie, hypotonia, ataxia, dysarthria, mental retardation) has also been seen in patients with GPI deficiency.[58] Splenectomy reduces the transfusion requirement in most patients.[59–62]

In addition to PK deficiency and GPI deficiency, there are multiple even rarer glycolytic enzyme deficiencies (**Table 5**). These disorders have many similar features to PK deficiency, with a few of the differences highlighted in **Table 5**.

Abnormalities of Purine and Pyrimidine Nucleotide Metabolism

Mature RBCs are incapable of de novo purine or pyrimidine synthesis, although many enzymes of nucleotide metabolism are present in erythrocytes. Abnormalities in purine and pyrimidine metabolism are associated with inherited hemolytic disease.

Pyrimidine 5′ Nucleotidase Deficiency

Pyrimidine 5′ nucleotidase (P5′N) deficiency is a rare RBC defect but is the most common enzyme abnormality affecting nucleotide metabolism.[57,63–65] Ribosomal RNA in normal reticulocytes is degraded to 5′ nucleotides. The enzyme P5′N further catalyzes the degradation of cytidine and uridine mononucleotides to inorganic phosphate and the corresponding nucleoside. Whereas the mononucleotides are impermeable to the RBC membrane, after P5′N exposure, the nucleosides can passively diffuse from the cell. P5′N thus rids maturing reticulocytes of pyrimidine degradation products of RNA. Reticulocytes deficient in P5′N accumulate large

Table 5
Features of glycolytic and nucleotide enzymopathies

Enzymopathy	Approximate Fraction of All Enzymopathies	Mode of Inheritance	Clinical Features
Pyruvate kinase (PK)	80%–90%	AR	Moderate/severe CNSHA
Glucose phosphate isomerase (GPI)	3%–5%	AR	Moderate/severe CNSHA ± neurologic defects
Pyrimidine 5′ nucleotidase (P5′N)	2%–3%	AR	Moderate CNSHA
Hexokinase	<1%	AR	Mild/severe CNSHA
Phosphofructokinase (PFK)	<1%	AR	Mild CNSHA; ± myopathy
Aldolase	<1%	AR	Mild/moderate CNSHA; ± myopathy
Triosephosphate isomerase (TPI)	<1%	AR	Moderate/severe CNSHA; neurologic deficits
Phosphoglycerate kinase (PGK)	<1%	X-linked	Mild/severe CNSHA; ± neurologic deficits; ± myopathy
Adenosine deaminase (ADA) excess	<1%	AD	Mild CNSHA
Adenylate kinase (AK)	<1%	AR	CNSHA ± neurologic deficits

Abbreviations: AD, autosomal dominant; AR, autosomal recessive; CNSHA, chronic nonspherocytic hemolytic anemia.

Data from Glader B. Hereditary hemolytic anemias due to red blood cell enzyme disorders. In: Greer JP, editor. Wintrobe's clinical hematology. 13th edition. Philadelphia: Wolters Kluwer; 2014. p. 728–56.

quantities of cytidine and uridine compounds. The reason why P5′N deficiency leads to hemolytic anemia is not known.

P5′N deficiency is an autosomal recessive condition; patients have less than 10% normal P5′N activity. Diagnosis of this disorder is suggested by a screening test that demonstrates increased pyrimidine nucleotides in erythrocytes. Definitive diagnosis, after a positive screen, is obtained by molecular testing. Patients have lifelong hemolytic anemia associated with splenomegaly and intermittent jaundice. The classic blood smear finding is of marked basophilic stippling. P5′N is readily inactivated by heavy metals, such as lead, and it has been proposed that the RBC basophilic stippling seen in lead poisoning is secondary to acquired P5′N deficiency. Transfusions usually are not required, and splenectomy may not be beneficial. Neurologic changes have been noted in several patients.

SUMMARY

Disorders of erythrocyte metabolism should be considered when evaluating a child with chronic hemolytic anemia. Past medical history, physical examination, and the initial laboratory evaluation may provide important clues to the diagnosis, and specific enzyme assays and molecular testing will identify patients with specific RBC enzyme disorders. Patients with nonepisodic hemolysis require ongoing monitoring for complications. Suspicion for these disorders should be raised in the setting of neonatal jaundice and/or chronic nonimmune hemolysis, even in those with only mild or entirely compensated anemia. Diagnosis is key for appropriate supportive care, monitoring of both short-term and long-term complications, and treatment.

REFERENCES

1. Mason PJ, Bautista JM, Gilsanz F. G6PD deficiency: the genotype-phenotype association. Blood Rev 2007;21(5):267–83.
2. Beutler E. G6PD deficiency. Blood 1994;84(11):3613–36.
3. Nkhoma ET, Poole C, Vannappagari V, et al. The global prevalence of glucose-6-phosphate dehydrogenase deficiency: a systematic review and meta-analysis. Blood Cells Mol Dis 2009;42(3):267–78.
4. Chinevere TD, Murray CK, Grant E Jr, et al. Prevalence of glucose-6-phosphate dehydrogenase deficiency in U.S. army personnel. Mil Med 2006;171(9):905–7.
5. Nagel RL, Roth EF Jr. Malaria and red cell genetic defects. Blood 1989;74(4): 1213–21.
6. Luzzatto L, Nannelli C, Notaro R. Glucose-6-phosphate dehydrogenase deficiency. Hematol Oncol Clin North Am 2016;30(2):373–93.
7. Beutler E. The molecular biology of enzymes of erythrocyte metabolism. Philadelphia: W B Saunders,; 1993.
8. Boyer S, Porter IH, Weilbacher RG. Electrophoretic heterogeneity of glucose-6-phosphate dehydrogenase and its relationship to enzyme deficiency in man. Proc Natl Acad Sci U S A 1962;48:1868–76.
9. Reys L, Manso C, Stamatoyannopoulos G. Genetic studies on southeastern Bantu of Mozambique. I. Variants of glucose-6-phosphate dehydrogenase. Am J Hum Genet 1970;22(2):203–15.
10. Jiang W, Yu G, Liu P, et al. Structure and function of glucose-6-phosphate dehydrogenase-deficient variants in Chinese population. Hum Genet 2006;119(5): 463–78.
11. Piomelli S, Corash LM, Davenport DD, et al. In vivo lability of glucose-6-phosphate dehydrogenase in GdA- and GdMediterranean deficiency. J Clin Invest 1968; 47(4):940–8.
12. Rifkind RA. Heinz body anemia: an ultrastructural study. II. Red cell sequestration and destruction. Blood 1965;26(4):433–48.
13. Fairbanks V, Beutler E. A simple method for detection of erythrocyte glucose-6-phosphate dehydrogenase (G-6-PD spot test). Blood 1962;20:591–601.
14. Miwa S, Fujii H. Molecular basis of erythroenzymopathies associated with hereditary hemolytic anemia: tabulation of mutant enzymes. Am J Hematol 1996;51(2): 122–32.
15. Beutler E, Vulliamy TJ. Hematologically important mutations: glucose-6-phosphate dehydrogenase. Blood Cells Mol Dis 2002;28(2):93–103.
16. Luzzatto L, Mehta A, Vulliamy T. Glucose-6-phosphate dehydrogenase deficiency. In: Scriver C, Beaudet A, Sly W, et al, editors. The metabolic and molecular bases of inherited disease. New York: McGraw Hill; 2001. p. 4517–53.
17. Johnson L, Bhutani VK, Karp K, et al. Clinical report from the pilot USA Kernicterus Registry (1992 to 2004). J Perinatol 2009;29(Suppl 1):S25–45.
18. Kaplan M, Hammerman C, Feldman R, et al. Predischarge bilirubin screening in glucose-6-phosphate dehydrogenase-deficient neonates. Pediatrics 2000;105(3 Pt 1):533–7.
19. Youngster I, Arcavi L, Schechmaster R, et al. Medications and glucose-6-phosphate dehydrogenase deficiency: an evidenced based review. Drug Saf 2010;33(9):713–26.

20. Burka ER, Weaver Z 3rd, Marks PA. Clinical spectrum of hemolytic anemia associated with glucose-6-phosphate dehydrogenase deficiency. Ann Intern Med 1966;64(4):817–25.
21. Galiano S, Gaetani GF, Barabino A, et al. Favism in the African type of glucose-6-phosphate dehydrogenase deficiency (A-). BMJ 1990;300(6719):236.
22. Kattamis CA, Kyriazakou M, Chaidas S. Favism: clinical and biochemical data. J Med Genet 1969;6(1):34–41.
23. Hamilton JW, Jones FG, McMullin MF. Glucose-6-phosphate dehydrogenase Guadalajara–a case of chronic non-spherocytic haemolytic anaemia responding to splenectomy and the role of splenectomy in this disorder. Hematology 2004; 9(4):307–9.
24. Kappas A, Drummond GS, Valaes T. A single dose of Sn-mesoporphyrin prevents development of severe hyperbilirubinemia in glucose-6-phosphate dehydrogenase-deficient newborns. Pediatrics 2001;108(1):25–30.
25. Schulz S, Wong RJ, Vreman HJ, et al. Metalloporphyrins–an update. Front Pharmacol 2012;3:68.
26. Glader B. Hereditary hemolytic anemias due to red blood cell enzyme disorders. In: Greer JP, Arber DA, Glader B, et al, editors. Wintrobe's clinical hematology. 13th edition. Philadelphia: Lippincott Williams & Wilkins; 2014. p. 728–45.
27. Tanaka KR, Zerez CR. Red cell enzymopathies of the glycolytic pathway. Semin Hematol 1990;27(2):165–85.
28. Eber SW. Disorders of erythrocyte glycolysis and nucleotide metabolism. In: Handin R, Lux S, Stossel T, editors. Blood: principles and practice of hematology. Philadelphia: Lippincott, Williams & Wilkins; 2003. p. 1887–920.
29. Beutler E, Gelbart T. Estimating the prevalence of pyruvate kinase deficiency from the gene frequency in the general white population. Blood 2000;95(11):3585–8.
30. Bowman HS, McKusick VA, Dronamraju KR. Pyruvate kinase deficient hemolytic anemia in an Amish isolate. Am J Hum Genet 1965;17:1–8.
31. Muir WA, Beutler E, Wasson C. Erythrocyte pyruvate kinase deficiency in the Ohio Amish: origin and characterization of the mutant enzyme. Am J Hum Genet 1984; 36(3):634–9.
32. Grace RF, Bianchi P, van Beers EJ, et al. The clinical spectrum of pyruvate kinase deficiency: data from the Pyruvate Kinase Deficiency Natural History Study. Blood 2018. [Epub ahead of print].
33. Keitt AS. Pyruvate kinase deficiency and related disorders of red cell glycolysis. Am J Med 1966;41(5):762–85.
34. Grimes A, Meisler A, Dacie JV. Hereditary non-spherocytic haemolytic anaemia. A study of red-cell carbohydrate metabolism in twelve cases of pyruvate-kinase deficiency. Br J Haematol 1964;10:403–11.
35. Oski FA, Marshall BE, Cohen PJ, et al. The role of the left-shifted or right-shifted oxygen-hemoglobin equilibrium curve. Ann Intern Med 1971;74(1):44–6.
36. Mentzer WC Jr, Baehner RL, Schmidt-Schonbein H, et al. Selective reticulocyte destruction in erythrocyte pyruvate kinase deficiency. J Clin Invest 1971;50(3): 688–99.
37. Nathan D, Oski FA, Sidel VW, et al. Extreme hemolysis and red-cell distortion in erythrocyte pyruvate kinase deficiency. N Engl J Med 1965;272:118–23.
38. Nathan DG, Oski FA, Miller DR, et al. Life-span and organ sequestration of the red cells in pyruvate kinase deficiency. N Engl J Med 1968;278(2):73–81.
39. Tanaka KR, Paglia DE. Pyruvate kinase deficiency. Semin Hematol 1971;8(4): 367–96.

40. Zanella A, Fermo E, Bianchi P, et al. Red cell pyruvate kinase deficiency: molecular and clinical aspects. Br J Haematol 2005;130(1):11–25.

41. Bianchi P, Zanella A. Hematologically important mutations: red cell pyruvate kinase (third update). Blood Cells Mol Dis 2000;26(1):47–53.

42. Zanella A, Fermo E, Bianchi P, et al. Pyruvate kinase deficiency: the genotype-phenotype association. Blood Rev 2007;21(4):217–31.

43. Baronciani L, Beutler E. Prenatal diagnosis of pyruvate kinase deficiency. Blood 1994;84(7):2354–6.

44. Nathan DG, Oski FA, Sidel VW, et al. Studies of erythrocyte spicule formation in haemolytic anaemia. Br J Haematol 1966;12(4):385–95.

45. Oski F, Nathan DG, Sidel VW, et al. Extreme hemolysis and red-cell distortion in erythrocyte pyruvate kinase deficiency. N Engl J Med 1964;270:1023–30.

46. Raphael MF, Van Wijk R, Schweizer JJ, et al. Pyruvate kinase deficiency associated with severe liver dysfunction in the newborn. Am J Hematol 2007;82(11):1025–8.

47. Grace RF, Zanella A, Neufeld EJ, et al. Erythrocyte pyruvate kinase deficiency: 2015 status report. Am J Hematol 2015;90(9):825–30.

48. Iolascon A, Andolfo I, Barcellini W, et al. Recommendations regarding splenectomy in hereditary hemolytic anemias. Haematologica 2017;102(8):1304–13.

49. Salem HH, Van Der Weyden MB, Firkin BG. Iron overload in congenital erythrocyte pyruvate kinase deficiency. Med J Aust 1980;1(11):531–2.

50. Becker MH, Genieser NB, Piomelli S, et al. Roentgenographic manifestations of pyruvate kinase deficiency hemolytic anemia. Am J Roentgenol Radium Ther Nucl Med 1971;113(3):491–8.

51. Muller-Soyano A, Tovar de Roura E, Duke PR, et al. Pyruvate kinase deficiency and leg ulcers. Blood 1976;47(5):807–13.

52. Vives-Corrons JL, Marie J, Pujades MA, et al. Hereditary erythrocyte pyruvate-kinase (PK) deficiency and chronic hemolytic anemia: clinical, genetic and molecular studies in six new Spanish patients. Hum Genet 1980;53(3):401–8.

53. van Straaten S, Bierings M, Bianchi P, et al. Worldwide study of hematopoietic allogeneic stem cell transplantation in pyruvate kinase deficiency. Haematologica 2018;103(2):e82–6.

54. Kung C, Hixon J, Kosinski PA, et al. AG-348 enhances pyruvate kinase activity in red blood cells from patients with pyruvate kinase deficiency. Blood 2017;130:1347–56.

55. Grace RF, Rose C, Layton DM, et al. Effects of AG-348, a pyruvate kinase activator, on anemia and hemolysis in patients with pyruvate kinase deficiency: data from the DRIVE PK study. Blood 2016;128:402.

56. Garcia-Gomez M, Calabria A, Garcia-Bravo M, et al. Safe and efficient gene therapy for pyruvate kinase deficiency. Mol Ther 2016;24(7):1187–98.

57. Beutler E. Red cell enzyme defects as nondiseases and as diseases. Blood 1979;54(1):1–7.

58. Kugler W, Lakomek M. Glucose-6-phosphate isomerase deficiency. Baillieres Best Pract Res Clin Haematol 2000;13(1):89–101.

59. Baughan MA, Valentine WN, Paglia DE, et al. Hereditary hemolytic anemia associated with glucosephosphate isomerase (GPI) deficiency–a new enzyme defect of human erythrocytes. Blood 1968;32(2):236–49.

60. Beutler E, Sigalove WH, Muir WA, et al. Glucosephosphate-isomerase (GPI) deficiency: GPI elyria. Ann Intern Med 1974;80(6):730–2.

61. Hutton JJ, Chilcote RR. Glucose phosphate isomerase deficiency with hereditary nonspherocytic hemolytic anemia. J Pediatr 1974;85(4):494–7.

62. Paglia DE, Holland P, Baughan MA, et al. Occurrence of defective hexosephosphate isomerization in human erythrocytes and leukocytes. N Engl J Med 1969; 280(2):66–71.

63. Zanella A, Bianchi P, Fermo E, et al. Hereditary pyrimidine 5'-nucleotidase deficiency: from genetics to clinical manifestations. Br J Haematol 2006;133(2): 113–23.

64. Vives-Corrons JL. Chronic non-spherocytic haemolytic anaemia due to congenital pyrimidine 5' nucleotidase deficiency: 25 years later. Baillieres Best Pract Res Clin Haematol 2000;13(1):103–18.

65. Chiarelli LR, Fermo E, Zanella A, et al. Hereditary erythrocyte pyrimidine 5'-nucleotidase deficiency: a biochemical, genetic and clinical overview. Hematology 2006;11(1):67–72.

Acquired Aplastic Anemia
What Have We Learned and What Is in the Horizon?

Süreyya Savaşan, MD

KEYWORDS

- Acquired aplastic anemia • Hematopoietic stem cell • Autoimmunity
- Immunosuppressive therapy • Hematopoietic stem cell transplantation • Clonality
- Myelodysplastic syndrome

KEY POINTS

- Refractory cytopenias of childhood, inherited bone marrow failure syndromes, and familial disorders associated with myelodysplasia or immune dysregulation should be investigated during the diagnosis of acquired aplastic anemia.
- Although pancytopenia is the norm at diagnosis, it must be kept in mind that isolated cytopenias may be the predominant presenting symptom, along with milder decreases in other lineages in some cases.
- The role of autoimmune reaction targeting hematopoietic stem cells is well-understood in the pathogenesis of acquired aplastic anemia; however, alterations in stem cells leading to this response or, in other words, drivers of autoimmunity are not clearly identified.
- Although matched related donor hematopoietic stem cell transplantation is the treatment of choice with great outcomes, immunosuppressive therapy provides response in two-thirds of the patients who do not have matched family donors. Alternative donor transplants have been associated with much improved results in recent years.
- Acquired aplastic anemia can be associated with hematopoietic stem cell clonal disorders: paroxysmal hemoglobinuria can accompany at diagnosis or develop later. Clonal abnormalities leading to myelodysplasia and acute myeloid leukemia may follow immunosuppressive therapy.

Idiopathic acquired aplastic anemia (aAA) is a rare disorder with an estimated incidence of 300 to 600 cases in the United States annually; it is less frequent in children. It is characterized by peripheral pancytopenia and significantly decreased cellularity in the bone marrow (BM). Though isolated cytopenias may seem to be the only manifestation, all 3 lines are often affected at presentation. For instance, severe

Division of Hematology/Oncology, Pediatric Blood and Marrow Transplant Program, Children's Hospital of Michigan, Barbara Ann Karmanos Cancer Center, Wayne State University School of Medicine, 3901 Beaubien Boulevard, Detroit, MI 48201, USA
E-mail address: ssavasan@med.wayne.edu

Pediatr Clin N Am 65 (2018) 597–606
https://doi.org/10.1016/j.pcl.2018.02.006
0031-3955/18/© 2018 Elsevier Inc. All rights reserved.

thrombocytopenia may be the prominent finding; however, an increased mean corpuscular volume and/or mild decrease in other counts may accompany the thrombocytopenia. Therefore, close monitoring and keeping the possibility of aAA in mind is prudent because therapeutic approaches to thrombocytopenia significantly depend on the underlying cause and delay in aAA diagnosis establishment may be very consequential. Infections and bleeding are the most common causes of morbidity and mortality in the very severe and severe forms of aAA. Severe aAA is characterized by peripheral blood absolute neutrophil count less than 0.5×10^9/L and the very severe form by less than 0.2×10^9/L, in addition to platelets less than 20×10^9/L and reticulocytes less than 20×10^9/L with decreased hematopoietic and overall cellularity in the BM.[1]

Although phenotypic findings in inherited BM failure syndromes (iBMFS) are not uncommon, some patients may not have any. Ruling out an underlying iBMFS is a prerequisite for establishing the diagnosis of aAA. Whereas lymphocyte chromosomal breakage testing is standard and practical in investigating underlying Fanconi anemia (FA), telomere length assessment is used for detecting disorders characterized by shortened telomeres in both myeloid and lymphoid cells in peripheral blood.[2] Telomere length in residual granulocytes are shortened in aAA. Not infrequently, there is a fine line between aAA and hypoplastic myelodysplastic syndrome (MDS) or refractory cytopenia of childhood (RCC) due to similarities in clinical presentation and laboratory findings.[3] In that regard, cytogenetic analysis of BM cells using karyotyping and fluorescence in situ hybridization (FISH) technique may provide some help, though they are not sensitive or specific enough.

Beyond the previously mentioned iBMFS, such as FA and short telomere disorders, BM aplasia may be in the spectrum of some inherited or familial conditions that are associated with immune dysregulation and/or tendency to develop myelodysplasia or myeloproliferation. It has become reasonable to run large gene panels to investigate for these underlying disorders at the time of diagnosis of BM failure.[4–6] Whether the utility of this approach can be justified is debatable; however, discovery of such genetic background may significantly affect treatment decisions. Paroxysmal nocturnal hemoglobinuria (PNH) is caused by an acquired hematopoietic stem cell (HSC) defect, leading to intravascular hemolysis, anemia, and thrombotic complications closely associated with aAA. Therefore, investigating for PNH is also a necessary step in patients with newly diagnosed aAA. Clinically evident PNH may be present around the time of aAA diagnosis and would require additional interventions.[7] Even flow cytometric detection of small clonal PNH populations may indicate the need for closer monitoring for the development of symptomatic PNH down the road and also points to possibility of a greater response to immunosuppressive therapy (IST).[8]

HISTOLOGY AND PATHOGENESIS

The BM tissue in acquired severe aplastic anemia (aSAA) displays severely decreased cellularity with some degree of reactive changes. There is no histologic evidence of acute inflammation at the time of diagnosis. As seen in tissue atrophy, blood supply to BM is diminished. Microvascular density and vascular endothelial growth factor (VEGF) expression were found to be lower in aSAA BM tissue, along with decreased serum levels of VEGF, which were substantially improved following successful IST.[9] Despite severely decreased hematopoiesis, typically there is no accompanying fibrosis in the BM. Space emptied by the elimination of hematopoiesis appears to have been partially filled by adipocytes. Relative lymphocyte predominance, primarily of T lymphocytes, is characteristic of BM histology. Additionally, relative increase in mast cells, plasma cells, and histiocytes, some displaying hemophagocytosis, is common. Among these changes, visible mast cell presence has been thought to be related to their longer life span following HSC injury; however, the possibility of their compensatory effort to stimulate angiogenesis[10] has not been specifically investigated.

Though the knowledge on the pathogenesis of aAA has increased enormously in recent years, it still continues to be an enigmatic disease in many ways.[11,12] Research in aAA has been somewhat hampered by the lack of availability of a sufficient number of hematopoietic stem cells for experiments. This has led to focusing on the aAA BM microenvironment. Furthermore, studying the recovering BM tissue following IST in comparison with diagnostic samples has significantly contributed to the understanding of the disease process. With technological advancements, molecular genetic studies on stored samples have helped improve the understanding of the genetic basis and the heterogeneity of aAA, emphasizing the importance of storing samples after obtaining signed consents in such rare disorders.

Early observations of chemical (benzene and pesticides) or radiation exposure and idiosyncratic drug (chloramphenicol) reaction-associated BM aplasia cases thought to be pointing at a direct injury to HSC.[13–15] Incidental observation of autologous recovery of BM after allografting conditioned with antilymphocytic serum in aSAA patients led to use of IST in aSAA.[16] Moreover, this observation has also provided additional evidence for potential role of immune response in the disease pathogenesis. Furthermore, autologous recovery following failed allogeneic HSCT conditioned by high-dose cyclophosphamide pointed to the potential role of IST in aAA treatment.[17] Demonstration of oligoclonal expansion of cytotoxic CD8+CD28−T cells and production of helper type-1 T lymphocyte cytokines, such as interferon-gamma and tumor necrosis factor-alpha, by the lymphocytes and stromal cells in aAA BM microenvironment supported an immune reaction directed toward HSC. However, what triggers the autoimmune reaction is still not well-understood. Although an alteration in HSC population due to an infection inciting an autoimmune reaction could be speculated in hepatitis-associated aAA cases, there is no detectable history of recent infection at diagnosis in the majority of aAA cases.[18] Not surprisingly, hepatitis-associated aSAA cases also respond to IST. Even in some of the cases of aSAA associated with chemical or drug exposure, IST has been successful, again suggesting a potential role of autoimmune reaction to HSC in those patients.[15]

There seems to be a fine line between some cases of idiopathic aAA and MDS. BM dysplastic changes may provide an important clue in distinguishing idiopathic aAA from RCC and some inherited BM disorders associated with identified genetic defects.[19] In a third of the study population, somatic mutations in MDS or acute myeloid leukemia (AML)-associated genes with increasing prevalence by aging were detected; clonal hematopoiesis determined mostly by the presence of acquired mutations was observed almost in half of the cases in aAA.[20,21] The incidence of those mutations at diagnosis was much lower. Among the mutated genes, DNMT3A and AXSL1 showed an increasing clonal population and were associated with progression to MDS or AML. On the other hand, mutations in PIGA and BCOR/BCORL1 were stable or decreased over time and represented a better outcome. These observations are reminiscent of the recently described entity clonal hematopoiesis of indeterminate potential (CHIP), more frequently described with aging.[22] It might be interesting to see if detection of incidence of clonality would increase if methods other than detection of mutations were used.

Copy-number neutral loss of heterozygosity or uniparental disomy of the chromosome 6p (6pUPD) leading to HLA haplotype loss was seen in clonal aAA and escape form autoreactive T-cell attack due to lack of appropriate HLA class I molecule expression was proposed as the mechanism.[23] Furthermore, recurrent HLA class-I mutations suggested HLA class I-driven autoimmune reaction and also providing mechanistic evidence for clonal evolution.[24] In summary, observation of somatic mutations at diagnosis in some idiopathic aAA cases and preferential elimination of HSC without the mutations through autoimmune attack, leading to increased presence of HSC with the mutations following IST provides the explanation for clonal evolution.[25]

Several findings indicate heterogeneity of aAA. The reason for unresponsiveness to IST is not well-understood. Persevering autoimmune reaction due to inadequate immune suppression is possible because some cases, but not all, respond to other forms of IST.[26] Furthermore, a thrombopoietin mimetic agent, eltrombopag, has shown some efficacy in refractory patients,[27] pointing at the potential role of HSC stimulation, maybe overriding ongoing autoimmunity to a certain degree, similar to results with eltrombopag observed in another immune-mediated disorder, idiopathic thrombocytopenic purpura.[28] Although slow versus fast responses obtained with IST may be a consequence of the adequacy of the immune suppression provided, there may be more to this observation. One question is: are recovering HSC completely normal following IST in all cases? The author recently showed evidence for increased response to tunicamycin-induced endoplasmic reticulum (ER) stress in myeloid cells in aAA. Interestingly, there was no difference (albeit using small numbers) in induced ER stress in vitro between active disease and post-IST response state in culture-grown myeloid cells, raising the possibility of continuing altered HSC recovery despite improvements in BM cellularity and peripheral counts.[29] The health of the recovering HSC without detectable genetic abnormalities is another area of research that may expand understanding of aAA pathophysiology.

There are several similarities between hereditary iBMFS, such as FA, and idiopathic aAA BM tissue findings, including increased fat cells, mast cells, and lymphocytes, as well as a lack of significant fibrosis, pointing at common tissue reaction to depletion of the HSC compartment regardless of the cause in these disorders. Cellular stress, such as repeated infection, plays an important role in the development of BM aplasia in FA.[30] The evolution of a clinical picture is much more gradual in most iBMFS cases compared with idiopathic aAA. Often, isolated peripheral cytopenia, such as thrombocytopenia, is the first finding, followed by a long lag time to the development of significant pancytopenia.

Recipient origin of nonhematopoietic supportive cells, such as fibroblasts and mesenchymal stem cells (MSC), following successful allogeneic hematopoietic stem cell transplantation (HSCT) does not support a primary role for BM microenvironment defects in the pathogenesis of aAA.[31,32] Several aberrations have been described in hematopoietic microenvironment MSC, likely contributing to impaired quality and decreased quantity of hematopoietic BM niches, and indicating changes in nonhematopoietic cells.[33] However, this matter remains controversial because some investigators point to the preserved integrity of MSC in aAA.[34] Impaired hematopoietic niche in BM in aAA, and restoration of vascular and perivascular niches, are shown following successful allogeneic HSCT independent of donor-derived BM MSC.[35,36]

TREATMENT

Similar to basic research efforts, obtaining clinical data on aSAA cases has been challenging due to rarity of this condition. The great majority of published reports originate from review and analysis of the results retrospectively. The results often include data from both pediatric and adult cases. Spontaneous remissions have been reported infrequently, usually taking place within the first 2 months of diagnosis.[37] Pregnancy-associated aAA is an entity in which spontaneous remissions are seen more frequently.[38] Although a wait-and-see strategy is not practical, tests to investigate for underlying inherited BMFS or RCC with or without myelodysplasia and searching for potential related or family donors generally takes some time, during which the patients receive transfusion support. Prophylactic antimicrobials and good oral hygiene may be necessary based on the severity of aAA. Use of granulocyte-colony stimulating factor (G-CSF) can increase neutrophil counts marginally in some patients. Such supportive care measures, and red blood cell and platelet transfusions, continue during IST, increasing the possibility of transfusion-associated allergic reactions and alloimmunization to red blood cells and platelets. Treatment options and approaches in aAA were recently reviewed.[39] The 2 top choices for the treatment of idiopathic aSAA are allogeneic matched sibling donor (MSD) or matched related donor (MRD) HSCT. If such a donor is not available, IST including steroids, cyclosporine A (CSA), and antithymocyte globulin (ATG) is the preferred treatment form.

Immunosuppressive Therapy

The response to IST is generally assessed at 6 months of therapy. Due to incomplete response, some patients were kept on CSA for longer periods. In a retrospective analysis of 455 children, overall survival was superior statistically at 92% with equine ATG, including IST, compared with 84% rabbit ATG at 10 years.[40] Use of equine ATG in IST has been associated with improved response rates in the first 6 months in a systematic review and meta-analysis report.[41] One of the common and major shortcomings of retrospective studies comparing the effectiveness of equine with rabbit ATG has been the lack of equal dosing of the each of the ATG products. In a randomized prospective clinical trial comparing rabbit ATG (Thymoglobulin, Genzyme) and equine ATG (ATGAM, Pfizer), 60 pediatric and adult subjects were enrolled in each arm. Equine ATG was superior with a 6-month response rate of 68% to 37% in the rabbit ATG group. Furthermore, overall survival was also better in the equine ATG arm (96% vs 76%) at 3 years.[42]

Severe allergic reactions during ATG infusion may necessitate switching to another product. Attention should be given to controlling hypertension at the early stages of IST when CSA and steroids are administered together, owing to the possibility of posterior reversible encephalopathy syndrome (PRES). Some patients may not be able to continue CSA treatment due to recurrent PRES when challenged again following the first episode. Because IST containing tacrolimus has been shown to be as effective as the CSA-containing regimen,[43] in case of CSA intolerance, a trial of tacrolimus may be reasonable.

Approximately one-third of the cases do not respond to IST and other cases may recur after initial response. High-dose cyclophosphamide has been used with a certain degree of success associated with high incidence of infectious complications in children.[44] Alemtuzumab has been used as a single agent in refractory cases with a response rate of 37% and 56% in recurrent cases[45] and, therefore, it can be considered as an option for those cases.[26] Eltrombopag showed promising results in IST-refractory aSAA subjects.[27] It has also improved the outcome when added to standard IST regimen in untreated aSAA subjects.[46] Clonal cytogenetic evolution was seen in 7 subjects (8%) at a median 2-year follow-up; 5 occurred within the first 6 months and 2 later. The investigators reported that the incidence was not different from the historic cohort. Although these are encouraging results, one must be careful about the potential long-term MDS or AML risk of eltrombopag administration, given the recent findings of significant presence of somatic mutations in certain genes.

Hematopoietic Stem Cell Transplantation

Because BM is already aplastic, there is no need for myeloablative conditioning in aSAA HSCT. On the other hand, immune suppression is very critical for engraftment and prevention of graft-versus-host disease (GvHD). Exposure to repeated blood and platelet transfusions increase the risk of alloimmunization and sets the immune system in a more active state. Current commonly used conditioning regimens include various combinations of cyclophosphamide, fludarabine, and ATG or alemtuzumab, and/or low-dose total body irradiation.

A survival advantage was reported for marrow grafting over peripheral HSC in all ages in a report from European Group for Blood and Marrow Transplantation.[47] The risk of acute and chronic GvHD was lower in the BM graft group. Furthermore, inclusion of ATG in conditioning was associated with less incidence of both forms of GvHD and superior survival in the same study. Equine ATG and rabbit ATG have different biological and clinical properties in HSCT setting; rabbit ATG was associated with higher incidence of stable mixed chimerism.[48] Unrelated donor (UD) HSCT did not lead to a statistically significant different survival rate compared with MSD HSCT; however, it was associated with increased risk of both acute and chronic GvHD.[49] In a recent multiinstitutional retrospective analysis of 833 aSAA MSD or UD HSCT recipients, use of rabbit ATG in conditioning was found to be associated with lesser incidence of acute GvHD compared with equine ATG. Chronic GvHD was also higher in the equine ATG group without overall survival difference in MSD cases.[50] Greater lymphodepletion and enhancement of regulatory T cells following rabbit ATG were proposed as the mechanisms of the observed effects. UD HSCT has also been associated with successful outcomes in children.[51,52] Progression into MDS and AML was seen an average of 2.9 (1.2–13) years after aSAA diagnosis in 17 children and young adults; event-free survival in those cases following allogeneic HSCT for MDS or AML was 41%.[53]

Late graft rejection is a known experience in aSAA HSCT and a study revealed its close association with decreasing donor chimerism.[54] In MRD HSCT cases, a second attempt using the same donor was commonly done with or without donor leukocyte infusions. Alternative donor sources are also used for aSAA HSCT after failing IST or MRD HSCT in recent years, including umbilical cord blood cells and haploidentical family members.[55] In mismatched donors, investigating for anti-HLA antibodies is a common practice. Given the risk of graft failure in HSCT for aSAA, and increased risk in cord blood cell transplants in general, umbilical cord blood cell transplantation has a higher nonengraftment risk.[56] Haploidentical HSCT with postinfusion cyclophosphamide has shown promising results.[57] Although return to recipient hematopoiesis is the most common pattern in late graft failure, donor-derived recurrent aAA cases due to immune reaction have been described.[58] Treatment with ATG may resolve the late graft failure in such cases.

SUMMARY

Recent discoveries of clonal hematopoiesis due to identification of somatic mutations and other genetic changes at presentation, more frequently in the long-term following IST in some cases, and HLA class-I gene mutations playing a central role in the development of autoimmune reaction in some other cases, have shed light on the aAA pathogenesis, as well as pointing at aAA heterogeneity. MRD HSCT provides great outcomes in aSAA. However, in patients without a matched family donor, equine ATG in combination with CSA as IST has been associated with superior outcomes compared with rabbit ATG. Addition of eltrombopag to classic IST regimen has improved the response rate, opening a new dimension to medicinal treatment of aSAA because HSC stimulation with erythropoietin and G-CSF therapies had not been successful in the past. Alternative donor HSCT has been increasingly used in patients who failed IST or MRD HSCT, with improved results indicating the potential for it to be considered as a first-line approach in the future. There is still need for progress and long-term follow-up of recovered patients and out-of-box thinking would help open new avenues to better understanding and treatment of aAA.

REFERENCES

1. Guinan EC. Diagnosis and management of aplastic anemia. Hematology Am Soc Hematol Educ Program 2011;2011:76–81.
2. Townsley DM, Dumitriu B, Young NS. Bone marrow failure and the telomeropathies. Blood 2014;124:2775–83.
3. Niemeyer CM, Baumann I. Classification of childhood aplastic anemia and myelodysplastic syndrome. Hematology Am Soc Hematol Educ Program 2011;2011: 84–9.
4. Babushok DV, Bessler M. Genetic predisposition syndromes: when should they be considered in the work-up of MDS? Best Pract Res Clin Haematol 2015;28: 55–68.
5. Erlacher M, Strahm B. Missing cells: pathophysiology, diagnosis, and management of (pan)cytopenia in childhood. Front Pediatr 2015;3:64.
6. Bannon SA, DiNardo CD. Hereditary predispositions to myelodysplastic syndrome. Int J Mol Sci 2016;17 [pii:E838].
7. Narita A, Muramatsu H, Okuno Y, et al. Development of clinical paroxysmal nocturnal haemoglobinuria in children with aplastic anaemia. Br J Haematol 2017;178:954–8.
8. Narita A, Muramatsu H, Sekiya Y, et al, Japan Childhood Aplastic Anemia Study Group. Paroxysmal nocturnal hemoglobinuria and telomere length predicts response to immunosuppressive therapy in pediatric aplastic anemia. Haematologica 2015;100:1546–52.
9. Füreder W, Krauth MT, Sperr WR, et al. Evaluation of angiogenesis and vascular endothelial growth factor expression in the bone marrow of patients with aplastic anemia. Am J Pathol 2006;168:123–30.
10. Krystel-Whittemore M, Dileepan KN, Wood JG. Mast cell: a multi-functional master cell. Front Immunol 2016;6:620.
11. Young NS. Pathophysiologic mechanisms in acquired aplastic anemia. Hematology Am Soc Hematol Educ Program 2006;72–7.
12. Young NS. Current concepts in the pathophysiology and treatment of aplastic anemia. Hematology Am Soc Hematol Educ Program 2013;2013:76–81.
13. Aksoy M, Erdem S, Akgün T, et al. Osmotic fragility studies in three patients with aplastic anemia due to chronic benzene poisoning. Blut 1966;13:85–90.
14. Fleming LE, Timmeny W. Aplastic anemia and pesticides. An etiologic association? J Occup Med 1993;35:1106–16.
15. Malkin D, Koren G, Saunders EF. Drug-induced aplastic anemia: pathogenesis and clinical aspects. Am J Pediatr Hematol Oncol 1990;12:402–10.
16. Mathé G, Amiel JL, Schwarzenberg L, et al. Bone marrow graft in man after conditioning by antilymphocytic serum. Br Med J 1970;2:131–6.
17. Territo MC. Autologous bone marrow repopulation following high dose cyclophosphamide and allogeneic marrow transplantation in aplastic anaemia. Br J Haematol 1977;36:305–12.

18. Brown KE, Tisdale J, Barrett AJ, et al. Hepatitis-associated aplastic anemia. N Engl J Med 1997;336:1059–64.

19. Ganapathi KA, Townsley DM, Hsu AP, et al. GATA2 deficiency-associated bone marrow disorder differs from idiopathic aplastic anemia. Blood 2015;125:56–70.

20. Yoshizato T, Dumitriu B, Hosokawa K, et al. Somatic mutations and clonal hematopoiesis in aplastic anemia. N Engl J Med 2015;373:35–47.

21. Ogawa S. Clonal hematopoiesis in acquired aplastic anemia. Blood 2016;128:337–47.

22. Steensma DP, Bejar R, Jaiswal S, et al. Clonal hematopoiesis of indeterminate potential and its distinction from myelodysplastic syndromes. Blood 2015;126:9–16.

23. Katagiri T, Sato-Otsubo A, Kashiwase K, et al, Japan Marrow Donor Program. Frequent loss of HLA alleles associated with copy number-neutral 6pLOH in acquired aplastic anemia. Blood 2011;118:6601–9.

24. Babushok DV, Duke JL, Xie HM, et al. Somatic HLA mutations expose the role of class I-mediated autoimmunity in aplastic anemia and its clonal complications. Blood Adv 2017;1:1900–10.

25. Stanley N, Olson TS, Babushok DV. Recent advances in understanding clonal haematopoiesis in aplastic anaemia. Br J Haematol 2017;177:509–25.

26. Risitano AM, Schrezenmeier H. Alternative immunosuppression in patients failing immunosuppression with ATG who are not transplant candidates: campath (Alemtuzumab). Bone Marrow Transplant 2013;48:186–90.

27. Olnes MJ, Scheinberg P, Calvo KR, et al. Eltrombopag and improved hematopoiesis in refractory aplastic anemia. N Engl J Med 2012;367:11–9.

28. Bussel JB, Cheng G, Saleh MN, et al. Eltrombopag for the treatment of chronic idiopathic thrombocytopenic purpura. N Engl J Med 2007;357:2237–47.

29. Sidhu A, Callaghan MU, Gadgeel MS, et al. Evidence for increased response to induced endoplasmic reticulum stress in myeloid cells in acquired aplastic anemia. J Pediatr Hematol Oncol 2017;39:e163–6.

30. Longerich S, Li J, Xiong Y, et al. Stress and DNA repair biology of the Fanconi anemia pathway. Blood 2014;124(18):2812–9.

31. Golde DW, Hocking WG, Quan SG, et al. Origin of human bone marrow fibroblasts. Br J Haematol 1980;44:183–7.

32. Bartsch K, Al-Ali H, Reinhardt A, et al. Mesenchymal stem cells remain host-derived independent of the source of the stem-cell graft and conditioning regimen used. Transplantation 2009;87:217–21.

33. Balderman SR, Calvi LM. Biology of BM failure syndromes: role of microenvironment and niches. Hematology Am Soc Hematol Educ Program 2014;2014:71–6.

34. Bueno C, Roldan M, Anguita E, et al. Bone marrow mesenchymal stem cells from patients with aplastic anemia maintain functional and immune properties and do not contribute to the pathogenesis of the disease. Haematologica 2014;99:1168–75.

35. Wu L, Mo W, Zhang Y, et al. Impairment of hematopoietic stem cell niches in patients with aplastic anemia. Int J Hematol 2015;102:645–53.

36. Wu L, Mo W, Zhang Y, et al. Vascular and perivascular niches, but not the osteoblastic niche, are numerically restored following allogeneic hematopoietic stem cell transplantation in patients with aplastic anemia. Int J Hematol 2017;106:71–81.

37. Lee JH, Lee JH, Shin YR, et al. Spontaneous remission of aplastic anemia: a retrospective analysis. Haematologica 2001;86:928–33.

38. Kwon JY, Lee Y, Shin JC, et al. Supportive management of pregnancy-associated aplastic anemia. Int J Gynaecol Obstet 2006;95:115–20.

39. Bacigalupo A. How I treat acquired aplastic anemia. Blood 2017;129:1428–36.
40. Jeong DC, Chung NG, Cho B, et al. Long-term outcome after immunosuppressive therapy with horse or rabbit antithymocyte globulin and cyclosporine for severe aplastic anemia in children. Haematologica 2014;99:664–71.
41. Yang N, Chen J, Zhang H, et al. Horse versus rabbit antithymocyte globulin in immunosuppressive therapy of treatment-naïve aplastic anemia: a systematic review and meta-analysis. Ann Hematol 2017;96(12):2031–43.
42. Scheinberg P, Nunez O, Weinstein B, et al. Horse versus rabbit antithymocyte globulin in acquired aplastic anemia. N Engl J Med 2011;365:430–8.
43. Alsultan A, Goldenberg NA, Kaiser N, et al. Tacrolimus as an alternative to cyclosporine in the maintenance phase of immunosuppressive therapy for severe aplastic anemia in children. Pediatr Blood Cancer 2009;52:626–30.
44. Gamper CJ, Takemoto CM, Chen AR, et al. High-dose cyclophosphamide is effective therapy for pediatric severe aplastic anemia. J Pediatr Hematol Oncol 2016;38:627–35.
45. Scheinberg P, Nunez O, Weinstein B, et al. Activity of alemtuzumab monotherapy in treatment-naive, relapsed, and refractory severe acquired aplastic anemia. Blood 2012;119:345–54.
46. Townsley DM, Scheinberg P, Winkler T, et al. Eltrombopag added to standard immunosuppression for aplastic anemia. N Engl J Med 2017;376:1540–50.
47. Bacigalupo A, Socié G, Schrezenmeier H, et al, Aplastic Anemia Working Party of the European Group for Blood and Marrow Transplantation (WPSAA-EBMT). Bone marrow versus peripheral blood as the stem cell source for sibling transplants in acquired aplastic anemia: survival advantage for bone marrow in all age groups. Haematologica 2012;97:1142–8.
48. Atta EH, de Sousa AM, Schirmer MR, et al. Different outcomes between cyclophosphamide plus horse or rabbit antithymocyte globulin for HLA-identical sibling bone marrow transplant in severe aplastic anemia. Biol Blood Marrow Transplant 2012;18:1876–82.
49. Bacigalupo A, Socié G, Hamladji RM, et al, Aplastic Anemia Working Party of the European Group for Blood Marrow Transplantation. Current outcome of HLA identical sibling versus unrelated donor transplants in severe aplastic anemia: an EBMT analysis. Haematologica 2015;100:696–702.
50. Kekre N, Zhang Y, Zhang MJ, et al. Effect of antithymocyte globulin source on outcomes of bone marrow transplantation for severe aplastic anemia. Haematologica 2017;102:1291–8.
51. Samarasinghe S, Steward C, Hiwarkar P, et al. Excellent outcome of matched unrelated donor transplantation in paediatric aplastic anaemia following failure with immunosuppressive therapy: a United Kingdom multicentre retrospective experience. Br J Haematol 2012;15:339–46.
52. Yagasaki H, Takahashi Y, Hama A, et al. Comparison of matched-sibling donor BMT and unrelated donor BMT in children and adolescent with acquired severe aplastic anemia. Bone Marrow Transplant 2010;45:1508–13.
53. Yoshimi A, Strahm B, Baumann I, et al. Hematopoietic stem cell transplantation in children and young adults with secondary myelodysplastic syndrome and acute myelogenous leukemia after aplastic anemia. Biol Blood Marrow Transplant 2014; 20:425–9.
54. Lawler M, McCann SR, Marsh JC, et al, Severe Aplastic Anaemia Working Party of the European Blood and Marrow Transplant Group. Serial chimerism analyses indicate that mixed haemopoietic chimerism influences the probability of graft rejection and disease recurrence following allogeneic stem cell transplantation

(SCT) for severe aplastic anaemia (SAA): indication for routine assessment of chimerism post SCT for SAA. Br J Haematol 2009;144:933–45.

55. Onishi Y, Mori T, Kako S, et al, Adult Aplastic Anemia Working Group of the Japan Society for Hematopoietic Cell Transplantation. Outcome of second transplantation using umbilical cord blood for graft failure after allogeneic hematopoietic stem cell transplantation for aplastic anemia. Biol Blood Marrow Transplant 2017;23(12):2137–42.

56. Chan KW, McDonald L, Lim D, et al. Unrelated cord blood transplantation in children with idiopathic severe aplastic anemia. Bone Marrow Transplant 2008;42: 589–95.

57. DeZern AE, Zahurak M, Symons H, et al. Alternative donor transplantation with high-dose post-transplantation cyclophosphamide for refractory severe aplastic anemia. Biol Blood Marrow Transplant 2017;23:498–504.

58. Maruyama K, Aotsuka N, Kumano Y, et al. Immune-mediated hematopoietic failure after allogeneic hematopoietic stem cell transplantation: a common cause of late graft failure in patients with complete donor chimerism. Biol Blood Marrow Transplant 2018;24(1):43–9.

Management of Epistaxis in Children and Adolescents
Avoiding a Chaotic Approach

Peter Svider, MD*, Khashayar Arianpour, BS, Sean Mutchnick, MD

KEYWORDS

- Epistaxis • Nosebleed • Nasal packing
- Transnasal endoscopic sphenopalatine artery ligation
- Juvenile Nasopharyngeal Angiofibroma (JNA)

KEY POINTS

- Obtaining a comprehensive patient history may be useful in evaluation of patients with epistaxis, although timely management takes precedence for patients with significant and brisk hemorrhage.
- The differential diagnosis associated with epistaxis encompasses a wide range of etiologies, ranging from benign causes such as digital trauma and foreign bodies to life-altering entities including systemic hematologic disorders, locally destructive tumors, and sinonasal malignancies.
- The mean age at presentation is 7–9 years, and non-accidental trauma should be ruled out in children under two years of age.
- Epistaxis is controlled with conservative measures including application of topical decongestants, holding pressure appropriately (pinching the nostrils shut against the nasal septum) in the majority of cases. Chemical cautery and deployment anterior nasal packing are easily attainable skills and can be used by pediatricians, emergency physicians, and healthcare professionals as next line management. The trajectory of nasal packing deployment (aiming posteriorly towards the nasopharynx rather than superiorly towards the skull base) is critical for effective hemostasis.
- Implementation of standardized protocols involving otolaryngology consultation for minimally invasive endoscopic surgical management of recalcitrant epistaxis has demonstrated promise in reducing morbidity and cost at select centers, although further study is needed to clarify use in children.
- Juvenile nasopharyngeal angiofibroma is a vascular sinonasal tumor presenting exclusively in adolescent males. This should be ruled out in adolescent males with unilateral nasal obstruction and epistaxis.

Financial Disclosures and Conflicts of Interest: None.
Department of Otolaryngology–Head and Neck Surgery, Wayne State University School of Medicine, 4102 St. Antoine, 5E-UHC, Detroit, MI 48201, USA
* Corresponding author.
E-mail address: psvider@gmail.com

Pediatr Clin N Am 65 (2018) 607–621
https://doi.org/10.1016/j.pcl.2018.02.007
0031-3955/18/© 2018 Elsevier Inc. All rights reserved.

pediatric.theclinics.com

Commonly considered a minor nuisance by the lay public, epistaxis in the pediatric population harbors the potential for life-threatening hemodynamic instability and can present in a variety of settings. Significant hemorrhage may indicate serious underlying etiologic factors in select cases, making appropriate management and the understanding of when to pursue further workup of paramount importance. The differential diagnosis associated with epistaxis encompasses a wide range of etiologic factors, ranging from benign causes, such as digital trauma[1,2] and foreign bodies,[3,4] to life-altering entities, including systemic hematologic disorders,[5] locally destructive tumors, and sinonasal malignancies.[6-8] Although similarities exist on comparison with adults, numerous pathologic factors unique to children and adolescents must be considered; for example, epistaxis in infants and toddlers merits consideration of nonaccidental trauma or hematologic disorder, whereas certain neoplasms, such as juvenile nasopharyngeal angiofibroma (JNA), occur exclusively in adolescents (**Box 1**).[9-11] This article aims to provide an organized foundation that facilitates the management of acute epistaxis, as well as an understanding of features that merit further diagnostic workup.

Box 1
Differential diagnosis of epistaxis in the pediatric population: common considerations

Primary (idiopathic) epistaxis

Secondary epistaxis
  Congenital
    Arteriovenous malformation
    Hemangioma
  Inflammatory
    Wegener
    Systemic lupus erythematosus
  Allergic
    Allergic rhinitis
  Infectious
    Acute or chronic rhinosinusitis
    Upper respiratory infection
  Traumatic
    Digital trauma
    Septal perforation
    Foreign body
    Nasal instrumentation (ie, nasogastric tube, nasopharyngeal airway)
    Nasal bone fracture
    Septal fracture
    Nasoorbitoethmoid fracture
  Iatrogenic
    Medication (anticoagulants, nonsteroidal antiinflammatory drugs)
  Toxin
    Illicit drug (snorted)
  Neoplastic
    Rhabdomyosarcoma
    Lymphoma
    JNA
    Nasopharyngeal carcinoma
  Hematologic
    Idiopathic thrombocytopenic purpura
    Von Willebrand disease
    Hemophilia
  Hereditary hemorrhagic telangiectasia

HISTORICAL AND EPIDEMIOLOGIC CONSIDERATIONS

My plan is not only effectual, but is easy of application and absolutely painless, and can be probed in the smallest patients. The little device which I use is made of fifteen of the longest threads of patent lint...it is passed back upon the floor of the nasal cavity and pushed on till you reach the posterior nares...then slowly withdraw the probe and plug the anterior nares and you have arrested the bleeding...In persuading children to submit to the operation, I often pass the lint up my own nose to satisfy them it gives no pain. If lint is not at hand, I use the largest size spool cotton.

—W.W. Parker, MD, 1890[12]

Although the past century has witnessed myriad technological innovations, principles for the initial management of acute epistaxis remain unchanged. On failure of conservative measures, such as anterior pressure, standard management includes deployment of nasal packing, a seemingly innocuous intervention that may prove challenging in the face of poor patient cooperation or brisk bleeding. The past 2 decades have witnessed the development of absorbable packing materials, precluding the need for packing removal,[13] and advances in optical technologies have further facilitated minimally invasive endoscopic approaches in cases requiring surgical management.

Children with epistaxis mainly present between 2 and 10 years of age, with questionnaire-based and population-based analyses reporting the mean age of presentation is 7 to 9 years.[14,15] More than half of children older than 5 years of age have experienced at least 1 nosebleed.[16] One analysis of nearly 20,000 patients presenting to emergency departments reported that 6.9% ultimately required procedures, almost all of which included simple cauterization or packing.[15] In contrast, only a small fraction (<1%) required surgical intervention. Surgical ligation has been associated with decreased length of stay among patients who require inpatient hospitalization,[17] although further studies exclusive to children and adolescents may better help delineate its role. Importantly, implementation of standardized protocols involving minimally invasive surgical management of recalcitrant epistaxis has demonstrated promise in reducing morbidity and cost at select centers.[18] In the contemporary health care environment characterized by growing consciousness of the costs interventions have on health care delivery, treatment paradigms may change in coming years. Nonetheless, conservative treatment followed by simple bedside cauterization and/or packing remains the mainstay of epistaxis management.

OVERVIEW OF PATHOPHYSIOLOGY

A diverse array of etiologic factors and risk factors can promote epistaxis (see **Box 1**). Primary (ie, idiopathic) epistaxis comprises most cases.[16,19] Dry environments lacking humidification can lead to dried nasal mucosa[20,21] and associated fissuring of mucosal surfaces, subsequently leading to desiccation and exposure of blood vessels. Almost all bleeds stem from the rich anastomotic area of vessels located on the anterior nasal septum (**Fig. 1**). Bleeding can also originate elsewhere, including from the lateral nasal wall (as opposed to the nasal septum, which is medial), particularly the branches of the sphenopalatine artery. Posteriorly, bleeding can stem from posterior branches of the sphenopalatine artery, Woodruff plexus, and venous sources.

Any conditions that cause coagulopathies or platelet disorders, including systemic hematologic conditions and hematologic malignancies, lead to a greater risk of more frequent and more severe episodes. Specifically, recurrent episodes or a family history

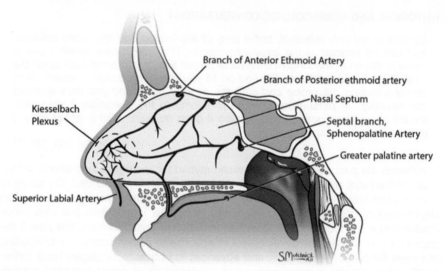

Fig. 1. Sagittal section depicting arterial contributions of Kiesselbach' Plexus on the anterior nasal septum.

of excessive bleeding should prompt further consideration of von Willebrand disease. (See Jorge Di Paola and Christopher J. Ng's article, "Von Willebrand disease: Diagnostic Strategies and Treatment Options," in this issue.) Other considerations are immune thrombocytopenia and hemophilia.[22] (See Stacy E. Croteau's article, "Evolving Complexity in Hemophilia Management," in this issue.) Notably, greater than half of patients with von Willebrand disease experience epistaxis. Other secondary etiologic factors should also be considered.[19,23] Patients with allergic rhinitis and chronic rhinosinusitis have a higher incidence of epistaxis.[20,21] These etiologic factors, along with upper respiratory infections, promote inflammation and subsequent hypervascularity of nasal mucosa.[16,24,25] Systemic factors can greatly increase the risk of developing epistaxis. Connective tissue and inflammatory disorders that lead to derangements in the formation of the walls of blood vessels increase vulnerability to epistaxis. Numerous medications, including anticoagulants, significantly increase the risk for epistaxis. Iatrogenic trauma, either from surgery or placement of appliances (nasogastric tubes, nasopharyngeal airways), can traumatize blood vessels anywhere in the nasal cavity. Traumatic facial injury, including nasal bone fracture or septal fracture, may present with significant epistaxis. Sinonasal neoplasms may present with epistaxis. Although rare, missing these lesions can lead to devastating impacts on morbidity and mortality; therefore, understanding when to pursue further diagnostic workup is critical. Rhabdomyosarcoma is the most common pediatric sinonasal malignancy; in addition to presenting with epistaxis, this lesion can spread to adjacent sites, including the orbit, skull base, and elsewhere in the head and neck region.[6] JNA presents exclusively in adolescent boys, usually presenting with unilateral nasal obstruction, epistaxis, and a mass involving the pterygopalatine fossa-nasopharyngeal area (**Fig. 2**).[26,27]

DIAGNOSTIC CONSIDERATIONS

Timely management of acute epistaxis takes precedence over exhaustive workup. For cases in which bleeding has stopped, as well as among patients experiencing recurrent or chronic epistaxis, several diagnostic steps should be considered. At a

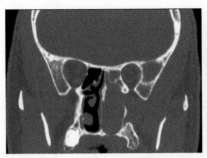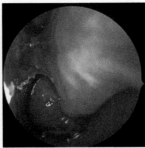

Fig. 2. Adolescent presenting with nasopharyngeal angiofibroma. Coronal computed tomography scan (bone window, *left panel*) depicting left-sided nasal mass. Endoscopic view (*right panel*) of nasal septum, located on left, and JNA, located posteriorly along floor (*grayish mass*). (*Courtesy of* W. Hsueh MD, J.A. Eloy MD, Department of Otolaryngology–Head and Neck Surgery, Rutgers New Jersey Medical School, Newark, NJ.)

minimum, without delaying care, vital signs and a complete blood count should be obtained during an acute episode with further consideration for a basic metabolic panel, prothrombin time, and partial thromboplastin time. Imaging is not indicated in initial evaluation, even on suspected nasal fracture. Nasal fractures are a clinical diagnosis made on history and physical examination (see later discussion) and radiographs harbor little to no value. If a significant likelihood of additional facial fractures (eg, orbital or midface injury) is suspected, then a computed tomography (CT) scan without contrast should be ordered for stable patients. Contrasted CT, MRI, and angiographic studies are considered with recurrent bleeds or other findings suggestive of a neoplasm or vascular entity, such as visualization during endoscopic examination (see **Fig. 2**). Genetic testing may be indicated for select cases in which there is a family history for an inherited disorder or associated physical findings that suggest a particular entity (see later discussion). The differential diagnosis for epistaxis is illustrated in **Box 1**.

PATIENT HISTORY

Obtaining a comprehensive patient history can be useful in evaluation of patients with epistaxis, although timely management takes precedence for patients with significant and brisk hemorrhage. When the epistaxis started, what the patient was doing when it started, and other inciting factors should all be taken into account. For example, facial trauma involving significant epistaxis suggests a high likelihood of nasal fracture, which is ultimately a clinical diagnosis not requiring ancillary tests such as radiographs.[28] When bleeding has already stopped on patient presentation, finding out which side the patient noticed the bleeding is helpful. Other components of the history that provide valuable insight into the underlying etiologic factors include whether the patient is on any blood thinning medications, past medical history (including details about prior episodes), past surgical history, a list of medications, social history (including snorting of illicit substances), and the presence of a family history of bleeding or systemic disorders. Among patients for whom this is a recurrent problem, learning what time of the year they experience epistaxis should also be considered. Importantly, learning about the interventions patients have undergone or what they have done for their epistaxis should be determined. For example, if a patient with epistaxis reports that it is not controlled with holding pressure on their nose, the patient should be asked to demonstrate how and where they hold pressure to determine whether they are doing so correctly (**Fig. 3**). Finally, it is important to rule out

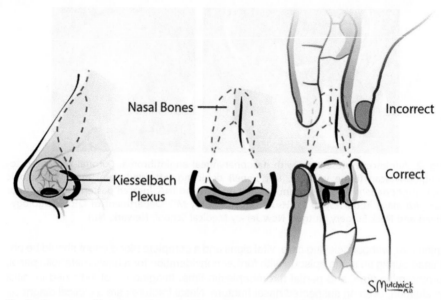

Nasal Bones

Kiesselbach Plexus

Incorrect

Correct

Fig. 3. Correct and incorrect strategies for holding nasal pressure to control epistaxis.

nonaccidental trauma,[29–31] a scenario considered in patients younger than 2 years old because spontaneous epistaxis is exceedingly rare in this cohort.[16]

PHYSICAL EXAMINATION

Vital signs and assessment of airway status should be completed in the initial survey of a patient presenting with epistaxis. Following this, appropriate physical evaluation encompasses a full head and neck examination with obvious focus on the nasal cavity. In many situations, detailed evaluation of the nose is not feasible while active bleeding is ongoing and control of hemorrhage is prioritized. In other instances, the bleed may have slowed and there is an opportunity for evaluation. During examination, the availability of a reliable light source and an appropriate suction apparatus is essential. Topical agents, such as neosynephrine or oxymetazoline, should be sprayed into the nose and anterior pressure should be applied and held, pinching the nostrils firmly onto the septum, for several minutes. These maneuvers can significantly slow or stop any bleeding and allow for a thorough examination.

Anterior rhinoscopy can be performed with an otoscope or, alternatively, a nasal speculum in conjunction with a light source. Most spontaneous nosebleeds stem from blood vessels located on the anterior nasal septum in Little area, also known as the Kiesselbach plexus. In epistaxis following facial trauma, it is critical to rule out a nasal septal hematoma because these can become infected and lead to subsequent cartilage destruction and long-term deformity.

Although most bleeds stem from the anterior nasal septum, identification of a posterior bleed can have important implications for management because posterior packing, or even surgical intervention, may be required (see later discussion). Fiberoptic endoscopy can be used to evaluate for a posterior source of bleeding when an obvious anterior source is not identified via anterior rhinoscopy (**Fig. 4**). Numerous reports have demonstrated this skill is easily taught and transferrable to health

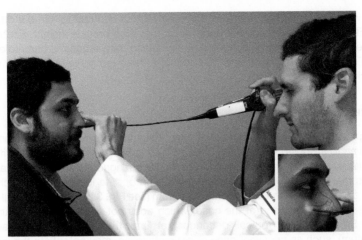

Fig. 4. Physician using fiberoptic endoscopy to perform transnasal endoscopy. (*Courtesy of* Mutchnick S, MD, Detroit, MI.)

care professionals.[32] Importantly, flexible fiberoptic endoscopes are universally available in emergency departments because these instruments are used by anesthesiologists and otolaryngologists for upper airway evaluation and fiberoptic intubation. If there is access to an endoscope, it is gently advanced posteriorly into the nasal cavity, maintaining the tip of the scope on the nasal floor and avoiding contact with structures such as the nasal septum, inferior turbinate, and middle turbinate. The nasal septum, in particular, can be especially sensitive. The exit point of the sphenopalatine artery can be evaluated, as well as the Woodruff area (the nasopharyngeal plexus) posteriorly because this is the most common posterior bleeding source.[33] Endoscopy can also be used to identify other less common etiologic factors facilitating epistaxis, including sinonasal tumors and telangiectasias, the latter of which can be a sign of a systemic disorder such as hereditary hemorrhagic telangiectasia (HHT).

In addition to a thorough nasal examination, the remainder of the head and neck examination can reveal important features guiding management. Palpable cervical lymphadenopathy should prompt consideration of occult malignancy because head and neck cancers drain to these lymph nodes. A thorough oral cavity examination is warranted because other signs of systemic disease can be noted. For example, petechiae can suggest thrombocytopenia, whereas HHT patients may have oral cavity telangiectasias. The otologic examination may reveal hemotympanum, whereas a cranial nerve examination may reveal deficits that could lead to further investigation of certain etiologic factors; for example, paresthesia in the distribution of the maxillary division of trigeminal nerve may be indicative of certain sinonasal neoplasm, a consideration also brought up among patients with proptosis or deficits in extraocular movements. Periorbital ecchymoses, nasal swelling, and external nasal deviation are consistent with nasal fracture in the setting of trauma. Of course, these symptoms and findings following direct nasal trauma clinically define a nasal fracture, and further imaging is not warranted to confirm this. Importantly, facial and nasal radiographs are obsolete in this era and provide no additional value for confirming a nasal fracture. Of course, other concerns in the setting of trauma and epistaxis, such as a patient who sustained a severe impact or is experiencing hypophthalmus, malocclusion, new onset paresthesias, extraocular movement restriction, or other cranial nerve deficits warrant further workup in the form of a facial CT scan without contrast to rule out other fractures. Findings outside of the head and neck may also provide insight. Ecchymoses elsewhere and signs and symptoms of a joint bleed may suggest a hematologic disorder. Furthermore, it is important to conduct a thorough survey to rule out signs of nonaccidental trauma.

NONSURGICAL MANAGEMENT

Although underlying etiologic factors certainly influence long-term management, priority is given to stopping hemorrhage and stabilizing the patient presenting with acute epistaxis, rather than performing a comprehensive diagnostic workup. Management includes making sure pressure is held in the appropriate location and pinching the nostrils closed against the anterior nasal septum (see **Fig. 3**). A common pitfall is holding pressure on the bridge of the nose, which does not provide pressure anywhere useful. Spraying of a topical decongestant into the nasal cavity (directed at the septum), such as neosynephrine or oxymetazoline, may potentiate the impact of holding appropriate pressure. Pressure should be held for a minimum of 10 minutes before checking to see whether this has slowed the bleed and, meanwhile, the physician can take the opportunity to obtain a patient history or pursue ancillary tasks, such as a blood draw to obtain a complete blood count and possible coagulation factors. In conjunction with vital signs and monitoring clinical status, these laboratory tests can identify derangements in coagulation and guide fluid resuscitation, as well as the administration of blood products, including whole blood, platelets, cryoprecipitate, fresh frozen plasma, and vitamin K, as appropriate.

After holding pressure, if bleeding has stopped or slowed sufficiently to allow for thorough examination of the nasal fossae, an attempt is made to identify prominent or bleeding vasculature on the anterior nasal septum that can be easily cauterized with topical silver nitrate. Importantly, use of silver nitrate cautery on both sides of the nasal septum in the same location can cause septal perforation and should be avoided.[34] If bleeding has not been controlled at this point, or if it has been controlled but the patient has a frequent or severe recent history of epistaxis, the next step customarily involves deployment of nasal packing, although recent paradigm shifts suggest more aggressive movement toward minimally invasive endoscopic surgery in select cases.

With appropriate knowledge of nasal geometry, nasal packing can be deployed by emergency department physicians, pediatricians, otolaryngologists, and other physicians and health care professionals (**Fig. 5**). It is important for individuals to appreciate that the nasal cavity actually leads posteriorly to the nasopharynx (rather than superiorly) (see **Figs. 1** and **5**). Choice of packing materials can be organized into absorbable and nonabsorbable, with the latter requiring removal in a follow-up appointment 5 to 7 days later. Greater consideration should be given to absorbable packing in patients with a higher risk of recurrent epistaxis, such as those with bleeding diatheses or taking blood thinning drugs. When placing packing, it is important to have the following available: a working suction apparatus, a light source (either headlight or an assistant holding a pen light), a nasal speculum, and forceps (preferably bayonet forceps) (**Fig. 6**). The nasal speculum can be used to expand the nostril, and the packing should be placed aiming straight back (not superiorly) along the nasal floor (see **Fig. 5**). This technique is appropriate for stopping anterior-based nosebleeds and, depending on packing, can help with posterior epistaxis in certain instances. After successful deployment of nasal packing, a patient can be observed for a short period in the emergency department or outpatient setting, if there is no further bleeding. There is no indication for inpatient observation if the patient is stable and has laboratory tests that are

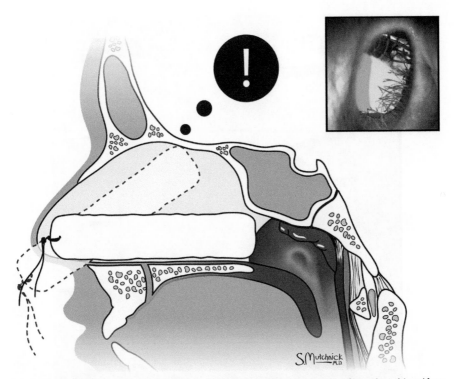

Fig. 5. Correct and incorrect (*dotted lines*) trajectories for placement of nasal packing (*foreground*). Nasal packing placement as viewed from inside the nose (*inset, upper right*); the viewing physician is deploying the nasal packing.

normal. Traditionally, prophylactic antibiotics (first-generation cephalosporins or penicillins) have been prescribed for the duration of planned packing placement to prevent superinfection and toxic shock syndrome, although this practice is not supported by contemporary literature. Recent prospective trials and systematic reviews have demonstrated a paucity of evidence supporting this practice.[35,36] Nonetheless, prescription of prophylactic antibiotics while packing in place remains standard practice at many institutions.

Another important consideration for classifying epistaxis that carries significant implications for management relates to the blood vessels responsible for the bleeding. Although almost all bleeds stem from the anterior blood supply, a small proportion of cases involve posterior-based epistaxis. Consequently, conservative measures and packing techniques aimed at controlling anterior epistaxis may not be effective, necessitating posterior-packing or even surgical management (see later discussion). When not controlled with anterior packing, a posterior bleed should be suspected and an otolaryngologist should be consulted in institutions with otolaryngology coverage. There are several commercially available packing devices intended for posterior bleeds, many of which use an inflatable balloon to allow for pressure along the choanae. In settings where such devices are not available, a Foley catheter can be used with the balloon inserted past the choanae and into the nasopharynx. The balloon is then inflated and the entire device gently pulled anteriorly to make sure it is secured. Any contact such devices have with the nostrils anteriorly should be protected with padding to prevent alar necrosis, a preventable

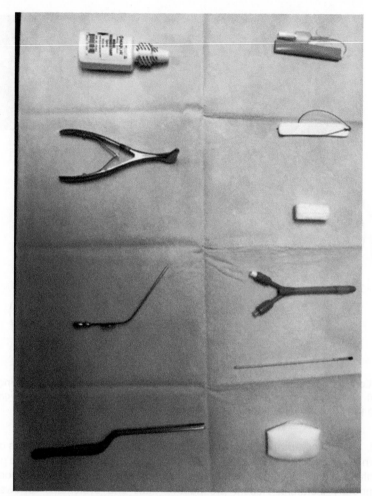

Fig. 6. Commonly used materials in the management of acute epistaxis. (*First column, from top down*) topical spray (oxymetazoline), nasal speculum, suction tip, and bayonet forceps. (*Second column*) Rapid Rhino Nasal pack, nasal pack, Bioabsorbable Pack, posterior nasal pack with balloon port, silver nitrate cautery applicator, and nasal dressing.

complication that may necessitate considerable reconstructive surgery.[37] Patients with a posterior pack require close monitoring with pulse oximetry, usually in an intensive care unit, due to the potential for activation of the nasopulmonary reflex, which can cause severe arterial hypoxemia and subsequent mortality. Despite several studies suggesting that these findings may be anecdotal,[38,39] intensive care unit or stepdown monitoring for patients with posterior packing remains standard practice in most institutions.

The utility of embolization in epistaxis has been examined in several settings, although trials focusing on pediatric subjects are limited.[40] Embolization is increasingly considered in specific etiologic factors associated with uncontrolled hemorrhage, such as in patients with sinonasal tumors. This modality also has utility in preoperative optimization of select vascular tumors, such as JNAs.[10,41] Embolization may be considered in cases with intractable bleeding or in patients who are unable to undergo general anesthesia. Despite the minimally invasive nature of this intervention, there are several challenges to consider, including radiation exposure, limited availability in smaller institutions, and increased costs. Furthermore, embolization of the ethmoidal arteries is contraindicated because these are derived from the ophthalmic artery and occlusion can cause blindness.[42] There is also a risk of unintentional embolization of the internal carotid artery and ophthalmic artery.

MINIMALLY INVASIVE SURGICAL MANAGEMENT

Historically, surgical management of epistaxis has involved several approaches, including those requiring sublabial (upper gingival) incisions to approach the internal maxillary artery and facial incisions to approach the ethmoidal arteries. With the refinement of endoscopic technologies, minimally invasive transnasal control of epistaxis has been increasingly performed and is now considered regularly in severe and recurrent epistaxis. Transnasal endoscopic sphenopalatine artery ligation (TESPAL) is routinely performed at many institutions, and epistaxis stemming from other sources (including the ethmoidal arteries) can be endoscopically addressed. Although these procedures can be performed with local anesthesia and sedation, the significant bleeding many patients are already experiencing necessitates general anesthesia and intubation for airway protection. These procedures do not involve any external incisions, can be done on an outpatient basis, and do not result in a considerable amount of pain. There have been myriad studies demonstrating adequate postoperative analgesia using nonopioid medications in patients undergoing endoscopic sinonasal procedures.[43–45]

In addition to utility in particularly severe or recurrent epistaxis, several centers have explored endoscopic epistaxis control to minimize the morbidity and discomfort associated with nasal packing. Physicians at the University of Pittsburgh explored the implementation of a clinical care pathway using TESPAL for epistaxis not controlled with conservative measures and anterior packing.[18] Implementation of this algorithm decreased costs, length of stay, and days of packing. Other cost-effectiveness analyses have demonstrated TESPAL is cost-saving first-line therapy for patients with posterior epistaxis (ie, episodes not controlled with simple anterior packing).[46,47] These cost-effectiveness analyses and algorithms exploring the use of minimally invasive surgical management have been studied in adults, and further exploration of their use exclusively in children and adolescents is warranted. Furthermore, there has been controversy on whether exposure to general anesthetics has long-term impact on neurocognitive development in children,[48–50] and these potential risks must be considered in the decision-making process.

SUBSPECIALTY COLLABORATION

The appropriate role of subspecialty consultation differs based on underlying etiologic factors and clinical setting (**Table 1**). In patients for whom systemic inflammatory or connective tissue disorders are suspected, collaboration with rheumatology may be invaluable for identifying a specific diagnosis and subsequent management. Similarly, in patients for whom entities involving specific organ systems are suspected, subspecialty referral is essential; for example, in HHT, seeking evaluation from gastroenterology, pulmonary, and neurology or neurosurgery colleagues is critical for identifying involvement of these organ systems. In patients with hematologic disorders, including those with coagulopathies, platelet disorders, and hematologic malignancies, close collaboration with a pediatric hematologist is important for long-term management.

Table 1
Suggested management of epistaxis for physicians in various settings

Intervention	Outpatient Pediatrics	Inpatient or Emergency Department Physician	Otolaryngologist
Pressure	X	X	X
Decongestants (Topical)	X	X	X
Anterior Packing	X	X	X
Silver Nitrate Cautery	X	X	X
Nasal Endoscopy	—	X	X
Blood or Reversal Agents	—	X	X
Posterior Packing	—	X	X
Endoscopic Ligation	—	—	X
Recurrent Epistaxis	—	—	X[a]

[a] For controlled acute bleeds, recurrent epistaxis can be generally worked up and managed via outpatient otolaryngology referral for most stable patients.

Otolaryngology consultation should be considered for the successful management of patients with severe, recalcitrant, and recurrent epistaxis. Familiarity with appropriate conservative management, including the correct way to deploy nasal packing, may be sufficient for addressing most bleeds without expert consultation. Otolaryngology consultation is warranted in patients with recurrent, severe, or posterior-based bleeds, as well as in those in whom there is early consideration of minimally invasive endoscopic ligation. All otolaryngologists should be comfortable in the diagnosis and management of epistaxis, including employment of conservative measures and surgical management. Fellowship-trained pediatric otolaryngologists have subspecialty training dedicated to the unique considerations specific to the pediatric population. Fellowship trained rhinologists focus on minimally invasive treatment of the nasal cavity, paranasal sinuses, and anterior skull base, including endoscopic management of sinonasal and skull base tumors.

SUMMARY

Prompt management of acute epistaxis takes precedence over comprehensive diagnostic workup. A standardized approach should include conservative measures such as holding pressure and using nasal packing. Severe, recurrent, and posteriorly based bleeds should prompt consideration of alternate interventions and expert consultation, particularly because the importance of minimally invasive endoscopic intervention has increased in recent years. Although most episodes stem from idiopathic causes, consideration of secondary etiologic factors is important in select cases.

REFERENCES

1. Bequignon E, Teissier N, Gauthier A, et al. Emergency department care of childhood epistaxis. Emerg Med J 2017;34(8):543–8.
2. Burton RD. Nasal bleeding in children. Calif Med 1961;94:366–8.
3. Svider PF, Johnson AP, Folbe AJ, et al. Assault by battery: battery-related injury in the head and neck. Laryngoscope 2014;124(10):2257–61.
4. Svider PF, Sheyn A, Folbe E, et al. How did that get there? A population-based analysis of nasal foreign bodies. Int Forum Allergy Rhinol 2014;4(11):944–9.

5. Mittal N, Naridze R, James P, et al. Utility of a paediatric bleeding questionnaire as a screening tool for von Willebrand disease in apparently healthy children. Haemophilia 2015;21(6):806–11.
6. Chung SY, Unsal AA, Kilic S, et al. Pediatric sinonasal malignancies: a population-based analysis. Int J Pediatr Otorhinolaryngol 2017;98:97–102.
7. Dutta R, Dubal PM, Svider PF, et al. Sinonasal malignancies: a population-based analysis of site-specific incidence and survival. Laryngoscope 2015;125(11): 2491–7.
8. Svider PF, Setzen M, Baredes S, et al. Overview of sinonasal and ventral skull base malignancy management. Otolaryngol Clin North Am 2017;50(2):205–19.
9. Alshaikh NA, Eleftheriadou A. Juvenile nasopharyngeal angiofibroma staging: an overview. Ear Nose Throat J 2015;94(6):E12–22.
10. Boghani Z, Husain Q, Kanumuri VV, et al. Juvenile nasopharyngeal angiofibroma: a systematic review and comparison of endoscopic, endoscopic-assisted, and open resection in 1047 cases. Laryngoscope 2013;123(4):859–69.
11. Leong SC. A systematic review of surgical outcomes for advanced juvenile nasopharyngeal angiofibroma with intracranial involvement. Laryngoscope 2013; 123(5):1125–31.
12. Parker WW. A simple substitute for Bellocq's cannula and all other methods for controlling epistaxis. Medical Record 1890;38(14):379.
13. Weber RK, Hosemann W. Comprehensive review on endonasal endoscopic sinus surgery. GMS Curr Top Otorhinolaryngol Head Neck Surg 2015;14:Doc08.
14. Davies K, Batra K, Mehanna R, et al. Pediatric epistaxis: epidemiology, management & impact on quality of life. Int J Pediatr Otorhinolaryngol 2014;78(8):1294–7.
15. Shay S, Shapiro NL, Bhattacharyya N. Epidemiological characteristics of pediatric epistaxis presenting to the emergency department. Int J Pediatr Otorhinolaryngol 2017;103:121–4.
16. Record S. Practice guideline: epistaxis in children. J Pediatr Health Care 2015; 29(5):484–8.
17. Sylvester MJ, Chung SY, Guinand LA, et al. Arterial ligation versus embolization in epistaxis management: counterintuitive national trends. Laryngoscope 2017; 127(5):1017–20.
18. Vosler PS, Kass JI, Wang EW, et al. Successful implementation of a clinical care pathway for management of epistaxis at a tertiary care center. Otolaryngol Head Neck Surg 2016;155(5):879–85.
19. Melia L, McGarry GW. Epistaxis: update on management. Curr Opin Otolaryngol Head Neck Surg 2011;19(1):30–5.
20. Morgan DJ, Kellerman R. Epistaxis: evaluation and treatment. Prim Care 2014; 41(1):63–73.
21. Purkey MR, Seeskin Z, Chandra R. Seasonal variation and predictors of epistaxis. Laryngoscope 2014;124(9):2028–33.
22. Qureishi A, Burton MJ. Interventions for recurrent idiopathic epistaxis (nosebleeds) in children. Cochrane Database Syst Rev 2012;(9):CD004461.
23. Schlosser RJ. Clinical practice. Epistaxis. N Engl J Med 2009;360(8):784–9.
24. Abrich V, Brozek A, Boyle TR, et al. Risk factors for recurrent spontaneous epistaxis. Mayo Clin Proc 2014;89(12):1636–43.
25. Whymark AD, Crampsey DP, Fraser L, et al. Childhood epistaxis and nasal colonization with *Staphylococcus aureus*. Otolaryngol Head Neck Surg 2008;138(3): 307–10.
26. Martins MB, de Lima FV, Mendonca CA, et al. Nasopharyngeal angiofibroma: our experience and literature review. Int Arch Otorhinolaryngol 2013;17(1):14–9.

27. Neel HB 3rd, Whicker JH, Devine KD, et al. Juvenile angiofibroma. Review of 120 cases. Am J Surg 1973;126(4):547–56.

28. Kelley BP, Downey CR, Stal S. Evaluation and reduction of nasal trauma. Semin Plast Surg 2010;24(4):339–47.

29. Boscardini L, Zanetta S, Ballardini G, et al. Epistaxis in children under the age of two: possible marker of abuse/neglect? A retrospective study in North-Eastern Piedmont hospitals. Minerva Pediatr 2013;65(1):71–5.

30. McIntosh N, Mok JY, Margerison A. Epidemiology of oronasal hemorrhage in the first 2 years of life: implications for child protection. Pediatrics 2007;120(5): 1074–8.

31. Walton LJ, Davies FC. Nasal bleeding and non-accidental injury in an infant. Arch Dis Child 2010;95(1):53–4.

32. Dewitt DE. Fiberoptic rhinolaryngoscopy in primary care. A new direction for expanding in-office diagnostics. Postgrad Med 1988;84(5):125–6, 131-125, 138 passim.

33. Chiu TW, Shaw-Dunn J, McGarry GW. Woodruff's plexus. J Laryngol Otol 2008; 122(10):1074–7.

34. Lloyd S, Almeyda J, Di Cuffa R, et al. The effect of silver nitrate on nasal septal cartilage. Ear Nose Throat J 2005;84(1):41–4.

35. Lange JL, Peeden EH, Stringer SP. Are prophylactic systemic antibiotics necessary with nasal packing? A systematic review. Am J Rhinol Allergy 2017;31(4):240–7.

36. Pepper C, Lo S, Toma A. Prospective study of the risk of not using prophylactic antibiotics in nasal packing for epistaxis. J Laryngol Otol 2012;126(3):257–9.

37. Judd O, Gaskin J. Securing the posterior nasal pack; a technique to prevent alar necrosis. Ann R Coll Surg Engl 2009;91(8):713–4.

38. Jacobs JR, Levine LA, Davis H, et al. Posterior packs and the nasopulmonary reflex. Laryngoscope 1981;91(2):279–84.

39. Loftus BC, Blitzer A, Cozine K. Epistaxis, medical history, and the nasopulmonary reflex: what is clinically relevant? Otolaryngol Head Neck Surg 1994;110(4): 363–9.

40. Goldman JL, Winstead W, Ganzel TM. Embolization as the definitive treatment of epistaxis in the pediatric patient. Ear Nose Throat J 1995;74(7):490–2.

41. Shukla PA, Chan N, Duffis EJ, et al. Current treatment strategies for epistaxis: a multidisciplinary approach. J Neurointerv Surg 2013;5(2):151–6.

42. Willems PW, Farb RI, Agid R. Endovascular treatment of epistaxis. AJNR Am J Neuroradiol 2009;30(9):1637–45.

43. Church CA, Stewart C 4th, O-Lee TJ, et al. Rofecoxib versus hydrocodone/acetaminophen for postoperative analgesia in functional endoscopic sinus surgery. Laryngoscope 2006;116(4):602–6.

44. Koputan MH, Apan A, Oz G, et al. The effects of tramadol and levobupivacaine infiltration on postoperative analgesia in functional endoscopic sinus surgery and septorhinoplasty. Balkan Med J 2012;29(4):391–4.

45. Sanders JG, Dawes PJ. Gabapentin for perioperative analgesia in otorhinolaryngology-head and neck surgery: systematic review. Otolaryngol Head Neck Surg 2016;155(6):893–903.

46. Dedhia RC, Desai SS, Smith KJ, et al. Cost-effectiveness of endoscopic sphenopalatine artery ligation versus nasal packing as first-line treatment for posterior epistaxis. Int Forum Allergy Rhinol 2013;3(7):563–6.

47. Rudmik L, Leung R. Cost-effectiveness analysis of endoscopic sphenopalatine artery ligation vs arterial embolization for intractable epistaxis. JAMA Otolaryngol Head Neck Surg 2014;140(9):802–8.

48. Andropoulos DB, Greene MF. Anesthesia and developing brains - implications of the FDA warning. N Engl J Med 2017;376(10):905–7.
49. Jevtovic-Todorovic V. General anesthetics and the developing brain: friends or foes? J Neurosurg Anesthesiol 2005;17(4):204–6.
50. Sun L. Early childhood general anaesthesia exposure and neurocognitive development. Br J Anaesth 2010;105(Suppl 1):i61–8.

Moving?

Make sure your subscription moves with you!

To notify us of your new address, find your **Clinics Account Number** (located on your mailing label above your name), and contact customer service at:

Email: journalscustomerservice-usa@elsevier.com

800-654-2452 (subscribers in the U.S. & Canada)
314-447-8871 (subscribers outside of the U.S. & Canada)

Fax number: 314-447-8029

Elsevier Health Sciences Division
Subscription Customer Service
3251 Riverport Lane
Maryland Heights, MO 63043

*To ensure uninterrupted delivery of your subscription, please notify us at least 4 weeks in advance of move.